THE

NATURAL WAY
TO A HEALTHY
HEART

THE
NATURAL WAY TO A HEALTHY HEART

LESSONS FROM ALTERNATIVE AND CONVENTIONAL MEDICINE

Stephen Holt, M.D.

M. EVANS AND COMPANY, INC.
New York

Copyright © 1999 by Stephen Holt, M.D.

M. Evans and Company, Inc.
216 East 49th Street
New York, New York 10017

Library of Congress Cataloging-in-Publication Data

Holt, Stephen, 1950–
    The natural way to a healthy heart / Stephen Holt.
        p.   cm.
    ISBN 0-87131-966-7
    1. Heart—Diseases—Popular works. 2. Heart—Diseases—Prevention.
  3. Naturopathy. I. Title.
RC672.H64 1999
616.1'2—dc21   99050398

Book design and typesetting by Rik Lain Schell

Printed in the United States of America

9   8   7   6   5   4   3

CONTENTS

We, in the very late twentieth century, are on the verge of witnessing the total transformation of health care in the United States. Perhaps nowhere is this more evident than in the traditional medical community. Skyrocketing health-care costs are bankrupting the individual, the family, and the entire country. In today's disease-oriented society, most physicians will wait until symptoms occur and then treat patients with hospitalization, surgery, and expensive drugs. According to recent statistics, Americans annually spend over eighteen billion dollars on coronary artery bypass surgery alone. By the year 2000, cancer may surpass heart disease as the number one cause of death. Heavy metals, auto emissions, insecticides, pesticides, and industrial pollutants of all sorts are giving birth to a whole new assortment of ills, from immune dysfunction to allergies and chemical sensitivities. Living in this age of chemicals will present many challenges to today's physicians. But what is the alternative?

The alternative, quite simply, involves a paradigm shift from disease to health and prevention, and the creation of new medical specialties to prevent and treat emerging threats. As a board-certified cardiologist, I have worked with thousands of cases of heart disease, but my introduction to true healing emerged during my training as a psychoanalyst. After twelve years of study in both Gestalt and bioenergetic psychotherapy, it became clear to me that pathology (becoming ill) is often a form of disease that emerges from the chaotic imbalance of mind, body, and spirit.

To restore this balance and maintain health, many new healing modalities have been created, and ancient therapies have been reintroduced. Rigidity, the Achilles heel of mainstream medicine, is finally showing some flexibility.

Many physicians have experienced a gradual shift in the philosophy and psychology of healing and are now incorporating complementary and alternative care techniques. They, like the patients they treat, have become disenchanted with our modern medical systems. However, if physicians are to survive in today's climate, they must heed the message and listen to the outcry of the public. Starving for information, they are consulting alternative therapists and visiting book and health food stores in record numbers , thus creating a multi-billion-dollar industry—completely outside of the mainstream medical community!

One cannot think of the story of Nero fiddling while Rome burns. Whose responsibility is it to examine all options that have the potential to ease human suffering? Who is best to partner with patients in their quest to take charge of their health and well-being? Who could be better qualified than our highly-trained medical professionals to test the efficacy and safety of alternative and complementary therapies, under strict peer review, thus protecting the patient from quackery and snake oil? And, once empowered with the knowledge of a wide variety of healing modalities, who is better able to provide them with the best possible care?

As we move into a new century, key aspects of our world are being forced to re-invent themselves. Driven by changes in the population (such as the aging of America), environmental disturbances, and technological breakthroughs, the physician of the future will need to be like a chameleon: flexible and adaptable, ever ready to meet the needs of a new tomorrow. As those who have embraced the biomedical model of the last century are now learning, it is inadequate to carry us into the future. Women's health and environmental, behavioral, nutritional, and energy medicine are knocking at the door with an increased urgency. It is up to each and every one of us to accept the challenge of integrating all aspects of health and healing into a cohesive, viable entity, working in harmony for our own future generations.

It is with great pleasure that I introduce Dr. Stephen Holt's book, *The Natural Way to a Healthy Heart*. Seven years ago, I met Dr. Holt at a National Nutritional Food Association meeting where we were keynote speakers on the scientific program. We traded our own books and discussed our interests, resulting in a professional relationship. Dr. Holt is a physician, scientist, and author whose work has become revered in the modern movement of complementary medical practice.

This book demonstrates Dr. Holt's original thoughts about ways to combat the epidemic of cardiovascular disease. An epidemic of alarming proportions in our modern society, cardiovascular disease strikes both men and now increasing numbers of women as well. He emphasizes that modern high-technology medicine is to be applauded, but no standing ovation can occur without the paradigm shift that is now impacting cardiovascular disease prevention.

As a conventional/contemporary cardiologist, I am intrigued by the recommendations of Dr. Holt, a board-certified gastroenterologist with special training in cardiology twenty years ago. Dr. Holt has a meritorious background in academic medicine and research and these qualities show in his writings. He stresses the notions of body/mind or mind/body and is unwilling to dissociate behavioral medicine from the prevention or treatment of cardiac disease. In his usual eloquent style, he picks apart the best of conventional and alternative medical approaches with piercing accuracy. Dr. Holt has not turned his back on conventional medicine and he cannot be regarded as completely embracing alternative medicine. His thoughts are truly pluralistic, matching his call for "medical pluralism": lateral thinking and new approaches to cardiac disease treatment and prevention in the next millennium.

Like all questioning physicians, Dr. Holt's opinions are unlikely to be music to the ears of institutionalized medicine, managed care, or the pharmaceutical industry. He presents powerful evidence that remedies of natural origin and nutritional treatments have a great deal to offer in the quest for ideal cardiovascular health. His messages are powerful, backed by scientific methodology.

Stephen Holt, M.D., has made many contributions to the evolving discipline of alternative and complementary medicine. His background is firmly entrenched in conventional medicine, as evidenced by his hundreds of contributions to the scientific and medical literature. As a highly credentialed conventional physician, he brings a refreshing balance to alternative medicine. He is poised at the cutting edge of nutritional medicine, remedies of natural origin, biotechnology, complementary medicine, and conventional medicine. His eclectic interest and abilities make him one of the most valuable thought leaders in the new domain of integrated medical practice.

The Natural Way to a Healthy Heart offers a leading-edge approach to cardiovascular prevention. The messages in his book are timely, given the changing landscape in today's medical environment.

Stephen T. Sinatra, M.D., F.A.C.C., F.A.C.N., C.B.T.
Author of Optimum Health, Heartbreak and Heart Disease,
The CoEnzyme Q10 Phenomenon, *and* HeartSense for Women

This is not just another book about lowering blood cholesterol, nor does it offer a single program or philosophy that guarantees positive results. Rather, *The Natural Way to a Healthy Heart* presents information from diverse health-care philosophies. I wrote this book for all adults who are concerned about their overall health, and it is intended to inform the layperson and the health-care professional alike. It provides my opinions about the best options offered by natural (and conventional) medicine in the quest for cardiovascular health. What I present is not alternative, conventional, or complementary medicine—it is medicine, *period*: the best of all worlds.

Some may consider the material I present here to represent "integrative" medicine. However, I reject the terms integrated or integrative medicine because either exemplifies the dichotomy that exists in medicine between conventional and alternative treatments. If we are sensible enough to look at the trends developing in our culture today, we clearly see that the physician of the future will offer "what works." Just think, obsessing about the source of the treatment will be a thing of the past.

As we enter a new millennium, medical breakthroughs are positioned at the intersection of health-care disciplines. I have frequently used the term "pluralistic medicine," and the age of this type of health care is at last being ushered in. As health-care consumers, it is our right to "have it all."

The advantages of pluralistic medicine are never more apparent than in the area of prevention and treatment of cardiovascular disease. Although I have written books about many health-care topics, promoting cardiovascular wellness is my answer to the devastating effects of cardiac disease on my family and friends. Is there any family in our culture that is not familiar with heart disease and the emotional "heartache" that goes along with it? Perhaps you and I share our disappointment with results of the current treatment and many futile attempts to prevent coronary heart diseases. Now, however, *the story of the causes of heart disease and what constitutes effective prevention of this life-robbing process need to be told.* There is power in the telling when the story is correct, complete, and told from the heart.

Many books on cardiovascular health make false promises or adopt a narrow focus on the problem. Others sell products or services, and several offer misguided or even dangerous advice. But this book provides you with a heart-healthy lifestyle that you can live with and make your own. It helps guide you through both the advantages and limitations to the use of dietary supplements to promote cardiovascular health.

If you are like many health-care consumers, you may be confused by seemingly conflicting information that fills print and electronic media. It is true that medicine is at a crossroads in its approach to cardiovascular health. Conventional medicine beats a high-technology drum while some "alternative" practitioners hype poorly researched natural remedies. The point is, of course, that we must demand quality from both disciplines. We deserve the best of both worlds. An integrated medical approach may risk rejection by both conventional and alternative health-care givers, but I believe that this is a chance worth taking because it is a goal worth pursuing.

Real progress most often occurs at that cutting edge that separates disciplines. Many people are disenchanted with both conventional and alternative medicine; the constant dogfights between the conventional and alternative practitioners of medicine leave us wondering about the competence of both. Every health-care consumer should have the right to receive the best treatment and the best preventive care. Anyone who truly needs cardiac bypass surgery should have it and not have to resort to untried or untested interventions. However, one good option may be to put the cardiac surgeon out of business by preventing heart disease through an "alternative" approach. Only part of this "alternative" approach is likely to be alternative medicine. I believe that these kinds of options should be available.

During my work with the Institute of Medicine Task Force in Washington, D.C., in the late 1980s, the importance of lifestyle change as a key to health was embraced by all assembled health experts. The concept of disease prevention by lifestyle adjustment was not a new idea. The conclusions of the task force were accepted by the U.S. Congress, but not completely enacted. Certainly, for more than thirty years, innovative scientists, politicians, and physicians have demonstrated the benefits of correcting adverse lifestyles. (Theologians and philosophers have recommended this approach from time immemorial, so there really isn't anything radically new about the current advice.) But as we enter a new millennium, lifestyle plans are still not part of mainstream health care. Several European countries have taken a lead in preventive health strategies; unfortunately, the U.S. lags far behind.

This book is meant to overcome some of the complacent attitudes that exists in health care and among many health-care consumers about enacting beneficial lifestyle adjustments for the purpose of promoting cardiovascular and general health. I have examined and included credible scientific information about natural medicines to support my recommendations and conclusions about its integration into current medical practice. I strongly believe it is about time to get past caring about whether a therapy is considered alternative or conventional and go with what works!

Another goal—or ambition—for this book involves my hope to motivate health-care providers to embrace obvious but overlooked solutions to cardiovascular wellness. Because it helps the "medicine go down," I have attempted to keep this book light in tone. However, it is serious, too, not just because the subject matter is serious, but because it is necessary to present valid scientific information. Without it, it would be impossible for you to gain the full knowledge you need to understand the intertwined risks of cardiovascular disability and death.

In short, what I offer is a marriage of conventional medicine and effective natural options for cardiovascular health. When health-care givers and patients read this book with optimism, they may gain a new perspective on the use of combined approaches to tackle humankind's number one enemy and killer—cardiovascular disease.

Stephen Holt, M.D.

THE OPTIMAL WAY

The objectives of my approach are to achieve a reduction in undesirable forms of cholesterol, control body weight, improve general well-being, and make a contribution to longevity. In my book *The Weight Control Revolution*, I stress the idea of one diet that serves both weight loss and health goals. The concept is good, but the need for tailored nutrition will always prevail. *The Natural Way to a Healthy Heart* stresses the importance of the normalization of blood lipids as a primary target of programs for cardiovascular wellness, but this should not be the only objective of a "heart-smart" way of life. There are many other health benefits that can accrue from the selection of natural cholesterol-lowering options and other changes in body chemistry that are discussed in later chapters of this book. These natural options are versatile, and they have significant benefits for other health concerns. Many recent scientific studies demonstrate conclusively that lifestyle interventions in mature adults and the elderly are beneficial. It is now time to bring the level of preventive strategies to childhood and even in utero.

MODIFYING YOUR RISK

The tools to change some key risk factors are within your reach—and your continuing control. An overweight person can resolve to lose weight and seek help to support the effort, thereby modifying this risk factor. A smoker can do whatever it takes to quit smoking. *You are not helpless in the face of risk factors—that is one of the major messages of this book.*

While there are unchangeable risk factors, such as your genetic profile and your sex, *most cardiovascular risk factors are changeable.* Even if an individual has atherosclerosis, there are contributing factors to advancing disease that are readily controllable. It may come as a surprise that based on statistical observation, growing older is not an independent risk factor for coronary artery disease. However, chronological age does not always coincide with biological age. Poor lifestyle can add years, and a healthy lifestyle can slow down the progression of biological aging. You have probably seen forty-year-olds who seem like they are fifty-five or sixty. Conversely, the remarkable men and women at age seventy or more often appear special and notable because they seem so energetic and youthful, as if they actually had sipped from a fountain of youth.

There are several readily identifiable risk factors that can be changed, and many bear some relationship to cholesterol (see Table 1.1, Chapter 1). Equally, there are several simple goals that underlie such changes. Do not feel discouraged or that you are unique in facing these challenges—you have many companions in the same boat!

WHO IS THIS BOOK FOR?

The Natural Way to a Healthy Heart is virtually for all health-conscious adults, whether or not they have known heart disease or identified risk factors. As you will see, much of the discussion focuses on prevention. Without question, preventing an illness beats treating one—hands down. However, the information presented here is equally important for those undergoing treatment for heart disease. For all the available high-tech surgeries and sophisticated drugs, individuals have the greatest impact on the course of their own recovery. Optimal treatment for heart disease is a partnership between health-care providers and patients. This partnership focuses on halting progression of the disease, preventing its recurrence, and, to any extent possible, reversing it.

For some people, a diagnosis of heart disease serves as a kind of alarm bell that goes off suddenly, and the "big bang" loudly proclaims that they must make changes in their life. Rather than signaling the end of something, illness sometimes serves as a new beginning. Perhaps you are in the process of making a fresh start in your approach to health and wellness. If that is the case, I congratulate you. I also congratulate you if your primary motivation is a deep desire to maintain your health and avoid future illness. Adopting healthful behavior can be uncomfortable sometimes, but in the long run, it will help you *feel* better.

THE IMPORTANCE OF FAMILY AND LOVED ONES

Hospital waiting rooms are lonely places, yet for many people, their first introduction to cardiac disease involves waiting for physicians and nurses to deliver *the news* about their loved one. One of the best discussions about what it is like to be a "cardiac spouse" is presented in *Heartmates: A Survival Guide for the Cardiac Spouse*. Author Rhoda F. Levin explores the world of the cardiac spouse by drawing on her own experience as the wife of a man whose heart disease led to bypass surgery. Why, for example, do spouses often feel guilty when their partner suffers a heart attack—or even has high cholesterol readings? How much responsibility should the spouse have in monitoring compliance with the treatment plan? What about the ongoing anxiety experienced by cardiac patients and their families? Many spouses experience ongoing fear that their lives will never be "normal" again.

I highly recommend Levin's book because she brings her background as a psychotherapist to this work. More than just a story of her personal journey, *Heartmates* offers practical suggestions and guidelines for the recovering spouse, who traditionally is not given the attention he or she needs. As Levin points out, the crisis for the cardiac spouse usually begins suddenly and often without warning. These men and women suddenly find themselves in unfamiliar territory—often chaotic and always frightening. In addition to advice about day-to-day adjustments and coping with the natural anxiety inherent in the experience, this book also discusses the sensitive issue of sexuality from the point of view of the cardiac spouse.

If you are coping with a partner's diagnosis, you need the information presented in this book to maintain your own well-being, including the chapters on lifestyle, stress, and diet (Chapters 5, 6, and 7). Most health-care providers agree that when one family member is ill, the stressful event may put other family members at increased risk for illness, too. This is the time to take very good care of yourself, and you can use the principles in this book to help you.

HOW TO GET THE MOST FROM THIS BOOK

As you will see, this book offers a wide range of information, some of which may seem a bit too technical for some readers, but which will be exactly what other readers need and want. Some people would like to understand, at a fundamental level, the reasoning and the science behind the information and recommendations in this book. I hope to provide the largest number of readers with beneficial and highly usable information.

I invite you to use this book as both a foundation and a tool. It is a foundation because you can build a healthy lifestyle program upon its principles; it is a tool because it can be used again and again to help you sculpt your heart-healthy lifestyle—the true "fountain of youth."

Ideally, the information in this book should be presented "holistically," meaning that the issues are best viewed as unified and fundamentally inseparable. Can we legitimately separate lifestyle issues such as weight control from our understanding of beneficial fats? Should stress be discussed separately from suggestions for an optimal diet? Though, by necessity, the issues must be discussed individually in order to be presented clearly, remember the important principle: *the whole is greater than the sum of its parts.* As much as possible, think of this information as a fundamentally cohesive whole.

This book is organized to logically move through the key topics. In Chapters 2 and 3 you will find a comprehensive discussion of cholesterol and other blood lipids, as well as explanations of other theories about the cause of heart disease, including a discussion of the homocysteine theory. Chapters 5 and 6 are devoted to the critical areas of lifestyle risk factors, including stress. No one should skip these chapters, no matter how conscientious about prevention and health one may be. From there we move on to the complex—and often confusing—topics of nutrition and diet. We live in an exciting era and, more than ever before, data about the therapeutic benefits of nutrients are rapidly accumulating. Some of these nutrients have an important role in preventing and treating heart disease. For example, recently acquired information about coenzyme Q10 has shown its great potential as a natural option in prevention and treatment plans. Nutritional information also is key to understanding the homocysteine theory.

In recent years, low fat has become the new mantra of heart-healthy nutrition. However, we now have greater understanding about "good" and "bad" fats. I have devoted a chapter to an explanation of the need to include healthful fats in your diet. I also explain the way in which these fats promote health and how many fats that are plentiful in the Western diet contribute to heart disease.

The Natural Way to a Healthy Heart would be incomplete without information about plant-based remedies for heart disease. Therefore, a chapter is devoted to descriptions of a variety of botanical therapies. Because they are so important for cardiovascular health, I also include a chapter about the benefits of soy food products and nutritional supplements. Finally, I have added a chapter about weight control, because it is such a common—and serious—risk factor.

As you read about steps you can take to promote a healthy heart, you may notice that these guidelines also promote overall health. This book could just as easily have been called "Natural Ways to Improve Your Health." Consider this book a roadmap for your self-care journey—and do not stop here. The valuable resources I mention throughout this text are listed in the back of this book.

CHOOSING HEALTH-CARE SERVICES

I did not write this book to proffer medical advice. Your health-care provider is the person with whom you should consult in a quest for health. However, I trust that the content of this book will stimulate your thinking about the lifestyle changes you can make that will promote cardiovascular wellness. Understanding the principles of a natural path to health may help you make wiser choices about health-care services.

When I use the term "health-care services," I mean everything from the use of a weight-loss clinic to the need for advanced cardiac life support. If this book pushes at-risk individuals toward health-care providers who can steer those persons away from risk, it will have achieved its objective. I encourage readers to engage their physicians in debate and share the contents of this book with them.

CHAPTER ONE

THE SECRET TO YOUTH?

The proverbial quest for the "fountain of youth" did not start with the Spanish explorer, Ponce de León, and it certainly has not ended with him. Men and women always have been on a perpetual search for the one potion, elixir, or alchemist's formula that guarantees eternal youth. In our own time, this search has taken on a new twist. Men and women may put their faith in lotions and creams and even expensive plastic surgery to make them look younger. Those on a quest for external beauty and a perpetually youthful appearance often overlook the need for health from within—specifically, cardiac wellness.

Given the current emphasis on "antiaging," it would seem that baby boomers do not want to grow old. Frenetic antiaging tactics do not always recognize that the eradication of heart disease will add at least ten to fifteen *useful* years to our lifespan. Let us face the important fact that industrialized communities are plagued by cardiovascular disease. Coronary heart disease remains the number one killer in Western society, and its prevention and treatment remain the priority in health care for the new millennium. True, there is a minor trend for reduction in death rate from heart disease in several Western countries. However, this is balanced by observations of increasing cardiac death rates in developing nations and Eastern Europe. Loaded with risk factors for premature cardiac death, there are millions of people waiting for their first sign of heart disease. The heart disease bomb is scattered throughout the human population, and it is waiting to detonate.

Youth-oriented lifestyles are marketed to all age groups in an ill-advised attempt to help everyone *feel young!* It is unfortunate that so many of us search for the ever-elusive fountain of youth, but ignore the known steps we can take to stay well and active for as long as possible. The fact is, a healthy heart is as close to a true fountain of youth as you will ever get. When you think about the signs of aging and what will cause you to lament that your youth is over, poor health is at the top of the list. And there is no question that heart disease can rob you of your vitality and interfere with your quality of life. However, for the most part heart diseases are preventable, and you are not simply at the mercy of advancing years.

While no one can live forever, there are natural ways to improve the odds that you will live fully and prevent cardiovascular diseases. Heart disease is not a single condition with a simple answer. Rather, it is a complex process that takes place over years—even decades—which is why understanding heart disease is the first step on the path to cardiovascular wellness.

UNDERSTANDING THE HEART-DISEASE "BOMB"

As we enter a new century, given all that we know about cardiovascular disease, anyone who questions the role of high blood cholesterol (hypercholesterolemia) as an important cause of coronary heart disease should probably join the Flat Earth Society. However, despite the massive amount of attention it receives, high cholesterol is not the only issue relevant in a discussion of cardiovascular wellness. Other factors make up what I call a "bomb."

The concept of a bomb provides a useful way to view the heart disease issue. While most time bombs tick and provide some warning before they go off, unfortunately the heart disease time bomb has no tick. It can, however, be spotted before detonation. A high cholesterol level, one among many ingredients in the heart-disease bomb, is a primary clue that points to developing disease.

Remember that high cholesterol is not a disease in itself; however, it is often a marker that heart disease may be developing or is present, with varying degrees of severity. This is the reason why so much attention is focused on cholesterol numbers.

One component of this book provides a comprehensive description of the most important factors that determine the risks of atherosclerosis and coronary artery disease. Regardless of what risk factors—or lack of them—you are able to identify at this time, be mindful that cardiovascular disease is always a serious health issue. Elevated blood cholesterol is *one* major finding that is inextricably linked to other risk factors.

Medical research has shown that stress, obesity, cigarette smoking, and genetic predispositions also are often linked to high blood cholesterol and the risk of coronary heart disease. (See Table 1.1 for a comprehensive list of risk factors.) These factors operate together in compounding the risk of heart attack and ischemic heart disease, caused by reduced blood flow to the heart muscle and compromised circulation. Despite the advances in medical research and treatment, millions of men and women are affected by this killer disease.

Sadly, many people have developed a sense of complacency, perhaps counting on medical "miracles" to save them should heart disease strike. "Look around," they may say, "many people live for years—or even decades—while being treated for heart disease." Perhaps they point to drugs designed to lower cholesterol, or they count on sophisticated, lifesaving procedures to keep them alive and functioning. "After all," they say, "bypass surgery has given millions a new lease on life." Sure, numerous treatments exist, but prevention is always preferable to treatment—and it is significantly less expensive—no matter how many advances in treatment appear. Rest assured, your quality of life will be influenced by the presence of heart disease in all its manifestations. No heart medication or surgery developed to date can completely restore cardiovascular health once it has been damaged. In fact, several recent scientific studies have questioned the value of cardiac medicine and interventions in terms of their ability to alter the course of cardiac disease.

Tragically, many people are not aware that cardiovascular conditions are largely preventable. Or, even if they are aware of some common prevention measures, they may have difficulty implementing

Table 1.1: Risk Factors for Coronary Artery Disease.

Although alcohol and caffeine have been claimed by some to be independent risk factors, they have not been established to be clear risks. However, obesity acts by increasing the severity of hypertension, hyperlipidemia, and diabetes mellitus, and it has an important influence on the development of coronary artery disease.

FACTOR	SIGNIFICANCE
Diet	A high lipid (fat) content in diet contributes to coronary artery disease. Saturated fat is bad; essential fatty acids are good.
Blood lipids	Risk of atheroma is directly proportional to the increase in concentration of total cholesterol and of low-density lipoprotein (LDL) and inversely proportional to concentration of high-density lipoprotein (HDL).
Blood pressure	Risk is directly proportional to the increase of systolic or diastolic blood pressure.
Cigarette smoking	Risk is proportionate to the number of cigarettes smoked per day (risk is three times control at a pack or more per day).
Personality type	A competitive, driven person (so-called Type A personality) is more prone to coronary artery disease. An aggressive, conversation-interrupting male is a great risk.
Sedentary lifestyle	Individuals who do not exercise regularly may have a greater risk of myocardial infarction than individuals who exercise regularly.
Diabetes mellitus	Risk is two times control in diabetic men, three times control in diabetic women.
Obesity	Overweight people have more coronary artery disease than those of normal body weight.

them and making these strategies a natural part of day-to-day life. Meanwhile, the bomb ticks on.

The concept of *time* for the bomb to detonate is important, too. Cardiovascular risks compound over time, day after day, year after year. If you want to prevent the bomb from exploding, you must begin an intervention program, and it is essential that you correct adverse lifestyle choices. No treatment, no matter how sophisticated and "high-tech," is a substitute for choosing a sensible, heart-healthy way of life.

Furthermore, just as it is never too late to implement positive changes in your life, it is never too early to begin your prevention program. If you are a parent, the information in this book is crucial; it is no exaggeration to say that heart disease often has its roots in childhood. The fact that high blood cholesterol affects our children and that atherosclerosis may have its early manifestations in teenagers is too often overlooked.

Large numbers of our society's teenagers smoke cigarettes, and excessive drinking among high school and college students is so common that it is considered a significant social problem by psychologists and educators. Many adults know very well what it is like to quit smoking, or have family and physicians urge them to cut back on their alcohol intake, or otherwise face a major lifestyle cleanup program. Certainly the best path is to never smoke at all, but despite efforts to discourage it, millions continue the habit. Heavy drinking is an important risk factor, one that often goes unnoticed until problems with professional and personal relationships emerge or the damage to the body can no longer be ignored. With any of the lifestyle risk factors, it goes without saying that the earlier an intervention is initiated, the better the prognosis.

The "Bouquet of Barbed Wire"

Risk factors for cardiovascular disease are tangled together—interdependent and, unfortunately, difficult to separate. Recent scientific research continues to provide evidence of close linkage among the risk factors. Many studies show that elevated blood cholesterol goes hand in hand with stress, smoking, and obesity. Obesity is linked with hypertension (elevated blood pressure) and sedentary occupations as well as sedentary leisure time. Smoking causes heart disease and may bring about a heart attack.

Adverse lifestyle factors largely determine your level of overall risk; together, they form the common thread running through this complex "bouquet" of risk factors within the bomb—a bomb that is

Table 1.2: Some Sure Tactics for Poor Health.

These are not recommendations for anyone to follow. They are written and expressed in a manner that is designed to stimulate thoughts about lifestyle change that could accrue to an individual's benefit.

Smoke heavily	Safe levels of smoking defy clear definition.
Drink too much alcohol	If you do not die of liver disease, you will succumb to trauma usually after very painful social isolation.
Stay fat	Significant obesity is clearly associated with chronic disease and early death.
Do not exercise	This assures many health problems and a lack of well-being.
Stress yourself	You may become mentally distraught, or constantly physically ill, and you may harm others.
Eat a lousy diet	This is a good way to make almost every organ in the body fail.
Disdain conventional medical practitioners	He or she could save your life.
Disdain nutritionally oriented physicians	He or she has a lot to offer and can enhance the quality of your life.
Do not have periodic health checks	You will never know much about your risks of illness or death. You will suffer or die in ignorance.
Self-medicate with pharmaceuticals	Over-the-counter medications are freely available for you to abuse; some are lethal when misused.
Use too many "health foods," dietary supplements, or "way-out" herbal cures	You can ruin your health with excessive vitamin intake. Many dietary supplements have purposely misleading health claims. Some herbs are great poisons.
Make your own diagnosis and ignore prolonged or serious symptoms	There are many serious diseases that can kill you slowly. Several are amenable to cure. Self-medication or diagnosis is a great way of denying yourself a good health outcome.

| Engage in risky lifestyles | It may be pleasurable to put your life at risk, but it is easy to die prematurely. |

ticking. Most individuals know if they are too fat, smoke too much, spend their lives feeling rushed and tense, or engage in other risky behavior. However, these same individuals may continue to live on a dangerous edge. They may realize that they are traveling on a path toward trouble, but find themselves continuing to delay concerted efforts to change.

Most of us find change difficult. Nowadays, it may seem as if everything changes so quickly we have a hard time catching up with ourselves. In such a stress-filled world, personal change seems all the more difficult to initiate. However, you chose this book, so you are therefore likely to be highly motivated to change.

The Natural Way to a Healthy Heart is designed to help you untangle the cardiovascular risk factors you may be facing. It is my hope that you will be motivated to honestly examine the high-risk elements of your lifestyle and take steps to change the way you live. Cardiovascular wellness is an area of health care in which you, the patient, are in charge. When you think about it, there is nothing more natural than taking responsibility for your own lifestyle. Being self-directed is one of the key *natural* ways to cardiovascular wellness.

If we put TNT into a bomb it will cause a big *bang*, but the addition of plastic explosives and atomic fission will result in a devastating explosion. In the same way, multiple cardiovascular risk factors add up to more serious cardiovascular risks and consequences. Put simply, the dangers of coronary heart disease and heart attack increase as the number of risk factors increase, and they have a synergistic (additive) effect.

Most popular books on health topics stress the changes that are necessary to promote well-being. However, sometimes this positive approach may not be as effective as pointing out the ways to ensure ill health, outlined in Table 1.2. Despite clear warnings, some elements of a fundamentally risky lifestyle are pleasurable to many people. Many adults love a hot fudge sundae as much as children do, and sometimes the couch looks a lot more appealing than the treadmill. Denial, projection, or rationalization are all-too-human characteristics. A smoker might say, "I know I should quit, but I can't do it now because my wife still smokes and so do my coworkers. Since they smoke, I can't quit—this just isn't the right time." This sounds logical—even reasonable—to the addicted smoker. But does the "right time" ever arrive? A heavy drinker might rationalize, "An occasional six pack of beer" (almost every day, as it turns out) "doesn't hurt. And the beer I buy is brewed with spring water and organic hops!" (Organic "junk food" is indeed all the rage.)

A large body of scientific evidence establishes the fact that most people don't care to see the dangers of their indulgence in risky behaviors. For example, individuals whose eating disorder is the root cause of their obesity and high cholesterol levels are very likely to underestimate the quantity and quality of food they consume. Those who regularly eat breakfast and lunch at fast food restaurants may talk about their habit as if it is a "now-and-then" indulgence. Their denial is so complete that they are genuinely shocked when their doctors give them the bad news about their dangerously high cholesterol levels. Unfortunately, fast food has become a staple diet for many people—not only in this country, but thanks to a few multinational corporations, across the planet, too. Undeniably, fast food is usually loaded with unhealthy types of fat, and it is often rich in refined sugar and cholesterol. Fortunately, some fast food is becoming healthy.

While it is normal to mentally suppress or at least minimize the significance of a pleasurable risk, evidence also suggests that we can break through denial and change our behavior. Positive change is not only possible—it is common. Many millions of Americans have quit smoking over the last two or three decades; every year, thousands of individuals address addiction problems, often using both medical intervention and personal support groups. Obesity is overcome in many cases, and based on the continuous entry into commercial diet programs, millions persist in their efforts to achieve a healthful weight.

Despite the recent interest in low-fat diets, the overall statistics on fat intake are not encouraging. We know that excessive intake of the wrong type of dietary fat is a major factor in developing coronary heart disease and that fat intake is closely related to obesity and overeating. It has been estimated in some surveys that the average daily intake of fat has increased up to about eighty-three grams per day over the last decade. Fats are a major source of unwanted calories. Who can really discuss the nutritional value of fast food and keep a straight face when examining its caloric and fat content? (See some examples in Table 1.3.) Once the veil of denial is lifted, can anyone continue to eat fat-laden, highly processed foods and justify this as a relatively benign vice? Knowledge may be power, but when it comes to your health, you must apply what you know before it has any power at all.

SPOTTING THE RISKS IS *YOUR* JOB

The medical profession has gone so far down the path of technology that the idea of prevention through self-care interventions is often overlooked. I, or any other health-care professional for that matter, would be lying if I claimed to offer a quick fix. Prevention strategies often take time, persistence, and patience. Weight-loss diets that also are likely to lower cholesterol levels require a commitment and

---

Table 1.3: Approximate Fat Content of Some of the Most Popular Fast Food Items.

The fat is largely of the saturated type, and the food contains a relatively large amount of trans-fatty acids that may be dangerous to health. These fast food items are not much different from many processed animal protein products that are found in all stores. Compositions of food vary with time, and salad bars have emerged in fast food restaurants as this industry responds to demands for better nutrition.

Popular Fast Food Items	Grams of Fat Per Average Serving
Burger King Chicken Sandwich	42
Burger King Whopper	38
McDonald's Sausage and Egg Biscuit	33
McDonald's Quarter Pounder with Cheese	28
KFC Chicken Sandwich	27
Wendy's Big Classic hamburger	23

Fat content values are from *The Complete Book of Food Values,* by Corinne T. Netzer (Dell, 1994).

---

steady implementation over months, not days. Health club member-
ships are worthwhile only if you regularly show up and take the classes or use the equipment. In other words, natural ways may take time;
they are not an easy way out. Most certainly, they do not conform
with our society's "quick fix" mentality when it comes to health care.

Many simple—and natural—preventive strategies are rarely perceived as effective when compared to pharmaceutical or surgical
interventions. This is unfortunate, because in the long run, prevention is extremely worthwhile. Equally unfortunate is the fact that in
many cases, individuals interested in prevention cannot expect much
in the way of guidance or support from the agencies that fund medicine. This is one reason why many health-care consumers are willing
to spend their own money for advice from the so-called alternative
practitioners, many of whom spend considerable time educating and
counseling their patients. It is also the reason why many people may
look for information in books such as this.

As I previously explained, I prefer the term "pluralistic" medicine, because it implies that there is room for all effective treatments. The term "alternative" implies a separation from what
Western medicine considers "true" health care. Because of this
implied separation, patients may not tell their conventional physician that they are receiving additional medical advice from a non-
conventional practitioner. However, in some contexts, for clarity, we
are essentially stuck with the term "alternative."

**Table 1.4: Cardiovascular Risk Factors That Are Readily
Changed and Simple Approaches to Reducing Risks.**

Cardiovascular Risk Factors Amenable to Change:
- High blood cholesterol
- Smoking
- Physical inertia
- High blood pressure
- Low levels of high density lipoprotein

Aims of a Simple Risk Factor Reduction Program:
- Decrease saturated fat intake
- Achieve and or maintain ideal body weight
- Reduce sodium intake
- Stop smoking

The old-style family doctor, who often could be relied on for lifestyle advice, seems like a quaint figure of the past. Today's doctor is dominated by corporate medicine—that is, managed care. As you may well know, managed care organizations frequently talk about preventive medicine strategies, some of which are touted extensively in their marketing campaigns. However, very few managed care organizations will foot the bill or pay directly for preventive medicine. The "new" physician may often have a no-talk, hands-off, investigational-intense attitude, perhaps combined with a quick reach for a prescription pad. When did a physician in the United States last make a house call? In recent memory, only the infamous Dr. Jack Kevorkian has made regular house calls!

As you have seen in Table 1.2, I summarized several ways of almost ensuring cardiovascular disease or premature death. You will notice that cardiovascular risk factors are quite often known risks for other common killer diseases, such as diabetes or cancer.

The Folly of Just Lowering Cholesterol

One reason I began this book with a discussion of the cholesterol issue is that dietary and lifestyle interventions to control cholesterol are among the most immediate adjustments that individuals can make. Indeed, most roads of cardiovascular risk lead to the concepts that surround the "cholesterol theory" of cardiovascular disease. I subscribe to the cholesterol theory, but I also recognize that this theory is valid only when the other risks of cardiovascular disease are linked with it. High blood cholesterol is not the whole story of cardiac disease.

Some physicians and scientists have rejected the notion that low cholesterol diets reduce the risk of developing *atheroma*, the fatty degeneration and hardening of the arterial walls. True, clinical trials exist that have failed to show a clear connection between dietary saturated fat or cholesterol intake and coronary artery disease. On the other hand, there are many studies that indicate a clear connection—no wonder the situation is confusing! Unfortunately, a plea of confusion is used by many people as a reason to remain complacent about their diets and make little effort to change the dietary component of their lifestyle.

The Multiple Risk Factor Intervention Trial (MRFT) performed in the mid-1970s provides a good example of the failure of the focused intervention aimed at the reduction of cholesterol alone. This trial examined the role of reducing dietary cholesterol and saturated fats as a means of preventing heart disease. The MRFT involved the study of 12,000 men who were considered at risk for cardiovascular disease. Divided into two groups, the first was advised to adopt a diet designed to reduce blood cholesterol levels, and the second was given no advice about specific dietary interventions. Both groups received normal supportive medical care, such as medication to reduce blood pressure. This prospective (meaning forward, or ongoing) study showed that the group that was advised to consume a low cholesterol diet was able to achieve overall lower serum cholesterol values and lower blood pressure readings than the group that did not receive a specific dietary intervention. However, no major improvement in the death rate from cardiovascular disease was noted as a consequence of the dietary intervention to lower cholesterol. Needless to say, this was a disappointing result.

Some researchers have gone further in their criticism of medical interventions to lower cholesterol. These individuals have questioned the use of drugs to lower serum cholesterol, and some physicians who are more nutritionally oriented have described the practice of lowering cholesterol with drug therapy as perhaps worthless and potentially quite dangerous! All this confusing information underscores the importance of the time-bomb concept. Focusing on one risk factor, one ingredient in the bomb, at the expense of considering the synergistic, negative health effects of all risk factors is a common mistake in medicine today. I do not believe that lowering blood cholesterol is an unnecessary pastime, but other risk factors *must* be addressed simultaneously.

Primary and Secondary Interventions

Primary prevention involves removing, at inception, factors that may contribute to the cause of a disease process. As we have seen, removing one risk factor, in isolation, is hardly the best way to heart health. In contrast, there are measured benefits of reducing blood cholesterol in patients who already have high cholesterol and established heart disease. This is an example of *secondary* prevention.

These concepts are somewhat difficult to understand, and I do not want you to think lowering blood cholesterol levels in the presence of coronary artery disease is not worthwhile. However, the results of primary and secondary preventive measures clearly indicate that the benefits, or lack thereof, of reducing total blood cholesterol are quite dependent on the overall risk that the individual has for developing coronary artery disease and its consequences. In simple terms, this means: *the higher the overall risk you have, perhaps the greater the benefit of reducing blood cholesterol levels.*

"Miracle" Drugs?

Many drawbacks appear when we look more closely at the approach of targeted therapy to *just* lower blood cholesterol, which may be an example of shortsighted or even foolish medicine. In the absence of a nutritional program to improve general health, it is not always safe, nor is it cost effective, to reduce cholesterol by excluding cholesterol intake in the diet and/or prescribing synthetic drugs that lower fats (cholesterol) in the blood.

In the early part of the 1980s, a considerable amount of research was performed on the role of cholesterol as a key factor in the cause of coronary artery disease. Many leading health-care institutions and the federal government of the United States endorsed the cholesterol and heart disease link: by the latter part of the 1980s, reducing cholesterol levels had become a primary health objective. Coincidental with this, multinational pharmaceutical companies invested millions of dollars in researching and developing synthetic cholesterol-lowering drugs. As a result, there is often an enthusiastic willingness among physicians to reach for the prescription pad and take a pharmacological approach to treating high blood cholesterol. In order for this to happen, however, there must be an equal willingness on the part of individuals with high blood cholesterol readings to take this easy way out. We are, after all, a society conditioned to respect "miracle" cures.

The ability of cholesterol-lowering drugs to reduce cholesterol has overshadowed the importance of their possible side effects. The side effects of some of these lipid-lowering drugs are unpleasant at best, and sometimes potentially serious. Nausea, bloating, abdominal pain, and gastrointestinal distress are frequently reported, and these drugs may interfere with normal liver function. These are the short-term side effects, but over the long-term, potential damage remains an unknown factor. Furthermore, these drugs are expensive.

Dean Ornish, M.D., whose revolutionary program to reverse heart disease is based on nutrition and lifestyle measures, estimates that about 100 million people in the U.S. have high cholesterol readings, and were we to treat all these individuals with cholesterol-lowering drugs, it would cost *200 to 300 billion dollars a year*! On an individual level, patients may pay several thousand dollars each year for treatment with these drugs. The potential side effects and the high cost combine to provide overriding reasons to seek safer, natural options to lower cholesterol, normalize blood lipids, and promote general wellness.

The role of dietary and lifestyle adjustment in lowering cholesterol has been apparent from the start. However, an assumption was made—and continues to influence medical treatments—that patients would not comply with advice about changing adverse lifestyle factors. Anticipating noncompliance fueled the quantum leap away from appropriate, noninvasive, and—yes—natural, first-line options for reducing cholesterol to the widespread application of drug therapy to accomplish the same goal. Unfortunately, this situation occurred at the expense of considering lifestyle change as a key to cardiovascular health, general health, and longevity.

It is important to point out that many therapeutic programs for cardiovascular wellness use options to treat obesity *and* lower fats in the blood. However, drugs for obesity treatment are often ineffective, frequently addictive and, overall, should be avoided. (See Table 1.5.)

Nutrition as the Key

In the long run, an ideal—and natural—approach is to lower cholesterol while simultaneously enhancing general health through good nutrition. This therapeutic approach is drug-free and frequently very effective. It is most certainly a preferable first-line option for health-conscious individuals who want to control cholesterol and promote more general health through natural and nutritionally sound means.

Nowadays, this group of individuals is large and growing, and they are demanding the safest therapies possible. Most important of all, they are willing to take responsibility for their health.

Several bestselling books have focused on programs to lower cholesterol. Recommending lifestyle change is a common thread in these books, but overall they tend to favor a short-term focus on lowering cholesterol to improve cardiovascular health. Some of these books have practical suggestions and valuable advice, so I have listed them in the suggested reading list at the end of the book. In many cases, such books do not provide a comprehensive review of natural options or they may focus on only a single natural option. Short-term approaches to lowering cholesterol are not as beneficial to your health as a more comprehensive—holistic—approach.

One pivotal factor in preventing atheroma (arteriosclerosis, coronary heart disease, etc.) is a well-balanced diet that provides an optimal array of nutrients. Unfortunately, the average Western diet is not

---

Table 1.5: Drugs Commonly Used to Lower Cholesterol and Treat Obesity.

The asterisks (*) denote amphetamine-like compounds that should not, in the author's opinion, be used for obesity management. Many of the drugs listed for obesity management are controlled substances, and they have adverse effects on cardiovascular function. Some have been withdrawn.

Drugs to Lower Lipids	Drugs for Obesity
Probucol	Benzphetamine*
	Dextroamphetamine*
Fibric Acids	Diethylprotion
Clofibrate	Fenfluramine
Gemfibrizol	Mazindol
	Methamphetamine*
HMG CoA Reductase Inhibitors	Phendimetrazine
Lovastatin	Phenmetrazine
Pravastatin	Phenylpropanolamine
Simvastatin	
Bile Acid Sequestrants	
Cholestyramine	
Colestipol	

well-balanced and rarely, if ever, provides an optimal amount of necessary nutrients. Solving this problem by using dietary supplements is a reasonable approach—however, there is probably as much misuse of dietary supplements as there is of prescription or over-the-counter drugs. In some circumstances, excesses of some unregulated dietary supplements may be more dangerous than the adverse effects of prescription drugs!

This discussion may be confusing. On the one hand, I am sounding a warning against prescription drugs, whereas on the other, I am strong in my belief that some dietary supplements require caution when used. The resolution to the confusion rests in the fact that self-medicators should take the time to be certain that they have educated themselves in the judicious use of dietary supplements or other natural medical options. An effective strategy is to seek the services of a qualified health-care giver who has a well-balanced and pluralistic approach. This kind of health-care practitioner is open-minded about options and less willing to reach for the prescription pad. Within their separate domains, all health-care givers have much to offer. In some specific instances, naturopaths, osteopaths, podiatrists, chiropractors, and nutritionists may have much more to offer than a physician. Today, millions of patients regularly seek the services of these professionals.

The Modern Dilemma in Health-Care

Some consumers who turn to natural medicine find that many "conventional" physicians may reject, out of hand, dietary supplements or other natural therapies. This rejection is rooted in the ignorance on the part of some physicians of the value of natural medicine. Very few medical schools focus on teaching nutrition, at least to a level that would permit average physicians to provide informed judgments about many of the proposed nutritional options that are available to combat disease.

While one may be critical of conventional medicine with its bent toward a pharmacological approach to lower cholesterol, even more criticism may be directed at alternative medicine practitioners who do not consider the *entire* array of available natural options to promote cardiovascular wellness. The muddle we find ourselves in today is not the fault of only one branch or form of health care. The fault is equally shared, and it has taken attention away from seeking scientific evidence that many noninvasive, natural therapies are effective. (I have addressed many of these issues in a previous book, *Miracle Herbs*.)

Add to the dilemma the fact that many theories or applications of natural medicine are flawed, or are empiric, meaning they are based on observation and anecdotal reports. Alternative medicine suffers from a chronic lack of controlled clinical studies that demonstrate safety or efficacy of the intervention. I realize that it may not be easy to find the appropriate practitioners to help you use a natural path to health, especially those who also are familiar with the judicious use of conventional therapies. You may need to do some research in your location in order to find suitable practitioners. However, I hope the information in this book will help you make decisions not only about the kind of treatment you seek, but also about your self-care program.

Antiaging Tactics and Antiaging Antics

The members of the "baby boomer" generation have reached a point where they face the prospect of growing old. Modern concepts of getting on with life rather than growing old gracefully have permeated our thinking. Conventional medicine failed to spot this health-care consumer need and permitted the evolution of dozens of antiaging societies and organizations that often lean toward alternative medicine. I make no judgment, but it puzzles me why conventional medicine continues to fiddle while Rome burns.

Aging is a function of lifestyle, which of course points us back to the identification of a host of risk factors for organ dysfunction that may be amenable to prevention. Antiaging tactics should first involve prevention, but this is a hollow statement for the aged members of society.

Promises of the "fountain of youth" are the oldest ploy used by the snake-oil salesman (though, ironically, snake oil is very healthy stuff). Alternative medicine has contributed greatly to antiaging medicine, principally by denying that aging is an inevitability. However, antiaging tactics have bred antiaging antics. One such antic is the troublesome panacea recommendation for self-administered hormone therapy. This recommendation has most notably been applied to growth hormone, DHEA, melatonin, testosterone, estrogen, and progesterone, sometimes in a reckless manner.

There is a credible body of evidence that hormonal supplementation can have beneficial "antiaging" benefits, but playing with hormones is not a safe pastime. One of the most effective ways of raising HDL for women is estrogen replacement therapy, but at what cost? Hormone replacement therapy reduces the risk of heart attack but increases the risk of venous thrombosis and uterine and breast cancer, and its general side-effect profile is not good. Progesterone, alone or in combination with estrogen, is popular but the effects of these hormones on the risk of heart disease remains unclear. It should be widely recognized that progesterone may counteract some of the favorable effects of estrogen on blood HDL levels.

Studies on the benefits, or lack thereof, of hormone precursors (such as DHEA) or growth hormone on an aging cardiovascular system are decidedly incomplete. The idea of growing young with growth hormone may have some merit, but individuals with excesses of growth hormone (as in acromegaly) commonly die of heart failure due to cardiomyopathy.

Hormone therapies are classic examples of the double-edged sword. As such, hormones cannot be considered safe for self-medication, but they may be valuable when used by a physician who is skilled in their application. I raise these issues because injudicious use of hormones in supplements may be more of a risk for heart disease than people think.

SUMMARY

You have the power to help prevent cardiovascular disease, the number one cause of death in our society. Because there is no single risk factor for heart disease, the best way to view the myriad contributing factors is as a "bouquet of barbed wire." Take a close look at Table 1.2 to determine the elements of your lifestyle that are entangled in this bouquet of barbed wire. Are you living your way to a premature death? Cardiovascular disease is a problem rooted in lifestyle issues, and you have the power over almost all the risk factors for heart problems.

What You Can Do

- The "cholesterol factor" is important, but it is not the only risk factor worth your consideration. Begin to consider and untangle the whole "bouquet."
- Cholesterol-lowering drugs are available—and they are often effective—but they often have detrimental side effects and are expensive. Remember, too, that they address only one risk factor. The first-line option to lower cholesterol is using soy protein containing isoflavones.
- Improved nutrition represents the first line of defense against high cholesterol. You are in charge of your risk factors, and it is up to you to educate yourself about a "heart-healthy" diet.
- Both conventional and alternative medical philosophies have much to offer in preventing and treating cardiovascular disease—begin thinking in terms of "pluralistic" health care. Not all alternative options that are presented as natural may be safe. I have concerns about widespread self-medication with hormones.
- Be prepared to take responsibility for *preventing* cardiovascular disease.

CHAPTER TWO

WHAT THE TERMS AND CHOLESTEROL NUMBERS MEAN

Scientific evidence exists that clearly documents the relationship between high blood cholesterol (hypercholesteremia) and heart disease, but cholesterol is not the only significant blood lipid. (Lipids are any of the various fatty substances in the blood.) The functions of these lipids and the way they form can easily become confusing—even to health-care professionals. Just to clarify the issues we are discussing, I have included the following list of basic definitions.

- **Cholesterol:** A substance that is waxy in consistency, found throughout the body, and essential to health. Cholesterol is found in animal foods, and the liver manufactures cholesterol primarily from saturated fats. The body needs cholesterol to make sex and adrenal hormones and other essential substances.
- **Lipoprotein:** The "envelope" of protein that transports cholesterol in the blood. There are many different types of lipoprotein fractions in the blood (summarized in Table 2.1).
- **Triglycerides (TG):** This is a blood lipid, but it is not chemically similar to cholesterol. It is routinely measured in cholesterol testing. Both plant and animal foods contain triglycerides, and the liver also manufactures it.

Table 2.1: Major Serum Lipoproteins.

Lipoprotein	Function
Chylomicrons	transport of dietary fat
"Bad Cholesterol" Very low-density lipoprotein (VLDL)	transport of endogenous fat
"Bad Cholesterol" Low-density lipoprotein (LDL)	transport of cholesterol to peripheral tissue
"Good Cholesterol" High-density lipoprotein (HDL)	reverse cholesterol transport

Triglycerides are used for energy or are stored in the body. High triglyceride levels often go hand in hand with high levels of "bad" cholesterol and low levels of "good" cholesterol.

- **High-Density Lipoprotein (HDL):** The so-called "good" cholesterol, HDL can remove cholesterol from the cells and transport it back to the liver, where it eventually makes its way through the digestive tract and is excreted from the body. Advantageous levels of HDL also help prevent blood clots and constriction of the blood vessels. Low levels of HDL are often associated with high triglyceride levels.

- **Low-Density Lipoprotein (LDL):** The so-called "bad" cholesterol, LDL is used to carry cholesterol to the cells, but when its levels are too high it creates problems by "sticking" to arterial walls. Damage or lesions in the protective layer of cells (endothelial cells) in the arterial walls give the LDL a place to settle or "invade." Carbon monoxide and other agents in cigarette smoke can cause lesions in this layer of cells, which is one reason why smoking is a serious and direct cause of heart disease. Oxidation of LDL (combining with oxygen) tends to cause precipitation of LDL in arterial blood vessel walls.

- **Very Low-Density Lipoprotein (VLDL):** This lipoprotein is converted to LDL.
- **Plaque:** A substance that could be called "debris" because it is comprised of cholesterol, minerals, and other material. Plaque may build up and cause blockages and clots in blood vessels, making it a hazardous substance in the body. However, plaque buildup may be reversed.

It is possible to help prevent coronary artery disease if we maintain lower overall levels of blood lipids. Or, looking at it another way, consider that:

- a *high* total blood cholesterol
- a *high* low-density lipoprotein (LDL)
- a *high* very low-density lipoprotein level (VLDL)
- a *high* triglyceride level (TG)
- a *low* high-density cholesterol level (HDL)

comprise an *adverse* cholesterol profile, but the important thing to remember is that this profile *can be changed*. A good profile is often as important as cholesterol numbers. You do not always need a miracle or a drug to change this lipid profile. Natural options to change it are first-line options.

WHERE THIS PROFILE LEADS

Heart disease is actually a misnomer, since it is actually a group of conditions and manifests in a variety of ways. The following list is just a sample of basic terms you will hear when heart diseases are discussed.

- **atheroma/atherosclerosis:** The condition that results when cholesterol-containing deposits form plaque on the walls of coronary arteries and vessels.
- **arteriosclerosis:** Commonly called "hardening of the arteries," which is actually the thickening of the arterial walls. The arteries lose elasticity; hence, they are described as "hardening" or "hardened."

- **arrhythmia:** As the term implies, this condition is characterized by irregular heartbeat, or a situation in which the heartbeat is too fast or too slow.

- **myocardial infarction:** The heart muscle is damaged during an episode in which one or more of the arteries is blocked and portions of the heart are deprived of oxygen. In common language, this is known as a *heart attack*. Every year, about 1.5 million Americans will experience a heart attack, and one third—500,000—will not survive. The other one million individuals are forever changed in that they are now "heart patients." For some—the fortunate—this is a reason to make positive lifestyle changes. For others, however, a heart condition becomes an ever-present cause of fear, hopelessness, and even depression.

- **thrombosis:** The formation of a blood clot. Obviously, the blood must be able to coagulate and form a clot when an injury occurs. However, clotting can occur within an artery, particularly when these structures are narrowed as a result of a buildup of plaque. Blood clots are the cause of many heart attacks and strokes. The blood has both clotting and anti-clotting factors. Medications (including aspirin) are often given to heart patients to keep the blood thin and discourage the formation of clots. As you will later learn, some nutrients and common plants have a similar effect to aspirin, and some may be safer and more versatile in their benefits for cardiac health.

- **congestive heart failure (CHF):** This is a condition that a layperson might describe as a "weak" or "tired" heart. In a sense, this is an accurate description. The heart muscle is weak and unable to efficiently pump blood throughout the body, which frequently leads to fluid accumulation in the lower legs and ankles and congestion in the lungs. One could say that the heart is suffering from a lack of energy, and that means that patients tire easily and are often short of breath after mild exertion. This "pump failure" is the cause of fluid accumulation in the body.

HOW ATHEROMA FORMS IN BLOOD VESSELS

The hallmark of atheroma is the development of cholesterol containing plaque in the lining and wall of the blood vessels. Injuries to the lining of the blood vessels and excessive amounts of circulating LDL play a major role in promoting the formation of plaque. The lining of the blood vessels can be injured as a consequence of several events or factors, including the presence of diabetes mellitus, high blood pressure, smoking, and alterations in the function of the immune system.

Blockages in the arteries result when fats (lipids) from LDL and VLDL deposit in arterial walls. Arteries throughout the body have many branches with decreasing diameters. For example, the internal diameter of a major human coronary artery is quite narrow, about two to three millimeters (½ of an inch), and it is easily blocked by debris formed from cholesterol and fats.

The last decade or so has brought increasing understanding of the mechanisms whereby lipids are deposited in arteries to cause atheroma. It appears that lesions in the lining of arteries (intima) make them vulnerable to LDL cholesterol deposits. When a lesion occurs, the body responds by attempting to repair it. Repair proteins, platelet aggregation (clots), calcium deposits, and additional fats can build up over a long period of time, thereby leading to arterial blockage.

For many years—or even a lifetime—the arteries can go through this process of "damming up" without symptoms. Sometimes, the first manifestation of a blockage is a heart attack, with or without prior symptoms. The blockage of the blood vessels supplying the heart—coronary arteries—results in a starvation of oxygen and nutrients to the heart muscle. When the vessel is rapidly blocked or closed (occluded), a heart attack may result. When this process happens slowly, a condition known as *angina pectoris* may result.

Angina: A "Heart Scream"

Angina pectoris is chest pain that occurs when there is a lack of blood supply to the heart. The word *angina* comes from the Greek and means "strangulation" or "choking." This is a most descriptive word

Table 2.2: Physical Manifestations of Coronary Heart Disease.

Clinical manifestations are related to the anatomical changes that occur in arteries that supply the heart.

Disorder	Physical Events
Sudden death	Abnormal heart rhythm or heart attack
Heart failure	Myocardial compromise due to infarction (heart attack due to lack of blood supply) or ischemia
Arrhythmias	Altered electrical conduction in the heart due to ischemia or infarction
Myocardial infarction	Sudden occlusion due to coronary thrombosis
Unstable angina	"On and off" obstruction due to plaque or arterial spasm
Stable angina	Fixed atheromatous narrowing of coronary arteries

when one considers that the heart essentially "screams out" in pain, especially if exercise or physiological stresses place a demand for increased blood supply to the heart. The heart cannot get the blood it needs because the diameter of the arteries is reduced by atheroma, the buildup of cholesterol and fats. In addition, atheroma reduces the "relaxability" of the arteries. Angina can be stable or unstable; in the latter situation, the risk of heart attack may be imminent.

Most frequently, angina is felt as a left-sided or central chest pain that is brought on by circumstances that stress the heart, thereby resulting in increased demands for oxygen. (See Table 2.3.) Many individuals with angina describe a sensation of tightness in the chest of varying severity. The pain is usually said to be constricting, sometimes likened to a sense that the chest is being compressed or a band is being tightened around the chest.

There are several circumstances that may commonly precipitate an anginal episode. Some of these circumstances can be inferred by understanding the mechanisms whereby the heart is stimulated to cause an increased demand for oxygen by increasing its blood flow.

Table 2.3: Angina Pectoris.

Factors that stress the heart and result in increased oxygen demand can precipitate angina. Several factors regulate oxygen supply to the heart, including flow of blood through the coronary arteries and the status of oxygenation of the blood. Cigarette smoking may decrease blood oxygenation and precipitate angina in the susceptible individual with narrowing of the coronary arteries by atheroma.

Stressors That Determine Oxygen Demand of the Heart	Regulators of Oxygen Supply to the Heart
Increased cardiac work	Blood flow through coronary vessels
Increased heart rate	Blood flow occurs during diastole of the heart (relaxation phase), which can be of variable duration
Blood pressure changes	Coronary artery tone
Heart muscle contraction	Hemoglobin saturation with oxygen

Table 2.4: Circumstances That Can Cause the Onset of Angina Pectoris or Precipitate a Heart Attack.

• Intense emotions
• Physical exertion, especially if "unconditioned"
• Exposure to excessive cold or heat
• Vivid dreams (nocturnal angina)
• Lying flat (decubitus angina)
• Exaggerated "fright and flight" reactions
• Heavy metal exposures
• Smoking cigarettes or marijuana
• Using stimulant drugs
• Concomitant illness; e.g., retching, vomiting, excessive defecation

Table 2.4 summarizes some circumstances that can trigger an episode of angina. In a person with coronary artery disease, these circumstances can signal the onset of a heart attack (acute myocardial infarction, coronary thrombosis). Some individuals with angina learn to avoid events that cause the episodes. Obviously, this can result in a crippling existence.

Angina comes in many guises, and breathlessness is commonly associated with it. Sometimes the pain moves down the arms, especially the left arm, causing dead feelings in the upper extremities, and pain may be felt in areas of the body other than the chest. Some individuals experience shoulder aches, arm aches, or pain in the middle of the shoulder blades. Sometimes angina may occur only at the beginning of exercise and goes away with more strenuous exercise. This has been called "start-up" angina, and it may give an individual a false reassurance that initial niggling chest pains during exercise are not coming from the heart.

It is necessary to go into such detail in describing angina because the symptoms may be quite subtle, and unless a thorough medical history is taken, it can be missed. A careful analysis of a patient's symptoms is the most important way to make a correct diagnosis. In these days of high technology medicine, where speaking to patients has been superseded by testing procedures, an early diagnosis of mild angina can easily be overlooked.

Because effective interventions to reverse atheroma are available, early diagnosis of angina may be more important than once supposed, and early and effective intervention results in an improved prognosis. To wait for intervention while angina and blockage of the coronary arteries progress is a crime, one in which the punishment is doled out to the innocent sufferer.

Hypertension: The Silent Disease

Hypertension, commonly called "high blood pressure," is a condition that overlaps with many of the risk factors for cardiovascular disease. It is both a result of and a factor in the cause of heart diseases. High blood pressure is a primary risk factor for stroke.

As you probably know, blood pressure is expressed by using two readings. Systolic pressure is the maximum pressure reached as the blood surges into the arteries during rest or physical exertion; diastolic pressure is the lowest recordable point to which the pressure drops. When your blood pressure is measured, it is the resting blood pressure that determines conclusions about normal or high readings. A reading of 110 (systolic) and 70 (diastolic) is considered a normal—and favorable—reading for an adult. Fixed rises in diastolic blood pressure seem to carry more risk than rises in systolic pressure.

Hypertension is diagnosed when readings of systolic blood pressure consistently reach 150 or higher, and diastolic over 90 or higher. Blood pressure readings tend to move into higher ranges as we age, and there may be an adjustment in elderly individuals, for whom normal readings may regularly be as high as 150 over 90.

A single high reading is not sufficient to diagnose hypertension. Your blood pressure may increase when you are under stress or during exercise. This is a sign that you are alive, not necessarily an indication of the disease of hypertension. In addition, there is often some elevated blood pressure in a physician's office, simply because there is a degree of apprehension during an appointment with a health-care provider. True hypertension can be diagnosed when high blood pressure readings persist and remain consistently high.

Each year, almost two million adults in North America are detected with high blood pressure; as the population ages, this number is likely to rise. Currently, about sixty million Americans may have hypertension of variable degrees of severity. Many people do not realize they have high blood pressure, which is why it is called the silent killer. African Americans of all ages tend to be at a higher risk for developing high blood pressure, and men are more at risk than women. However, all adults must be vigilant about watching their blood pressure readings, and everyone can benefit from prevention and treatment programs based on improving their nutrition and lifestyle. Fixed hypertension must be treated.

Increased awareness about hypertension has been a good development. In fact, because lifestyle habits can contribute to the development of hypertension, there is some evidence that the overall prevalence of high blood pressure in adults has actually been reduced. This trend is the result of public education and greater awareness of ways to prevent hypertension.

The rush to use prescription drugs to lower blood pressure has had mixed results. In the short-term, blood pressure readings go down, but turning to medications as a first-line treatment can often lead to complacency about lifestyle and diet. Hypertension is common among those with a sedentary lifestyle and overweight individuals, and normalizing weight and increasing exercise can lead to consistently lowered blood pressure readings. Similarly, smoking and drinking alcohol can contribute to hypertension; when individuals eliminate these types of substance abuse, blood pressure readings may become normal. Though in some cases drugs that reduce blood pressure may be necessary, these drugs are not without risk. Natural approaches, which include the diet and lifestyle recommendations in this book, should be considered the first-line options in circumstances where rapid reductions of blood pressure are not mandatory.

MORE ABOUT "BAD" CHOLESTEROL

Low-density lipoproteins (LDL) are believed to be the major problem in causing coronary artery disease. In general, the higher the LDL reading, the greater the risk of developing coronary artery disease.

Remember that LDL carries cholesterol in the bloodstream, but that is not the whole story. When LDL attaches to the endothelial cells in the arteries, it undergoes a chemical process called *oxidation*, which attracts more LDL—and the process starts again. (You may have heard about "antioxidants." Certain nutrients that can prevent this oxidation in the arteries are discussed in later chapters.) In short, oxidized LDL is more likely to be deposited in the lining of arterial vessels, thereby leading to atheroma.

Very low–density lipoproteins (VLDL) enter the picture. Remember that the liver uses VLDL to produce LDL, thereby making VLDL the precursors of LDL. Higher levels of VLDL will tend to leave more available "material" for LDL production by the liver.

MORE ABOUT GOOD CHOLESTEROL

In simple terms, HDL has the important job of drawing cholesterol into the circulating blood and away from sites in arterial blood vessel walls where it can deposit. HDL has a complex function. It is responsible for directly protecting the lining of blood vessels from smaller remnants of fat that have been enzymatically digested in the bloodstream. It is important to note that very convincing studies show that HDL is raised by consistently giving attention to certain lifestyle choices, especially exercise and stress reduction.

HDL is mainly made in the liver and intestines, and it enters the bloodstream where it binds with cholesterol. This bound cholesterol is returned to the liver for reprocessing or elimination. In this manner, HDL functions to prevent the accumulation of cholesterol in the walls of blood vessels. HDL seems to have the added advantage of protecting LDL from oxidation. Remember, oxidized LDL is very damaging to the vascular tree.

HDL screening appears to be a valuable activity in medical practice (I would add a need for screening for high triglycerides as well). Drug therapy is not the principal answer to raising HDL. In fact, many cholesterol-lowering drugs (except niacin and gemfibrozil) actually reduce HDL. Modifications to "statin" drugs, used for lowering cholesterol, have less deleterious effects on HDL, but low HDL is best approached with the first-line options of diet and exercise.

The HDL "story" explains why people with normal blood cholesterol and few, if any, risk factors can get heart attacks. A low HDL with high triglycerides may often be more precarious than high total blood cholesterol levels.

Ratios of HDL to LDL

The ratio of the amounts of HDL to LDL is a reasonable measure of coronary artery disease risk, and the ratio of HDL to total cholesterol is an important measure of the risk of heart diseases. The most desirable ratio favors a preponderance of HDL. As you may know, ratios can be confusing. For example, looking at ratios of total cholesterol to HDL leads to a desirable ratio of less than 4:5. This ratio can be altered by raising LDL or lowering HDL, which tends to push the ratio higher. In contrast, lowering LDL and raising HDL tends to push the ratio lower. One of the best predictors of the presence of coronary artery disease is the ratio of total cholesterol to HDL, especially in women.

There is still some debate about the optimum total blood cholesterol level. Less than 200 mg/dL, or a ratio of total cholesterol to HDL cholesterol of less than 4:5 are probably generous allowances given current knowledge. The acceptable level of total blood cholesterol tends to be revised substantially downwards these days, but very low cholesterol numbers are not necessarily healthy!

Table 2.5: Conditions or Agents That Alter High-Density Lipoprotein (HDL) Cholesterol Levels.

Note low overall fat intake, as occurs in the presence of a strict vegan diet, lowers all types of blood lipids, including HDL. This has been used as an argument against the proposed healthfulness of the strict vegan diet.

Decrease HDL	Increase HDL
Vegetarian diet	Oral estrogens (females)
Cigarettes	Exercise
Sedentary lifestyle	Alcohol (moderate intake)
Obesity	Lean body mass
Menopause	Insulin
Progestogens	Androgens (balanced)

Table 2.6: Lipoprotein Fractions That Affect Blood HDL Levels.

A list of plasma lipoproteins which have varying functions and occur in varying concentrations in the blood. Alterations of the amount and pattern of these lipids occurs in abnormal circumstances of lipoprotein metabolism resulting in hyperlipoproteinemia.

Lipoprotein Fractions

- Chylomicron
- Very low–density lipoprotein (VLDL)
- ß-very low-density lipoprotein (ß-VLDL or $VLDL_2$)
- Intermediate density or remnant lipoprotein (IDL)
- Low-density lipoprotein (LDL)
- High-density lipoprotein (HDL)

Table 2.7: Healthy Levels of Blood Lipids.

Total cholesterol	less than 200 mg/dL
LDL cholesterol	less than 130 mg/dL
HDL cholesterol	greater than 35 mg/dL
LDL to HDL ratio	less than 4:5
Triglycerides	50 to 150 mg/dL

Exercise and moderate alcohol intake are associated with modest elevations of HDL. However, the recommendation of alcohol intake even in modest amounts is not often mentioned by health-care givers. I believe that moderate alcohol intake is safe—no more than one or two standard drinks a day (see pages 98–99 for the definition of a standard drink)—even accepting the oxidant and free-radical producing effects of alcohol. Several other conditions or factors affect blood HDL levels. (See Tables 2.5 and 2.6.)

MORE COMPLEX LIPIDS AND THEIR ROLES

Much concern has been expressed in the literature about the relative importance of a low LDL or a high HDL. Part of modern scientific evidence seems to imply that the ratio of LDL:HDL cholesterol appears to be more important than a consideration of either LDL or HDL alone. Controversy continues about triglycerides; specifically, about the risk of high triglyceride levels in the blood (hypertriglyceridemia) as an independent risk factor for coronary artery disease. I believe that hypertriglyceridemia alone is a risk factor. However, some current treatment recommendations suggest that this condition be specifically managed only if there is a marked elevation of triglycerides. Obviously opinions are divided.

Although I find that it is not possible to provide precise information about optimal levels of blood cholesterol and other lipids, Table 2.7 offers a guide to the levels that can be considered healthy. Remember that there is always a variation among individuals, and healthy cholesterol levels should probably be expressed in ranges rather than in absolute numbers. On occasion, individuals with high blood cholesterol may live to a ripe old age without cardiovascular problems. Conversely, those with low blood cholesterol may die prematurely. Remember, the cholesterol theory is not foolproof because factors other than cholesterol play a pivotal role in causing heart disease and other cardiovascular problems.

It is known that the overall average range of total blood cholesterol levels of adult Americans and Western Europeans is 210–225 mg/dL,

Table 2.8: The Main Groups of Lipoprotein Disorders.

Abnormalities	Changes in Blood Levels	Characteristics	Type of Disorder
Hypercholesterolemia	High cholesterol	High LDL cholesterol	Type II
Mild problem	200-239 mg/dL	130-159 mg/dL	
Moderate problem	240-300 mg/dL	160-210 mg/dL	
Severe problem	≥ 300 mg/dL	≥ 210 mg/dL	
Hypertriglyceridemia	High triglycerides		
Moderate Problem	250-500 mg/dL	High VLDL	Type IV
Severe Problem	>500 mg/dL	High VLDL + High chylomicrons	Type V
Mixed hyperlipidemia	High cholesterol (>240 mg/dL) High triglycerides (>250 mg/dL)		
Combined hyperlipidemia		High LDL + High VLDL	Type III
Dysbetalipo-proteinemia		High β-VLDL	Type IIB
Chylomicronemia		High VLDL + high chylomicrons	Type V
Low HDL	None	Low HDL (<35 mg/dL)	

Table 2.9: Blood Cholesterol Risk Levels.

This simple classification of risk, based on blood cholesterol levels, was proposed by the adult treatment panel of the National Cholesterol Education Program. Healthy levels are now revised downward.

Total Cholesterol	LDL Cholesterol
Desirable: Less than 200 mg/dL	Less than 130 mg/dL
Mild to Moderate Risk: 200–239 mg/dL	130–159 mg/dL
High Risk: Greater than 240 mg/dL	Greater than 160 mg/dL

and statistical studies clearly demonstrate that the death rate from coronary artery disease increases with increasing blood cholesterol levels. When the blood cholesterol level is 240 mg/dL, mortality from cardiovascular diseases increases fourfold above the average rate, and at 260 mg/dL, the risk of death is about sixfold or greater. (Remember that it is the total lipid profile, particularly LDL levels, that determines risk.)

In general, blood cholesterol levels in affluent countries are higher than those in third world countries. However, in affluent societies it is the lower socioeconomic groups that may be particularly at risk because foods that contain high cholesterol, high fat, low fiber, and high sugar contents are relatively cheap and abundant. Frankly, we have our taste preferences—met by the fast food industry—to thank for this. However, to be fair, this industry is tracking the trend to reduce fats in the diet and is making efforts to improve general nutrition, in part by including more vegetables in their menus. Later we will learn about the dangers of unhealthy fats in the diet (saturated fat, hydrogenated oils, and undesirable trans-fatty acids).

THE BOUQUET OF DISEASES AND DIETARY FAT

High blood cholesterol is a principal contributing factor to a variety of cardiovascular diseases including: heart attack, stroke, peripheral vascular disease (compromised circulation to the extremities), arteriosclerosis, and vascular causes of dementia. Other common and serious diseases that may be associated with high blood cholesterol include conditions of the prostate, kidney (renal) diseases, pancreatic disease, and certain cancers. It is well documented that hypercholesterolemia is an important association, or perhaps a cause of these diseases.

Although blood lipid abnormalities, including high blood cholesterol levels, have complex causes, diet frequently makes the most significant contribution to this problem. This has led groups such as the American Heart Association and the National Cholesterol Education Program to recommend reducing dietary fat to 30 percent or less of the total daily intake of calories and limiting animal fats, which are saturated fats. I agree with these recommendations, but I must note that these organizations have not placed enough emphasis on the health benefits of omega-3 types of essential fatty acids, which are found in certain fish and marine mammals. Essential fatty acids are discussed later in this book. They are called "essential" because they *are* essential, just like vitamins!

GENDER, ETHNICITY, AND SOCIOECONOMIC FACTORS

It is true that certain risk factors for coronary artery disease cannot be readily abolished. Being male is an obvious example. Men are more likely to develop heart disease at earlier ages than women. This is due in part to the lack of the female hormone estrogen, which is a heart-protective hormone. These protective effects in women last until menopause, at which point levels of estrogen in the blood tend to drop. The lower occurrence of heart disease in *premenopausal* women is quite striking and is approximately equivalent to that found in men who are about fifteen years younger. However, this should not lead to complacency. Do not forget that coronary artery disease is the most common cause of death in women, as it is in men. Recently, concern has increased about the management of coronary artery disease in women because evidence has emerged that it may be often underdiagnosed and managed in a much less assertive manner than in male patients. (The fixed risks and modifiable risks for heart disease are shown in Table 2.10).

Risk factors for coronary artery disease in the U.S. appear to be almost the same in African Americans, Hispanics, and Caucasians. However, it is apparent that coronary artery disease deaths have not declined to the same degree in African Americans or Native Americans as they have in Caucasians. I believe that this is due in part to a situation in which Native Americans and African Americans have less access to intervention strategies to reduce the risks of cardiovascular disease. In addition, it is well-known that the percentage of African Americans in the United States who do not have health insurance is higher than the percentage of white Americans without such coverage. This means that economically disadvantaged individuals, a group that includes a disproportionate number of African

Table 2.10: Fixed and Modifiable Risk Factors for Heart Disease.

An expanded list of "risk" factors for coronary heart disease. Arguments prevail about the true role of some of these items in the risk of cardio-vascular disease.

Amenable to Modification	Fixed Risk
Smoking	Age
Elevated blood pressure	Being male
Blood lipid disorders	Family history
Diabetes mellitus	Being a post-menopausal female*
Clotting disorders	
Behavioral issues	
Lack of exercise	
Obesity	
Deficiency of essential fatty acids	
Lack of other nutrients	

* The post-menopausal risk is forgotten by many but it may be amenable to modification by soy isoflavones or hormone replacement therapy.

Americans, do not have ready access to the most modern treatment facilities. There are some reports that African Americans tend to consume more fast food and their disposable income is on average less, perhaps resulting in greater consumption of less expensive, refined, fat-laden foods.

Even recipients of government-funded health care, such as Medicaid, do not have access to all practitioners. Some practitioners perceive that the reimbursement levels of public health-care programs are too low, and therefore they do not open their practices to these patients. In addition, many treatments that fall within the "alternative" health-care arena are not reimbursed by insurance nor are they paid for through publicly funded programs. Obviously, the latter situation is a disadvantage for all but the wealthy!

ARRIVING AT RECOMMENDATIONS

The modern concept of what constitutes a high blood cholesterol level grew out of data on blood lipids that were collected from more than 60,000 individuals in ten different population groups in the United States. A summary of data on blood lipid levels and the relevance of considering age and sex in the interpretation of normality is shown in Tables 2.11 and 2.12.

Many scientists have scrutinized safe levels of cholesterol and other blood lipids, and various interpretations of safe levels exist. In general, the incidence of coronary artery disease starts to climb with blood cholesterol levels greater than 200 mg/dL. Overall, it has been accepted that 200 mg/dL is the maximum acceptable "normal" total cholesterol level, regardless of age or sex. Some authorities have placed the maximum acceptable total blood cholesterol level at 180 mg/dL for adults.

The true significance of looking at cholesterol numbers relates to their use as a measure of risk. *It has been estimated that for each one percent of reduction in blood cholesterol levels, there is a two-percent reduction in coronary heart disease.* Perhaps if more individuals understood the difference incremental changes can make, they would be more highly motivated to take steps to improve their health. Small changes can result in significant gains. This principle is important in prevention. As an aside, small increments in physical activity may have more impact on cardiovascular disease prevention than minor reductions in blood cholesterol. However, there is not much money in measuring the benefits of exercise, while there is gold in drug therapy, at least for pharmaceutical companies.

CHOLESTEROL TARGETS DEFINED: THE ROLE OF COMBINED RISK AND MOVING DOWN CHOLESTEROL NUMBERS

There has been continuing argument as to the optimal levels of blood cholesterol that are desirable for good health. Higher blood cholesterol levels can be tolerated in individuals who have no other significant risk factors. Currently it is acceptable, following standard guidelines, for an individual to have a blood cholesterol level of up to 165 mg/dL, in the absence of any other cardiovascular risk factors. When multiple risk factors are present, it is advised that the target blood cholesterol level be less than 130 mg/dL. A large portion of individuals fall into a high-risk category, and achieving a blood cholesterol of this level is often quite difficult for individuals in Western society.

I do not believe that there is clear-cut evidence that reducing blood cholesterol to this level is necessarily advisable. I do recommend that blood cholesterol be lowered to less than 160 mg/dL if you have other cardiovascular risk factors in addition to elevated blood cholesterol. This advice is contrary to some accepted guidelines, and some health-care providers may believe it is too lax.

The benefits of taking aggressive steps to lower blood cholesterol in patients with coronary artery disease are much clearer than in the healthy person. It is advisable for a person with established coronary artery disease to shoot for the lowest cholesterol level possible; the optimal target is still a guess. The person with diagnosed coronary artery disease should be quite diligent about strategies to elevate blood HDL levels. This can prove to be difficult, however, because lowering cholesterol in the diet tends to result in reduced LDL *and* HDL cholesterol.

There are some natural remedies that can help achieve a better balance of LDL and HDL. Incorporating soy protein containing isoflavones into the diet can offer a solution to this problem, because some elevation of HDL is recorded with reasonable consistency in patients taking soy protein diets. (The potential benefit of soy protein to promote health and lower cholesterol is so important that I have devoted Chapter 10 to it.) Those with coronary artery disease are advised to try to get their blood HDL level to above 35 mg/dL.

Just Remember—A High HDL and a Low for the Rest

It is easy to become obsessed with cholesterol numbers. In my clinical experience, patients place too much emphasis on the apparent "magic numbers" of blood tests. A healthy adult would ideally have a blood cholesterol in the range of 120-180 mg/dL, but under 200 is often considered quite acceptable. However, there is little point in having a blood cholesterol number of 120 mg/dL if you continue to smoke, drink alcohol excessively, or attempt to cope with unrelenting stress—and do nothing to change your lifestyle.

To change blood lipid levels to promote cardiovascular health, you want to achieve a low LDL, a low VLDL, low triglycerides, a high HDL, a low total cholesterol, and good cholesterol ratios. Always keep

Table 2.11: Total Blood Cholesterol and LDL, by Age and Sex.

Tables 2.11 and 2.12 are modified from Kowalski, 1989. 5% and 95% are percentiles. The risk of heart disease relates to values above the 50th percentile.

	Age (Yrs.)	Average	5%	95%
Total Cholesterol				
Male				
	0-19	155	115	200
	20-24	165	125	220
	25-29	180	135	245
	30-34	190	140	255
	35-39	200	145	270
	40-44	205	150	270
	45-69	215	160	275
	70+	205	150	270
Female				
	0-19	160	120	200
	20-24	170	125	230
	25-34	175	130	235
	35-39	185	140	245
	40-44	195	145	255
	45-49	205	150	270
	50-54	220	165	285
	55+	230	170	295
LDL				
Male				
	5-19	95	65	130
	20-24	105	65	145
	25-29	115	70	165
	30-34	125	80	185
	35-39	135	80	190
	40-44	135	85	185
	45-69	145	90	205
	70+	145	90	185
Female				
	5-19	100	65	140
	20-24	105	55	160
	25-34	110	70	160
	35-39	120	75	170
	40-44	125	75	175
	45-49	130	80	185
	50-54	140	90	200
	55+	150	95	215

Table 2.12: Total Blood HDL and Triglycerides, by Age and Sex.

	Age (Yrs.)	Average	5%	95%
HDL				
Male				
	5-14	55	35	75
	15-19	45	30	65
	20-24	45	30	65
	25-29	45	30	65
	30-34	45	30	65
	35-39	45	30	60
	40-44	45	25	65
	45-69	50	30	70
	70+	50	30	75
Female				
	5-19	55	25	70
	20-24	55	35	80
	25-34	55	35	80
	35-39	55	35	80
	40-44	60	35	90
	45-49	60	35	85
	50-54	60	35	90
	55+	60	35	95
Triglycerides				
Male				
	0-9	55	30	100
	10-14	65	30	125
	15-19	80	35	150
	20-24	100	45	200
	25-29	115	45	250
	30-34	130	50	265
	35-39	145	55	320
	40-54	150	55	320
	55-64	140	60	290
	65+	135	55	260
Female				
	0-9	60	35	110
	10-19	75	40	130
	20-34	90	40	170
	35-39	95	40	195
	40-44	105	45	210
	45-49	110	45	230
	50-54	120	55	240
	55-64	125	55	250
	65+	130	60	240

in mind that cardiovascular disease caused by atheroma is at the root of the number one cause of death in Western society.

Concern about cholesterol readings results from the belief that the cholesterol theory of cardiovascular disease is correct. While evidence exists that clearly shows that the cholesterol theory is important, it is not the only relevant theory. Medicine has become preoccupied with cholesterol at the expense of considering other important factors in the course of heart disease. This may be one reason why modern attempts to eradicate heart disease are working slower than is optimal. In the next chapter, I will discuss other important issues that influence cardiovascular wellness.

SUMMARY

There is a clear relationship between high cholesterol levels and heart disease, although it is not the only important risk factor. Keep in mind that high-density lipoprotein (HDL) is considered the "good cholesterol," while low-density lipoprotein (LDL) is considered the "bad" cholesterol.

Cardiovascular disease is not a single entity, but rather, manifests in various ways. *Atheroma* occurs when plaque, a mixed fatty substance that deposits in tiny lesions on arterial walls, builds up and causes blockages, sometimes leading to clots in arteries and blood vessels. *Arteriosclerosis* is a condition known as "hardening of the arteries" because the arterial walls thicken and lose elasticity. *Angina pectoris* is chest pain that occurs when the blood supply to the heart is blocked. *Hypertension*—high blood pressure—is one of the key risk factors for developing cardiovascular problems. There is current evidence that it is possible to not only prevent these conditions, but perhaps reverse them as well, and the efforts made by you and your health-care providers may lead to vastly improved health.

What You Can Do

- Damage to the lining of blood vessels and arteries can be caused by, among other things, smoking, diabetes mellitus, and high blood pressure. Do not put your head in the sand about these issues.

- For many adults, a cholesterol level of under 200 mg/dL may be acceptable, although 120-180 mg/dL is considered ideal. Aim for the lower end of the range if you have established heart disease.
- HDL cholesterol should be the only "high" cholesterol number.
- Cholesterol readings are not "magic numbers." Addressing other risk factors is just as important as lowering cholesterol.
- All adults should have regular screening for hypertension. Blood pressure tends to rise as we grow older, but remember that regardless of age, when consistent readings reach 150, or higher, over 90, or higher, a diagnosis of hypertension is usually reached.
- Hypertension and high cholesterol levels may improve with the lifestyle changes, dietary recommendations, and natural therapies discussed in this book. Talk with your health-care provider about what you can do to help yourself.
- If your blood pressure is normal and your cholesterol levels low, focus *now* on prevention and correct lifestyle problems that may be doing their damage "silently."

CHAPTER THREE

THE KEY CULPRITS:
CHOLESTEROL, TRIGLYCERIDES, AND HOMOCYSTEINE

FRAMINGHAM, OSLO, AND ZUTPHEN: THE PIVOTAL CHOLESTEROL STUDIES

The post-World War II era in the United States was often summed up with the sentiment, "We never had it so good." This was true in many ways, but the era of celebration brought with it increased risks of cardiovascular diseases. Throughout the 1950s, similar conditions also developed in Western Europe. It is ironic that the rapid rise in standard of living, with its broad access to new convenience foods and the pervasive cigarette smoking of that era, also coincided with the initiation of the Framingham Study by the National Institutes of Health, so-named because its participants lived in Framingham, Massachusetts. It represents one of the most complete and longest prospective forward-looking studies of heart disease, clearly establishing *lifestyle issues* as important in the cause of coronary heart disease and stroke.

So strong was the association of high blood cholesterol and coronary artery disease in the Framingham Study that William Castelli, M.D., and his associates were able to publish in 1983 a now-classic paper, "Summary Estimates of Cholesterol Used to Predict Coronary Heart Disease." Data from this study characterized the typical heart attack victim as having an average blood cholesterol of 244 mg., with a range of 220–260 mg. So well-popularized was this notion that society was striken with cholesterol-lowering fever, at the expense of considering other risk factors for cardiovascular disease.

Other studies also related high blood cholesterol to coronary artery disease. What may be more important, however, are the results of the Oslo Study, performed in Norway, and the Zutphen Study, performed in Holland. These studies provide evidence that coronary artery disease can be prevented to some degree by lowering a high blood cholesterol.

The Olso Study included 1,234 mature males, split into two groups. One group modified their diet and adverse lifestyle with an emphasis on lowering blood cholesterol, whereas the other group formed a control group and received no such interventions. After five years, the incidence of heart attacks was 47 percent lower in the group with the lifestyle and dietary interventions when compared with the control group.

The twenty-year Zutphen Study assessed diet and lifestyle factors in 852 middle-aged males before they entered a prospective study for the development of coronary artery disease. This study showed that fish in the diet has a protective effect against cardiovascular disease, a finding that becomes important when we consider the issue of beneficial fats of marine origin (omega-3 fatty acids). The medical profession has been hit over the head with data on the benefits of omega-3 fatty acids, but often fails to consider fish oil. The Zutphen Study also expanded knowledge about the impact of adverse lifestyle factors and their role in determining eventual disability and death from coronary diseases.

The Framingham, Oslo, and Zutphen studies underscore the importance of reducing cholesterol, but they also offer additional incentives to quit smoking, bring blood pressure under control, and maintain a normal weight. Again and again, smoking, hypertension, and obesity emerge as risk factors for heart disease. This probably comes as no surprise. These are not complex risk factors, but if you smoke and/or are obese and have elevated blood pressure, the handwriting is on the wall. I advise taking immediate corrective action for a healthy lifestyle, and all adults should have regular screening for hypertension, since it is a silent disease.

LOOKING BEYOND CHOLESTEROL

To date, we know that several well-controlled scientific studies demonstrate unequivocally that individuals who are able to reduce blood cholesterol levels experience less heart disease. The converse seems to be true as well: overall, individuals who do not lower their blood cholesterol into the healthier ranges will tend to have *more* heart disease. Data derived from such studies show that reducing total blood cholesterol levels by a factor of one-third or more reduces the risk of coronary artery disease by about 50 percent. Animal experiments indicate that atherosclerosis will not occur in the absence of high blood cholesterol. In other words, high cholesterol and atherosclerosis go hand in hand. Extensive studies, such as the Lipid Research Clinics Coronary Primary Prevention Trial, have indicated that males who lower blood cholesterol with diet and cholesterol-lowering drugs suffer fewer heart attacks than those in whom blood cholesterol remains elevated. Far too often—in my opinion—these results have led to a premature prescription for lipid-lowering drugs.

Moved by all of the data, the American Heart Association recommended reducing fat intake in the diet to less than 30 percent of the total calories. I do not doubt that the American Heart Association was correct about the wisdom of lowering cholesterol given the available information at the time of this early recommendation—the mid-1980s—but, as you have already seen, this is not the whole story. Several dietary experts and enthusiasts of both the alternative and conventional medical persuasion have lost sight of the importance of good fats in the form of essential fatty acids and a switch to vegetable sources of protein, especially soy.

JUMPING THE GUN

Dietary modifications and synthetic drugs tend to be recommended together, often before the results of altered diet alone can be seen. This has meant that very few natural options are recommended to patients prior to drug interventions. Furthermore, much, if not most, of the research on blood lipids and cardiovascular research has been funded by multinational pharmaceutical companies, who clearly have a vested interest in promoting the efficacy of synthetic drugs. Yet, through all the studies, the concept of a normal range for cholesterol still defies accurate definition.

In general, it is considered that achieving a safe range may mean lowering blood cholesterol levels to targets below 160 mg. and triglyceride levels to below an unknown number. Dr. Castelli, of the Framingham Study, claimed that he had never encountered a case of coronary artery disease in a subject with a cholesterol level below 150 mg.

Another body of opinion is that the levels of cholesterol and blood lipids that traditionally are accepted as normal are, in fact, too high. Individuals who subscribe to this theory believe that the so-called "normal" range of blood lipids has been a passport to disability and death for many people. Taking this view at face value, this would mean that many "heart-smart" diets are not constructed to bring optimal results.

There are those still who reject the "cholesterol theory." These individuals argue that cholesterol consumption in Western society has remained reasonably constant for much of this century, while cardiovascular death rates have skyrocketed; therefore, there must be another explanation. However, in the past decade or so, cholesterol consumption has actually risen quite significantly in children. This is not difficult to see because billions—literally—of meat and dairy items have been sold in fast food restaurants. What will happen to these children in thirty or forty years? It seems rational to predict that the risk of developing cardiovascular disease is on the rise among the fast food generation. Fat children tend to eat fatty foods and have fatty deposits in their arteries. Fat children become overweight adults who have higher risks of fatal cardiovascular disease. For these reasons, I maintain that we should not become overly preoccupied with lowering cholesterol or blood lipids while disregarding more general health-building strategies, such as altered diets and exercise programs.

TRIGLYCERIDES AND SUGAR

A strong relationship exists between elevated blood triglyceride levels and cardiovascular disease. It has been pointed out that during this century there has been a steadily increasing consumption of foods that cause a rise in blood triglyceride levels. This coincides with the increase in cardiovascular disease and mortality. Foods that cause a rise in triglycerides include refined carbohydrates (sugars and starches) and saturated or hardened nonessential and essential fats. In addition, an overall increase in the number of calories in the diet, obesity, and lack of exercise all cause a rise in blood triglycerides.

To some people, mentioning the role of refined sugar consumption as a factor in developing cardiovascular disease can sound downright Puritanical. After all, white bread, ice cream, and pastries—all manner of desserts—are as favored a part of the Western diet as burgers and french fries. So, in addition to being told that you should cut back on certain types of unhealthful fats, including saturated animal fats, now your favorite snacks are under attack, too!

These refined carbohydrates have received considerable attention in the scientific and lay press. Potentially, refined sugar (sucrose) has a number of undesirable effects on the body's metabolism, including:

- Increased tissue damage caused by mechanisms of oxidation (see page 58)
- Interference with the body's ability to use vitamin C
- Interference with normal immune system functions

Some physicians would add that sugar increases the risk of developing the "Candida Syndrome" or even chronic fatigue syndrome. Although this may be a stretch of the imagination, the fact remains that if you eat a sugar-laden meal, your blood will show a prompt increase in triglycerides. Eliminating refined sugar in the diet, along with incorporating essential fatty acids and micronutrients, may prevent or reverse cardiovascular and other degenerative diseases. Chomping on sweet snacks (junk foods) effectively delivers a good dose of unwanted refined sugar, saturated fats, hydrogenated oils, and trans-fatty acids.

THE NECESSARY OMEGA-3 FATTY ACIDS

Cardiovascular disease cannot be shown clearly to be directly caused by dietary deficiencies. However, lack of essential nutrients may play a major role in its development. In some circumstances, increasing

57

intake of vitamins, minerals, essential fatty acids, and dietary fiber helps reduce blood cholesterol and triglycerides. The omega-3 fatty acids, found in fish oil, have significant benefits for cardiovascular health. They are antithrombotic and appear to be important, but modest, cholesterol-lowering agents, and—perhaps more important-ly—they show the ability to promote a healthy balance of blood lipids.

While it is still controversial to talk about vitamin deficiency in the affluent West, some experts estimate that as much as 85 percent of the population of Western societies may not have a consistent, optimal intake of vitamins, minerals, essential fatty acids, or fiber. It may come as a shock to many, but many scientists have observed that one of the most common deficiencies in Western diets is omega-3 fatty acids, found in fish oil. Put another way, if you are not consci-entious about your diet, the chance of deficiency of one or more of these nutrients is 100 percent! To use an aphorism of alternative medicine, high blood cholesterol is not due to a deficiency of lipid-lowering drugs in Western society.

OXIDATION AND THE IMPORTANT ANTIOXIDANTS

The concept of oxidation is important for completing an understand-ing of how atherosclerosis develops. You will remember that LDL cholesterol attaches to the wall of the artery if a "space" is provided in the form of a microscopic tear or lesion. Once there, a chemical process called *oxidation* takes place. Oxidation is linked to the pres-ence of *free radicals*, which are unstable and destructive molecules that can cause damage to the body, including contributing to impaired immune function. *Antioxidants* are substances that prevent free rad-icals from doing their damage. Therefore, antioxidants can play a major role in preventing coronary heart disease.

In essence, when an LDL molecule reacts with oxygen, it sets off a chain of events that results in attraction of more LDL. Meanwhile, the immune system sends in special cells, *macrophages*, whose job it is to neutralize the LDL molecules. However, if LDL levels are too high, these cells are, figuratively speaking, overwhelmed and eventually die or per-haps transform and cause damage to the wall of the artery. Platelets, the

Table 3.1: Summary of the Types of Damage to Cells and Molecules That Can Be Produced by Free Radicals.

Damage to cellular membranes that protect all cellular functions:

- Cross-linking of protein or DNA molecules. Genes are comprised of DNA, which can result in mutations.

- Lipid peroxidation, where fat is attacked—resulting in further free-radical release.

- Damage to cellular lysosomes, which contain damaging enzymes that are released inside cells.

- Free radicals cause lipofuscin (age pigment) deposition in cells.

blood cells involved in coagulating the blood and forming clots, become involved in this process, too, which eventually leads to scar tissue in the artery and the buildup of plaque. The artery diseased with atheroma has collections of small "garbage dumps" of cholesterol and fat.

As you can see, oxidation of fats has a central role in the genesis of atherosclerosis. It appears that oxidation of cholesterol and triglycerides is an important prerequisite for, and promoter of, fat deposition and the formation of cholesterol deposits in arteries.

Fortunately, oxidation can be prevented by nutrients that are antioxidants, most notably vitamins C and E, the carotenes, selenium, coenzyme Q10, and phytochemicals such as soy isoflavones. Oxidized fat is abundant in aged foods or meat, especially if they are poorly manufactured or stored. This is also where refined sugar plays a role because, as previously mentioned, it interferes with the antioxidant actions of vitamin C. The situation becomes even more complex—and interesting—when we consider that certain chemicals in some plants (phytochemicals) are also powerful antioxidants. Examples of such antioxidant phytochemicals are soy isoflavones, such as genistein and daidzein, or bioflavanoids such as pycnogenol, which are discussed in later chapters. It is important to emphasize phytonutrients, meaning nutrients of plant origin, because these agents are abundant in fruits and vegetables. They are key to understanding the health benefits of the current trend toward a more vegetarian diet. Many Westerners can benefit from fewer animal sources of protein in their diets. Meat and dairy products provide essential protein, but they associate with unwanted types of fat and cholesterol.

THE DANGERS OF A LACK OF VITAMIN C

It is not necessarily clear that vitamin C deficiency is part of the cause of heart disease. However, many scientific studies provide information that corroborates the importance of vitamin C and other compounds such as bioflavonoids, which facilitate the action of vitamin C in promoting cardiovascular wellness. Those who believe that a deficiency of vitamin C can cause heart disease maintain that a lack of adequate vitamin C causes repair proteins to be deposited in the arteries. As the name implies, repair proteins are substances that provide a protective coat over a lesion in the arteries—the body's way of protecting itself against damage. However, these repair proteins also become part of the plaque buildup. Vitamin C is an important antioxidant nutrient and helps prevent the oxidation of cholesterol and other lipoproteins. An apple—or, preferably, an orange—a day really can help keep the doctor away.

The protective role of vitamin C actually fits the theory of elevated cholesterol and triglycerides as major factors in the cause of cardiovascular disease. Some research has related an increased intake in vitamin C with a reduction in deaths from cardiovascular disease. There is no question that vitamin C is an important nutrient, particularly in its role as an antioxidant—the American Heart Association may be right in loaning their emblem to orange juice.

THE HOMOCYSTEINE THEORY

In the next few years, you will hear more about the "homocysteine theory" of heart disease, in part because it represents a different—and important—view of the cause of atherosclerosis. Homocysteine is an amino acid that is produced through the breakdown of other proteins in the body. The essential amino acid, methionine, found in a variety of animal proteins, is indirectly the source of homocysteine.

Homocysteine normally is present in very low concentrations because it is converted to another breakdown product, cystathionine, but please do not get bogged down in these terms. High levels of homocysteine in the body have been linked to arteriosclerosis and atheroma. In addition, high levels of homocysteine are also linked with increased clotting activity in the blood.

In an uncommon congenital (hereditary) condition called *homocysteinuria*, the body lacks an enzyme to break down and metabolize certain proteins and hence, the blood contains abnormally high levels of homocysteine. Enzyme deficiencies have been noted in certain types of mental retardation, and homocysteinuria has been linked with premature cardiac death of children with these disorders. One piece of the homocysteine puzzle emerged when, during autopsies, severe coronary artery disease was found to be present in these children. These were, by the way, "incidental findings" arising from research into possible enzyme deficiencies as a causal factor in mental retardation. This information was first noted in research conducted in Northern Ireland in the 1960s, but its significance has only recently become clear. The link between elevated homocysteine levels among a small group of young children and the progression of heart disease in the general population was discovered in a process that reads like a complex medical "whodunit." Starting in the late 1960s and into the 1970s, research pathologist Kilmer McCully, M.D., gathered together what was known about homocysteine and homocysteinuria, conducted independent research, and eventually made the important link between elevated homocysteine levels and the presence of atherosclerosis. Of course, the conventional medical profession shunned the observations at the outset.

A key piece of the puzzle involves the role of B vitamins in metabolizing homocysteine and efficiently preventing high levels of homocysteine from accumulating in the body. For example, an animal study conducted in 1949 had demonstrated that a diet adequate in all ways, except for a deficiency in vitamin B6, led to atherosclerosis and a corresponding high level of homocysteine in the bloodstream.

Dr. McCully conducted additional animal research and added to the body of evidence that established that high levels of homocysteine are implicated in the development of heart disease. Over the next decades, other researchers eventually linked deficiencies of *folic acid, B12,* and

B6 with high homocysteine levels and the progression of atheroma.

It is important to understand that the homocysteine theory, which could be called "the high levels of homocysteine" theory, is not in direct opposition to the cholesterol theory, but rather helps to complete a picture of the link between diet and heart disease. It helps to explain why, for example, heart attacks may occur even when cholesterol levels are low and blood pressure is normal. This is illustrated in a study in which a group of Swedish researchers examined men under the age of fifty-five who, prior to a first heart attack, had no warning signs that heart disease was present (*i.e.*, they did not have high cholesterol levels or hypertension). The common link between these men was elevated homocysteine levels and correspondingly low levels of folic acid, along with levels of B12 in the lower end of the normal range.

Elevated homocysteine levels have been linked with increased risk of stroke and of peripheral arterial disease, a condition in which arteriosclerosis affects the arteries in the extremities. While evidence exists that the enzymes involved in breaking down homocysteine may be defective or inefficient in some individuals as a result of a faulty gene profile, diet can make up for this deficiency. In other words, more folic acid and vitamin B6 in the diet will help the defective enzyme break down homocysteine.

McCulley: Politics and Science

One would suppose that Dr. McCully's research would have been considered so important that the "reputation" of the B vitamins would have been greatly enhanced. We could also suppose that Dr. McCully would have been viewed as a medical research hero. Sadly, this did not happen. In 1978, after about a decade of research on homocysteine, Dr. McCully's contract with Harvard University Medical School was not renewed. At the time it was believed that his theories had not been proved and probably never would be.

Dr. McCully continued to believe in his theory and conducted research in a new position as a pathologist at the Veterans Affairs Hospital in Providence, Rhode Island. However, for the next few years, the homocysteine theory went "underground." Today, as a result of a body of research, the homocysteine theory is recognized and respected. In 1997, Dr. McCully's book, *The Homocysteine*

Revolution, was published and continues to receive wide attention. The book discusses the importance of the B vitamins in promoting a healthy heart and reinforces the idea that the nutrient-stripped, highly processed food that lines the shelves of modern supermarkets does not promote a healthy heart. Furthermore, a diet rich in animal protein is higher in the amino acid methionine than are plant-based diets. Excessive methionine may then lead to elevated homocysteine levels in the blood. Again, it all comes back to diet!

Dr. McCully's book also chronicles the way in which the homocysteine theory initially seemed to go against the tide of prevailing opinion that high cholesterol was the key to understanding heart disease. It may seem odd that a serious research scientist would need vindication, but that is exactly what has happened with Dr. McCully and his work, which perhaps is best described as going beyond the cholesterol theory.

I recommend that you read *The Homocysteine Revolution* not only because the information can help you improve your health and lower your risk of heart disease, but also because it offers insight into the way in which medical research works. Theories go in and out of favor and it is often difficult—and expensive—to follow a clue through the maze of related information and reach a logical conclusion. A theory that is related to B vitamins, essentially a nutritional theory, does not lead to synthetic pharmaceutical "cures." One cannot obtain a patent on a natural substance, such as a vitamin. The fact is, the homocysteine theory is compatible with the idea that cardiovascular disease has its roots in lifestyle issues, with an emphasis on diet. Of course, this is why it is exciting to so many people, including many among the medical establishment who are interested in natural ways to improve health.

AN INTEGRATED THEORY

I have summarized the principal hypotheses of the nutritional causes of cardiovascular disease in Table 3.2. Clearly the cholesterol theory holds water, but it is obvious that other nutritional factors play a major role. This is important because when we consider multiple theories, it is much easier to understand why a dietary approach is criti-

Table 3.2: Principle Nutritional Theories of the Causation of Coronary Artery Disease.

The cholesterol theory is not the whole story, and each of the other theories is somewhat incomplete.

Theory	Comments
Cholesterol theory	Convincing evidence implicates hypercholesterolemia as a major risk for cardiac disease. However, it is incomplete; when applied alone as the treatment objective, it may be ineffective.
Triglyceride theory	A good correlation exists between blood triglyceride levels and coronary heart disease. Triglycerides increase with high saturated fat and refined carbohydrate diets.
Sugar theory	Simple sugars raise triglycerides, increase oxidative damage, and have other adverse metabolic effects.
Oxidation theory	Oxidized cholesterol and triglycerides damage arterial blood vessels.
Deficiency theory	Deficiency of one or more essential nutrients; *e.g.,* vitamins, minerals, and essential fatty acids, may raise cholesterol and cause oxidative stress and heart disease.
Vitamin theory	Linus Pauling proposed a unified theory to explain the cause and cure of cardiovascular disease with vitamin C. The deficiency of vitamin C may result in the deposition of repair proteins in arteries.
"Wacko" theory	There is a dietary supplement or natural treatment that has panacea benefit in curing cardiovascular disease.

cal to preventing and reversing cardiovascular disease. An integrated approach is based on the idea that these theories are not necessarily in opposition to each other. Rather, they highlight the need for a comprehensive nutritional approach. In the absence of this pluralistic view of the issue, we are left with the prevailing obsession with cholesterol as the sole dietary culprit, and cholesterol-lowering drugs as a preferred solution. I hope that you now can understand how "fuzzy logic" creeps into medicine.

In general, a diet that is low in saturated fat, high in fiber, high in fruits and vegetables, low in refined carbohydrates, and abundant in vitamins, minerals, and micronutrients is considered ideal for lowering blood cholesterol. This dietary adjustment has the advantage of providing a host of other health benefits. I am passionate about the idea of one diet for general health, even though it is wishful thinking in consumer societies that are hammered by the media to eat junk food.

POPULATION STUDIES PROVIDE INSIGHT

Theories about the development of heart disease have emerged from certain epidemiological studies that look at ethnic and/or geographic differences in the incidence of coronary artery disease. These studies have observed that coronary artery disease is lower in Japan than in the United States or Western Europe. Studies of Seventh-Day Adventists, who for the most part are vegetarians, show lower death rates from cardiovascular disease among this religious group when compared to the rest of the population. In addition, multiple observations of the cardiovascular disease profile of the Inuit or Eskimo population, eating their traditional diet, show a lower incidence of arteriosclerotic disease than encountered in Westerners. Anyone knowledgeable about these ethnic variations in diet may be confused because Eskimos are meat and fat eaters. The answer lies in the types of fat they consume in their traditional diet.

What is interesting is that this reduced incidence of cardiovascular disease among the Japanese, Seventh-Day Adventists, and Eskimos is not explained by differences in dietary intake of fat or cholesterol. The Japanese may eat greater than 30 percent of their total calories from fat, but this may be from marine sources. Also, the traditional Japanese diet is high is soy protein. Omega-3 fatty acids in the fat of fish and soy protein containing isoflavones both lower cholesterol and exert other beneficial effects that promote cardiovascular health. Similar principles apply to the Eskimo population, whose diet is very high in saturated fat intake, but the fish or marine mammal origin of the fat is also high in omega-3 fatty acids. These essential fatty acids are associated with reduced cardiovascular mortality by mechanisms that include, but are not limited to, lowering blood cholesterol.

Seventh-Day Adventists follow a vegetarian diet, but it is not strictly vegan, because they may consume relatively large amounts of fat and cholesterol in milk and cheese. However, members of this group consume a greater quantity of omega-3 and omega-6 essential fatty acids of vegetable origin, which may offer protection against cardiovascular disease. While genetic predisposition may play a role in the lower incidence of cardiovascular disease in some ethnic groups, dietary factors most likely account for many of the observed differences in disease profiles. These dietary differences include well-defined roles for essential fatty acids and soy protein, both of which are discussed in later chapters. Both soy protein and essential fatty acid supplements are among the most important natural options available to you in your quest for a heart-healthy lifestyle.

SUMMARY

During the second half the twentieth century, several studies have identified risk factors for cardiovascular disease, and this research has paved the way not only for effective treatments, but for sound prevention principles as well. Cholesterol was "implicated" in the bouquet of risk factors in the well-known Framingham Study, a research project initiated in the U.S. Equally important, however, some *lifestyle* issues have been noted as risk factors. Studies performed in Norway and Holland have added to the knowledge about the link between high cholesterol and heart disease and helped establish the importance of a healthful lifestyle for preventing heart disease.

Research also has established that elevated triglyceride levels are an additional risk factor for cardiovascular diseases. Consumption of refined carbohydrates and saturated fats are believed to cause a rise in triglyceride levels, and during the twentieth century, Western societies have drastically increased their consumption of foods produced with white flour, refined sugar, and saturated fats (including hydrogenated oils).

Oxidation is a chemical process linked to the presence of unstable molecules called *free radicals*, and the oxidation of cholesterol and triglycerides promotes the buildup of plaque in the arteries. For this reason, adequate amounts of antioxidant nutrients are essential for preventing cardiovascular disease.

Over several decades, Kilmer McCully, M.D., a research pathologist, developed the "homocysteine theory" of heart disease; in essence, he linked high levels of the amino acid homocysteine with increased risk of cardiovascular disease. Dr. McCully also established that deficiencies of certain B vitamins—B6, B12, and folic acid—promote atherosclerosis. This pioneering work helps to establish an "integrated" theory of the cause of heart disease.

What You Can Do

- Pay attention to the triglyceride levels in your blood, as well as total cholesterol readings.
- Unfortunately, refined foods made with white flour, sugar, and saturated fats are staple items in many households. Advice to "change your diet" is not just an empty statement. Your diet is an important key to preventing and reversing heart disease.
- The antioxidant nutrients such as vitamins C and E, the carotenes, selenium, coenzyme Q10, and phytochemicals such as soy isoflavones help protect arteries and blood vessels from damage caused by oxidation.
- In the coming years, you will be hearing more about the "homocysteine theory" of heart disease, and adequate amounts of vitamins B6, B12, and folic acid help keep your homocysteine levels favorably low.

CHAPTER FOUR

LATERAL THINKING

"Lateral thinking" is the practice of looking at other illnesses in an attempt to find a connection between them and cardiovascular disease. Although lateral thinking is useful for exploring other venues of thought on the subject of cardiovascular disease, most of these ideas are not strictly rooted in "science," and therefore require further research. This chapter presentss some lateral thoughts about the causes of cardiovascular disease, with sections that are necessarily somewhat disjointed in their content. I do not claim that the ensuing ideas are my thoughts alone; they are collected from literature written by healthcare givers whom I admire. Admiration, however, should not be confused with science.

REINVENTING THE "MEDICAL WHEEL"

The modern epidemic of cardiovascular disease seems to tell us that endless discussions about what we already know about the causes of heart disease will not solve this modern scourge of humankind. Western medicine has concentrated on the correction of factors that are destructive to cardiovascular health. This "model of destruction" pays attention to the known risk factors that act overtly in adults, but it may blind our thinking.

Lateral thoughts emerge as we realize that cardiovascular disease really is a complicated, mixed-bag of dirty tricks. Recently, scientists have started to discuss the possibility that atheroma and arteriosclerosis may be caused by inflammation, disordered immunity, and even infection. In addition, touching, thinking, mind-body medicine, and body "oneness" have emerged as important factors in health. These factors are addressed in many disciplines of alternative medicine (*e.g.*, Ayurveda, chiropractic medicine, and homeopathy). As current approaches to cardiovascular disease fail to make a major impact, lateral thinkers are beginning to be heard. In my writings, I have pointed out that many medical innovations are "reinventions of the wheel." Let's explore some of these modern trends.

IS ATHEROSCLEROSIS AN INFECTIOUS DISEASE?

For many years, others and I have suspected that atherosclerosis may be caused by infection with several microorganisms. In 1977, I published two short case histories under the titles "Severe Mycoplasma Pneumonia" (*Thorax* 32:112–115, 1977) and "Cytomegalovirus Induced Hemolytic Anemia Following Cardiac Surgery" (*Thorax* 31:788–789, 1977). In patients with mycoplasma or cytomegalovirus infections in these clinical reports, cardiac changes were present on EKGs, implying myocarditis (or heart damage). I recall my colleagues casting some doubt on my projected thoughts that mycoplasma (*Chlamydia pneumoniae*) or viral infections with agents like cytomegalovirus could be important causes of common heart disease. I am not trying to indicate that I had made a novel discovery in the 1970s; in fact there were studies as early as the 1940s that might lead one to suspect "bugs" as a prelude to acute, subacute, and chronic heart problems.

Lessons for Cardiology from the Masters of Gastroenterology

We may learn a lesson about cardiovascular disease and infections if we return to the discovery of the role of bacteria in the cause of peptic ulcer disease. Gastroenterologists (stomach and bowel doctors) have arrived at the recognition of the importance of the presence of the stomach bug (bacterium) *Helicobacter pylori* in ulcer disease. However, a journey back over fifty years in medical literature is illuminating; it is sometimes important to look back in order to move forward. The fathers of modern gastroenterology—A. C. Ivy, M.D., M. I. Grossman, M.D., and W. H. Bachrach, M.D.—provide us with some very stimulating thoughts about potential infectious causes of peptic ulcer in their 1950 book, *Peptic Ulcer*. The following is a quotation from Ivy, Grossman, and Bachrach's book:

> Since we did not find it possible to produce ulcer by direct infection of the gastric mucosa of dogs with organisms isolated from human gastric ulcer by Rosenow's technique or by virulent organisms from other sources with all other possible factors controlled, we can only conclude that if chronic ulcer of the stomach is due to infection, either the dog has a high natural immunity, which we doubt, or a highly specific organism is required, or other essential factors must be associated with the infection. It is possible that an infection of the tissues about an acute ulcer may cause production of connective tissue or inhibition of proliferation of mucosal cells, which, in the presence of other factors conducive to chronicity, will result in a chronic ulcer.

We need to look carefully at the above statements. If carefully interpreted, they give us some clues to potentially infectious causes of common diseases. The authors talk about the need for highly specific organisms, altered immunity, and poorly defined "essential factors" that must be associated with the infection in order, in this case, to produce a peptic ulcer. I draw attention to their notes of tissue changes involving connective tissues and other cells. Without being a "Monday morning quarterback," I can state that these masters of gastroenterology did much of the work that took another fifty years to surface in medicine. One of their most important statements relates to the presence of other factors, in addition to infection, which are conducive to chronicity. Enter the realm of "the bouquet of barbed wire" in cardovascular disease, which has been the focus of my constant repetition in this book.

Infections Figure in Cardiovascular Disease

Much evidence seems to point to the possibility that infections with common pathogens may contribute to cardiovascular disease. Certain bacteria, viruses, pathogenic yeasts, and fungi could be more than casual bystanders in the cause of the epidemic of heart disease. Several studies show that something as common as gingivitis (periodontal disease) is clearly associated with heart disease. Good oral hygiene and the right toothbrush (or technique of brushing) emerge as important tools in the fight against heart disease.

Recent papers in leading scientific journals focus on inflammation in atherosclerosis and discuss "the vulnerable plaque." The vulnerable plaque refers to certain deposits of atheroma that are distinguished by their likelihood to cause adverse cardiovascular events such as thrombosis or detachment (embolism). A *New England Journal of Medicine* review article (vol. 34) in 1999 discusses in detail the role of inflammation in atherosclerosis; medical treatises are appearing that relate infection with agents like *Chlamydia pneumoniae* and retroviruses (cytomegalovirus and even herpes) to cardiovascular disease. A flurry of new diagnostic tests are being developed to detect "vulnerable plaque" using high-speed magnetic resonance imaging and other high-technology diagnostic techniques. Vulnerable plaque appears to have an inflammatory component that makes it more likely to undergo detachment or surface complications. Amidst this new knowledge, some proponents of alternative medicine have found a new weapon to attack the conventional medical options of cardiac bypass surgery and angioplasty.

The alternative medicine community has been quite quick to jump on the possibility that inflammation is a prime cause of vascular disease. There is some danger of "hype" transcending science when it comes to theories about infection and cardiovascular disease. There are alternative practitioners of medicine who have been shunned by their colleagues because they are convinced that all chronic degenerative disease is infectious in origin. Some of these physicians claim to see evidence of infection or its consequences in the blood of many patients, even using simple microscopy. These observations have not been taken seriously by mainstream medicine, but now they require reappraisal in the light of current knowledge.

I am concerned that some alternative practitioners are ordering rather expensive tests to detect evidence of inflammation, or past or current infections in patients with cardiovascular disease, without any real knowledge about the cost effectiveness of this testing. Examples of these tests, which are perhaps better considered part of research only, include the detection of *Chlamydia pneumoniae* by PCR (an accurate test of infection in the lab), all types of vascular antibodies, and some types of adhesion molecules. We do not need more reasons to escalate the outpatient cost of cardiac care without further studies.

I do not feel quite as alone today as I felt in the 1970s when I suggested that certain infectious agents may cause nonvalvar, cardiac, or vascular disease. Some contemporary, but debated studies suggest reversal of angina and perhaps even prevention of heart attacks by antimicrobial therapy. These are potential, new directions in cardiac care. Infections with Chlamydia and certain viruses (and other bugs) may be to arteriosclerosis what Helicobacter is to peptic ulcer disease.

The Immune Basis of Cardiovascular Disease

There is a well-established relationship between nutrition, immune function, and aging. Add cardiovascular disease to this medical cocktail. These fields of science are just beginning to interact. While the functions of the immune system are beyond the scope of a detailed discussion in this book, immune mechanisms have been shown to play a major role in the initiation and propagation of atherosclerosis. "Diminution" in immune function, like cardiovascular disease, is itself somewhat a function of age. Maybe we can make this situation less inevitable than we currently think!

It is well-recognized that the elderly have more frequent and more severe infections than the young and these changes in immune function with age may have a great deal to do with preceding lifestyle and environmental influences. It is the functioning of the immune system that becomes unregulated in the elderly, rather than the mere circumstance of "simple" immune deficiency. Leading researchers have started to use terms like "immune senescence." Decreased immune function in the elderly is clearly linked with an increased occurrence of chronic degenerative disease and cancer.

It is known from animal studies and limited human data that circulating immune complexes (antigens linked to antibodies) can be linked to the causes of arteriosclerosis. With advancing age, the body shows a tendency to attack itself with its own immune functions. This situation is called autoimmunity. Overt evidence of the development of autoimmunity with age comes from many studies that show the development of antibodies against several components of different body tissues in different organs of the body.

Advancing years are associated with the occurrence of autoantibodies (antibodies against self) in the blood against cell nuclei (antinuclear antibodies), against DNA (genetic material), against components of the thyroid gland (thyroglobulin antibodies), against antibodies themselves (*e.g.*, rheumatoid factor), and against blood vessel components. A striking number of elderly people have these antibodies. About 65 percent of all people over the age of sixty-five have these types of antibodies in variable combinations or amounts. Autoimmunity appears to be a function of age, and it may be linked quite strongly to cardiovascular disease.

Monkey Business Is Revealing

We can learn more about the far-reaching consequences of autoimmunity for the health of the cardiovascular system if we examine some very interesting studies in monkeys. When monkeys undergo vasectomy (cutting the ducts that deliver sperm from the testes, a common operation used for male sterilization), an increase in antibodies to sperm and the presence of circulating immune complexes occurs. When these monkeys are followed for more than ten years, they have well-established immunity against their own gonads (testicles), but they have much more atherosclerosis than monkeys that did not undergo the operation of vasectomy. This seems, at first sight, to be merely an "insular discussion," but we have recognized that older people often show evidence of autoimmunity and even minor components of autoimmunity appear to contribute to atherosclerosis. Of course, much science presents a conundrum, because studies of vasectomized humans do not seem to show increased risks of cardiovascular disease.

Aging: Not Just a Case of Depressed Immunity

Depression of immune responses clearly reduces the body's ability to combat cancer, infections, and atherosclerosis. There are many reasons why immunity wanes with age, but one of the most important correctable causes of disordered immune function appears to be adequate nutrition. Many natural approaches to enhancing immunity exist including good balanced nutrition, exercise, and the specific use of vitanutrients such as vitamin E, omega-3 fatty acids, beta glucan, and selected herbs such as *Andrographis paniculata* (see my book, *Miracle Herbs,* Birch Lane Press, 1998). However, the idea of boosting immunity without restoring its normal and ordered mechanisms of function may not be the correct approach. Balance is required. A quote from Professor Mark E. Weksler, M.D., of Cornell University Medical College, exemplifies this circumstance. Weksler states:

> While immune senescence is frequently linked to a tired old dog lying quietly in front of the fire place, I would suggest that immune senescence is more like an aggressive bulldog, overactive and without a predictable course. If this latter simile is correct, the approach to enhancing the adaptive function of the immune system in the elderly should be to re-regulate the elements that have thrown the immune system out of control rather than to add more biological "vitality" to the immune system.

Practitioners of alternative medicine have focused their activity on boosting immunity as an antiaging tactic. Large quantities of nonspecific immune stimulating agents have been used in dietary supplement format. Such agents include Echinacea, expensive fermented rice bran, herbs, and other botanicals. To boost immunity in a nonspecific or inappropriate manner may not be valuable.

Tactics that diminish the body's tendency to produce autoantibodies (manifestations of autoimmunity) may be very worthwhile in helping to correct predispositions to cardiovascular and other diseases. Thus, more of a balancing act in immune function is required, not just a "kick at the dog" to get it moving. Few physicians in conventional medicine would even pay lip service to the importance of regulated immune function in the prevention or treatment of cardio-vascular disease. More questions remain unanswered than have been asked.

BRING FORWARD THE LEVEL OF PREVENTION BY GOING BACKWARDS

I have discussed the subject of adverse lifestyle in adults that oper-ates strongly in the causation of atheroma (common cardiovascular disease). Clearly, preoccupation with this approach has failed to com-pletely explain the development of coronary artery disease, and its success in tackling the epidemic of heart disease has been somewhat limited. Improving cardiovascular health requires an understanding of the origin of the problem, be it infection, disordered immunity, or the obvious cardiac risk factors—about which we are tired of hearing. Faced with the knowledge that risks of heart disease develop in child-hood has not led to clear public initiatives to address the risks. As we turn the millennium, the U.S. contains the fattest and perhaps the most idle kids in the world. These are not un-American statements; I am proud of our culture, but we must face reality.

We have learned that during childhood cholesterol (and other fatty material) starts to become deposited in the lining of arterial blood vessels. The main blood vessels of children who are three to four years old may show evidence of early atheroma, manifested by "fatty streaks" on vessel linings.

We know that the risk factors for an adult to develop atherosclero-sis operate in children the same way as they do in adults, but overall they operate at a lower level of risk. This may have made us more com-placent about addressing risk factors for cardiovascular disease in childhood as a solid investment for the prevention of atherosclerosis in adult life. This has been a big mistake, especially when we can quosh the pundits who claim that reduction of fat and cholesterol intake may impair growth. We know that children over the age of two have no dele-terious effects when they consume fat-modified (low saturated fat) diets that are recommended as "heart-smart" in adulthood.

Therefore, I may shock some readers by suggesting very strongly that coronary heart disease may have its root in the fetus. Changes experienced by the embryo, in utero, appear to be important in determining the occurrence of heart disease in later life. There is much evidence to support the idea that coronary artery disease may be linked to impaired fetal growth.

Studies in England and Wales of death rates from coronary heart disease show a relationship with death rates among newborn infants in the early years of this century. More detailed population studies using statistics collected by the Medical Research Council (UK) show relationships between small weight at birth or disproportionate size of babies and coronary heart disease in later life.

Low birth weight has been associated with the "insulin resistance syndrome" that has been discussed in the previous chapter. This syndrome is a common disorder in adults that predisposes to heart disease. It involves impairments in the body's ability to handle sugar (impaired glucose tolerance), disturbances in cholesterol and fat metabolism, and elevated blood pressure. Low birth weight is not the only identified risk factor. Some research indicates that a newborn with a short body length in relationship to head size may have long-term abnormalities of cholesterol metabolism and blood clotting.

Much of the research in this uncharted area of medicine has been highlighted by Professor D. J. P. Barker of the Medical Research Council in England. He points to a new research focus in prevention of heart disease. I believe that the data are strong enough to send another strong message about good prenatal lifestyle in women to ensure optimal well-being of the infant (and the adult). Programmed changes that affect health occur very early in our development. These are "neglected" preventive strategies for cardiovascular and other diseases.

ANGIOGENESIS AND DISEASE

Angiogenesis can best be defined by dissecting the word to its Greek roots: *angio* and *genesis. Angio* is Greek for "a vessel, usually a blood vessel" and *genesis* means "to originate or create." Angiogenesis is thus the growth of new blood vessels, a process that can happen in normal or disease-state circumstances in the tissues of the body. This process is also called neovascularization (neo means "new"). The phenomenon of angiogenesis has attracted considerable interest in the scientific community. In the normal adult, angiogenesis occurs infrequently. Exceptions are found in the female reproductive system, where it occurs during the development of follicles during ovulation and in the placenta after pregnancy. These periods of angiogenesis are relatively brief and tightly controlled with regard to the extent of new vessel formation. Angiogenesis is a multistep event in which endothelial cells— those that form the walls of small blood vessels called capillaries— migrate and proliferate. The capillary formation is triggered by several agents thought to be released from tissues near proliferating capillaries.

Normal angiogenesis also occurs as part of the body's repair processes; that is, in the healing of wounds and fractures. Angiogenesis also plays a major role in a variety of diseases, including: cancer (the growth of solid tumors), arthritis, atherosclerosis, skin conditions, eye disorders, and inflammatory disease. In these cases, it can be an unwanted and detrimental phenomenon. By adding the word inhibitors to angiogenesis, we have a descriptive phrase for compounds that prevent or reduce the growth of new blood vessels (antiangiogenesis). The application of methods to manipulate angiogenesis has created fascinating therapeutic options, including the potential of natural-based compounds that may modify new blood vessel growth (*e.g.*, extracts of shark cartilage or soy isoflavones).

Angiogenesis: A Double-Edged Sword

There are circumstances where angiogenesis is necessary—including pregnancy, ovulation, and atherosclerosis—when there is a need to develop a collateral circulation (new vessels to bypass those that are clogged), such as occurs in coronary artery disease or peripheral vascular disease. These circumstances are examples of conditions where anti-angiogenic therapy is to be used with caution and vigilance—or even avoided.

Attempts to induce angiogenesis (new blood vessel growth) have helped to identify many substances (*e.g.*, cytokines) that may promote blood vessel growth, including: acidic fibroblast growth factor, epidermal growth, transforming growth factors alpha and beta-1, tumor necrosis factor alpha, vascular endothelial growth factor, platelet-derived endothelial cell-growth factor, angiogenin, and angiotensin. Angiogenic cytokines show promise in plastic and reconstructive surgery, and they may have a role in stimulating a collateral circulation in people with cardiovascular disease as a consequence of blocked arteries. Pretreatment of donor and receptor skin graft sites with angiotropin has prevented tissue necrosis in skin flaps. Cytokines have also been used to promote angiogenesis during surgical procedures.

The intriguing role that angiogenesis may play in the amelioration of disease has led to speculation that angiogenic promoters may be useful in treating such disorders as peptic ulcers, fistulae, and hypoxia-induced resistance of tumors to repeated irradiation treatments and chemotherapy. In addition, other patients with avascular disorders may benefit from inducing neovascularization, including those with aseptic bone necrosis and vascular occlusion of tissue organs, notably peripheral vascular disease and ischemic heart disease. Inflammatory bowel disease, in which blood-flow abnormalities and neovascularization may occur, has been reported to show some favorable response to bovine cartilage treatments. Several clinical trials of angiogenic compounds in the treatment of peptic ulcer and cardiovascular disease are underway. From basic science to behavioral science, lateral thoughts on the causation of cardiovascular disease move across many boundaries.

DOES LOVE HEAL DISEASE?

I can answer this question with a resounding, *yes!* But despite the recognition of the healing power of love and intimacy in ancient literature and modern scientific studies, there is little application of this knowledge in modern medicine. I have to turn to the work of Wilhelm Reich, M.D.

Dr. Reich was a student of Sigmund Freud. He fell out with Freud, wandered through Europe, and finished up in the U.S. Dr. Reich was labeled unethical, and he was accused of engaging in malpractice when he proposed his theories about the importance of orgasm in the promotion of physical and mental well-being. It is true that Dr. Reich's concepts on sex and well-being appeared to be too focused on "orgasm," but he had a broader message. Modern authors on sexual healing such as Paul Pearsall, Ph.D., and Dr. Dean Ornish are riding on the coattails of Dr. Reich with their books on the healing power of love and its contribution to survival and physical (or mental) well-being. Let me make a further trip on the coattails of Dr. Reich!

Malpractice: Forgotten Sexual Healing!

The notion in the early part of the twentieth century that equating sex with healing was malpractice has come a full turn as we approach the next millennium. In his book, *Love and Survival: The Scientific Basis for the Healing Power of Intimacy* (Harper Collins Publishers, 1998), Dr. Dean Ornish indicates that only a few healers (including physicians) are educated about the therapeutic benefits of love and intimacy. He likens the lack of the application of this knowledge in clinical practice as an example of modern malpractice. I heartily agree!

The idea that a lack of direction from physicians on the healing power of human relationships could be termed malpractice would be music to the ears of Dr. Reich. It would appear that I revere the work of Dr. Reich, but I see this persecuted physician as one of this century's examples of the unfortunate success of narrow-minded, nebulous bodies of medical opinion that can shape medicine incorrectly.

Let Sexual Healing Move to the Forefront of Therapy

I see the healing power of sex, love, and intimacy as exceedingly important in dealing with recalcitrant problems of chronic disease and premature death. Cardiovascular disease remains a number one killer, but one could hardly transplant hearts into all cardiac cripples and cardiovascular medications have often shown a distinct inability to alter the course of cardiovascular disease. Many types of cancer continue to beat the chemotherapist but cancer sometimes appears to show a dramatic, but inconsistent, response to some alternative medical therapies.

There is some very credible evidence that sexual healing (synonymous in my mind with love and intimacy) can offer at least adjunctive benefit in the treatment of many incurable diseases that afflict modern humankind. I propose to review some of this evidence, but I emphasize that these concepts are neither novel nor new; they have been recorded throughout history.

Dean Ornish, M.D., Speaks

Dr. Dean Ornish has proven something that has been deduced about cancer, immune dysfunction, inflammatory disease, or mental disease. Cardiovascular disease can be reversed by lifestyle adjustment. Science may not have shown this to be the case in a consistent manner. However, meticulous prospective research is required by the more hidebound physicians before they will act on the obvious.

Dr. Ornish's lifestyle approach to reversing or preventing cardiac disease has been considered by some to be a hard path to follow. The variable degree of benefit that can be achieved by lifestyle approaches is likely to be dependent on compliance with change. For example, eating one less hamburger a day may do little to lower blood cholesterol. He has recognized the contribution of diet and exercise in his holistic, cardiac treatment program, but he recognizes that the solution to reversal of heart disease is more complex. In his book *Love and Survival*, Dr. Ornish notes that "something else is going on."

The Something Else!

Dr. Ornish has concluded after his many years of excellent and successful research in cardiovascular disease that love and intimacy are at the root of health. Dr. Ornish comments on the healing power of love and intimacy in the following manner: "I am not aware of any other factor in medicine—not diet, not smoking, not exercise, not stress, not genetics, not drugs,not surgery—that has a greater impact on our quality of life, incidence of illness, and premature death from all causes."

Other thought-leaders in alternative and complementary medicine such as Deepak Chopra, M.D., and Andrew Weil, M.D., have provided much support for Dr. Ornish's conclusions in their own writings. It would be impossible to review the large amount of precedent to support the notion that love, intimacy, nurturing relationships, and sexual union are healthful.

The powerful message of Ornish is somewhat diluted, in my opinion, by his apparent unwillingness to provide a detailed description of the importance of sexual intercourse per se as an important contributor to health and well-being. Perhaps he wished to avoid the kind of beating that was dished out to Dr. Reich and others who have been more explicit in their opinions about sex and health?

Science Shows the Healing Power of Sexuality and Love

For the doubting Thomas who questions the presence of a scientific basis for the healing properties of optimal sexuality, there are hundreds of well-conducted research studies to change his or her mind. The common theme of this research is to choose one or more aspects of healthy sexuality (and its associated phenomena) and show a positive health benefit. Love, intimacy, and sexual encounters have been shown to improve the outcome of cancer therapy (lung and breast cancer), rehabilitation following strokes or injuries, and cardiovascular disease.

The important positive correlation between optimal circumstances of love and intimacy and well-being is found to be quite tenable when one recognizes the negative impact of absent or dysfunctional relationships on health. People with emotional problems from broken relationships who are isolated from love and intimacy tend to die at younger ages and have a worse prognosis in the presence of disease (*e.g.*, cardiovascular problems and cancer). Just having a partner, regardless of the quality of the relationship, may be healthy. Unmarried individuals with absent social ties are more often victims of disease and early death in many research studies.

Broken Relationships

If love and intimacy are at the root of health, then the termination of relationships would be expected to be damaging in many ways. Divorce or death of a spouse are prime risks for cardiovascular disease, but we do little to prevent divorce in our society. Adverse health circumstances arise when separation of loving partners is an inevitable event. Unfortunately, love and hate seem to be close together in human feelings. When a person evokes strong feelings of love or hate in another, good and bad things can happen. Close partners know generally how to push each other's buttons.

KNOWLEDGE TO CHANGE THE CAUSE OF DISEASE

We know that many medical tests can help the diagnosis and monitoring of disease states. These tests, however, become quite superfluous if they do not translate into a beneficial course of action for the patient. The same arguments apply to knowledge derived from research, or "lateral thoughts."

Modern medicine is not rewarding lateral thought among its membership. The current trend in conventional medicine is to work to recipes called "clinical practice guidelines." These guidelines consist of statements that are designed to help medical practitioners *and patients* make decisions about appropriate medical management in certain clinical circumstances. Whatever the impact of these guidelines on physician behavior, these guidelines are not often shared with patients, nor do many patients even recognize their own power in guiding therapy. I believe that these guidelines strip the art out of medicine, and they have clear limitations.

Dr. Jeoffrey K. Stross, M.D., of the University of Michigan School of Medicine (*Annals of Internal Medicine*, 131, 4, 304-306, 1999) has pointed to the limitations of practice guidelines in a recent editorial. Dr. Stross points out that modern medical practice behavior seems to be influenced by many factors. In particular, physician decision making seems to occur under the influence of social issues, learning abilities, and many factors that may or may not induce changes in behavior. Research findings do not seem to exert a major impact on clinical decision making, unless the communication is powerful (usually from a pharmaceutical company).

Physicians can only be predisposed to change with new findings in medicine. If physicians cannot easily change their approach to disease prevention and treatment, what chance does the patient have? Things are changing as consumers of health care take charge of their own health-care decisions. This newfound self-reliance among patients includes a repeated questioning of many current conventional medical approaches. There is an increasing predilection for more natural forms of treatment that may be safer and as effective as allopathic options in some circumstances. Unless new knowledge (or reinvention of the wheel) is put into action, chronic degenerative disease will prevail and cardiovascular disease, in particular, may remain rampant.

SUMMARY

Medicine has concentrated on the correction of factors that are destructive to cardiovascular health, which may blind us to the fact that cardiovascular disease is a very complicated issue. All lateral thoughts on the cause of cardiovascular disease cannot be reviewed. There are hundreds of branches of alternative medicine with widely differing opinions and philosophies. Careful scientific review of all these "lateral thoughts" is needed. This chapter is mainly useful as an exercise to expand our understanding of the heart disease epidemic.

Much evidence seems to point to the possibility that infections with common pathogens may contribute to cardiovascular disease. Certain bacteria, viruses, pathogenic yeasts, and fungi could be more than casual bystanders in the cause of the epidemic of heart disease. Gingivitis, for instance, has been shown to be clearly associated with heart disease.

Auto-immunity, the process by which the body develops autoantibodies (antibodies against self) against DNA, thyroid gland components, blood vessel components, and even themselves, appears to be a function of age and may be linked quite strongly to cardiovascular disease.

There is much evidence to support the idea that coronary disease may be traced back even as early as impaired fetal growth.

Angiogenesis, new blood vessel growth, may be a valuable tool in the future treatment of cardiovascular disease.

Dr. Wilhelm Reich and contemporary author Dr. Dean Ornish have both studied the therapeutic benefits of love and intimacy.

There is an increasing need for fresh ideas in the fight against cardiovascular disease. Lateral thinking is becoming more and more important as we continue to search out previously unthought of initiatives in this field.

CHAPTER FIVE

LOOKING AT YOUR LIFESTYLE

If you have read this far, you understand that cardiovascular wellness for most people is largely the result of the choices they make throughout their lives. Therefore, you have a significant role to play in preventing heart disease and controlling or even reversing it, should it develop. There is nothing more natural than individuals playing a role in their own health care, and therefore, exerting a degree of control over their destiny! As you have seen, the risk factors of cardiovascular disease seldom occur in isolation; they must be tackled together. This is the heterogeneous nature of cardiovascular disease, meaning that there are many contributing factors.

You may be thinking that lifestyle change is easier said than done, but you can systematically tackle each problem—or risk factor. Most people prefer to first take on the risk factor that is easiest to change, or one that, when eliminated or altered, yields the most benefit. What is easy for one person may be difficult for another, and there is no doubt great variation among individuals in the degree of difficulty involved in beneficial change. But no matter how great the challenge ahead may appear, remember that many other men and women are on the same path with you. I want you to feel encouraged, because being positive and feeling good is very beneficial for cardiovascular health.

THE LIFESTYLE CONCEPT

Lifestyle is a general term that defines the way we live and the relative level of our psychological, physical, and social well-being. Of course, depending on the context, the word "lifestyle" can mean many different things, from how we spend our money to the way we choose to spend our leisure time. Multibillion-dollar industries exist to analyze every detail of our consumer lifestyle, and carefully designed advertising campaigns attempt to influence—indeed, manipulate— every buying decision. It is ironic that some of this advertising is designed to lure us into choices that adversely affect our health with the message to "be good" to ourselves by eating one sugary, fat-laden treat after another. It has led to an enormous array of convenient snack foods, most of which do not build our health. It is not difficult to see that far less money is spent on promoting healthful lifestyle choices than is spent promoting products of dubious value for health.

By definition, a healthy lifestyle requires that you eliminate high-risk behaviors. The art of managing lifestyle issues is easy to overlook because the effects of poor lifestyle choices may not be immediate. A smoking addiction usually develops when a person is young and impetuous, and the ill effects may manifest years or even decades later. Even with vastly increased education about the risks involved in smoking cigarettes, some of our adolescents remain unconvinced that smoking damages their bodies and almost certainly has the potential to rob them of years of vibrant health in their adult life.

Adults are not immune from ignoring important issues either. They routinely justify their procrastination in making positive lifestyle changes because the rewards for their efforts are so often slow to manifest. Yet intellectually, these same adults know that physical and mental well-being are the greatest treasures we have in life. When we approach lifestyle issues, perhaps the most important goal is achieving congruency between what we *know* and what we *do*. Having smoked for some years, I fell into this trap. My behavior was incongruent with what I knew to be true about the dangers of smoking.

When evaluating your lifestyle issues, begin by assessing individual behaviors or areas, including psychological well-being. The way you think and feel about the quality and circumstances of your family relationships, your career, and your ties within your community are important for cardiovascular health and cannot be overlooked in any assessment. All the following areas have an important influence on physical and mental health and are interrelated—and, in many cases, interdependent:

- Alcohol, tobacco, and other substance abuse
- Nutrition/diet
- Sexual activity
- Physical activity/exercise
- Psychological well-being

Fortunately, most of us have a high degree of control over these lifestyle factors and the available ways that exist to evaluate our risk. The best method to measure or check lifestyle involves comparing an individual's behaviors with those of the general population. This method has the advantage of demonstrating that lifestyle is not an either/or, or an "all-or-nothing" phenomenon. For example, while obesity is a risk factor for heart disease, the degree of risk increases as the degree of obesity increases. Likewise, individuals who are heavy drinkers are at a higher risk for cardiovascular disease—and other conditions—than occasional social drinkers. Heavy drinkers are often heavy smokers, and these risks become inextricably linked and compounded.

Since evidence exists showing that your lifestyle is a major determining factor of your health, it makes sense to assess your risk factors and take effective corrective action. Clearly, the more you engage in beneficial lifestyle choices, the better you will feel!

Taking Stock

When it comes to lifestyle assessment, you have two choices. You can complete medical history forms and wait for a physician or a nurse to ask you the "right" questions in order to measure your level of risk. The second—and, probably, the best—method involves self-identification of a problem, with self-intervention. Nowadays, interactive computer software programs provide a method for patients to perform self-assessments. The program asks the questions and then statistically calculates the risk factors.

Together with my colleagues, I have developed a computer-assisted testing program that has been shown to be useful in assessing lifestyle in our medical clinic patients. Most patients find this method quite acceptable and, moreover, some evidence suggests that a patient may provide more information to a computer than to a doctor! We found that lifestyle testing prompted patients to discuss concerns with their doctor that they may otherwise have failed to bring up in a routine visit.

Self-Identification and Self-Intervention

Did you know that Benjamin Franklin was one of the earliest recorded self-watchers? In their book *Self-Watching*, authors Hodgen and Miller have reported that Franklin created a detailed plan for self-observation and for monitoring behaviors he considered ideal for a healthy and virtuous life. The remarkable Ben Franklin provides us with an early example that resembles current recommendations to keep a "self-watching" diary. Looking to an even earlier time, the same authors quote the inscriptions on the shrine of the Oracle at Delphi—"Know thyself"—with the added caveat, "Nothing to excess." Perhaps these simple statements serve as guideposts to the pivotal issues in maintaining health.

These authors have identified lifestyle problems, and they offer ways for individuals to monitor their own involvement in the behaviors. For example, if smoking is an issue, then the number of cigarettes smoked per day and the number of puffs per cigarette provide good estimates about the amount of nicotine and harmful chemicals taken into the body. Beyond that, smokers can begin to see patterns in their smoking behavior. Eating patterns, drinking, the number of hours spent working, drug use, and so forth can be monitored in the same way. You may wonder why *working* is on the list. After all, we usually think of work as a virtue, not a vice—Ben Franklin certainly did. However, workaholism—the problem of overworking—is without doubt an adverse behavior that contributes to cardiovascular disease. It may be one of the most underestimated risk factors for cardiovascular disease in modern society.

Using self-watching techniques may seem merely odd to some people and downright ridiculous to others. Surely the smoker realizes how many packs of cigarettes he or she "kills" every day. Is the drinker unaware of how many shots of bourbon he or she tosses back? As strange as it might seem to some, the answer is yes. Human beings have a great capacity for self-deception, and many individuals must scrupulously identify adverse lifestyle issues as a prerequisite to modifying behavior or overcoming addictions.

Recent advances in behavioral sciences shed light on the way habits are developed and become entrenched in a person's life. Hodgen and Miller have coined the phrase "the ABC approach" to understanding the way habits and addictions are formed and reinforced. The ABC component is a mnemonic device that helps us remember each area: "A" stands for Antecedent cues, "B" focuses on the Behavior itself, and "C" indicates the Consequences of the habit or behavior that may diminish or enhance it.

An antecedent cue is simply a fancier way to indicate a trigger for a behavior. A triggering event may be physiological or social. For example, an urge to smoke can result from the body's craving for nicotine or from a social cue. When they are trying to quit, smokers almost always report difficulty being around other smokers. The same is true for drinkers or drug users.

Antecedent cues—or triggers—tend to give signals, warnings, or promises of consequences—"payoffs"—that can result from the behavior that underlies the habit. For example, if Joe Hooch is sitting in a bar, he knows he is in a setting that is loaded with triggers to drink or smoke. The consequences could be good feelings, better social interactions, or just suppressing unpleasant physical withdrawal from nicotine or alcohol. Once Joe identifies the triggers and the subsequent potential "payoffs," he can decide how he will handle the triggers. Perhaps he can stay away from bars until the triggers to the behavior lose their power. Or, he can realize that although the triggers are present, no one is forcing him to act on them. He can make a different choice.

Behavioral scientists (not to mention storytellers, theologians, philosophers, and poets) have wrestled with attempts to understand why individuals persist in adverse lifestyle habits or patterns even though they know that the consequences of their behavior can be catastrophic. Alcohol abusers sometimes lose their jobs as well as their families, and smokers may develop heart disease or lung cancer. In the last decade or so, many smokers have become socially isolated, too, but even this may not be motivation enough to stop smoking. Drug users may end up committing crimes in order to support their expensive—and illegal—habits. Yet, they often seem unable to leave the addiction behind and start down a different road.

The answer to this enigma may lie in understanding the concept of immediate gratification. When Joe Hooch reaches for his friend's pack of cigarettes, he is acting on a short-term need. The immediate pleasure Joe gains from smoking far outweighs any considerations of long-term harm. When he leaves the bar—or even after the first cigarette—Joe may feel great remorse and wonder why he could have acted so foolishly. However, short-term gratification is a powerful reinforcer of adverse lifestyle. Until Joe understands this, he is likely to repeatedly fall back into old habits.

Smoking provides a dramatic example, and one that is familiar to anyone who has experience with an addiction to nicotine and the smoking habit. However, other behaviors are similar, even if not so obvious. For example, heading to the fast food restaurant because it is readily available and offers an easy choice means consuming food that is loaded with refined sugar and saturated fat. These meals may contribute significantly to the development of heart disease and are a factor in developing or maintaining obesity. However, these consequences are not apparent after one quick lunch, but will likely appear weeks or months after the behavior persists. In the U.S. alone, millions of individuals consume fast food on a regular basis, and I am quite sure that most are aware that much of this food does not promote health. However, like Joe the smoker, the lure of immediate gratification wins out.

Other reinforcements are more relative or intermittent. Serious alcohol drinkers may continue to drink in the face of criticism because they may believe they function better after a few drinks. These individuals may not get the desired feelings or outcome each time they drink, but they keep on consuming alcohol because of their desire to get the "buzz" they are looking for.

Hodgen and Miller explain the three kinds of reinforcement in terms of expected consequences. They use the terms *reward now*, *reward sometimes*, and *rewards of avoiding discomfort* to match the concepts of short-term gratification, intermittent reinforcement, and relativity of reinforcement, respectively. Table 5.1 provides a way to

Table 5.1: ABC Reinforcement.

Hodgen and Miller (1982) propose that cues lead to behavior with consequences (ABC Approach) and that the behavior is reinforced by short-term, intermittent, or relative elements.

The ABC Approach	Reinforcement of Behavior
Antecedent cues	Short-term gratification—reward now
Behavior	Intermittent reinforcement—reward sometimes
Consequences	Relative reinforcement—reward of discomfort avoidance

see these concepts more clearly. Self-identification of problems and actions to change lifestyle are two pivotal steps in the prevention of cardiovascular disorders and other chronic degenerative diseases.

Changing Behavior

Understanding adverse lifestyle habits is an important step, and we can learn much from the behavioral scientists. At the end of the day, however, awareness must lead to change or it is without value. Once you understand the mechanism that reinforces the lifestyle issues you want to change, you can and must develop action plans to fight the habits, compulsions, and addictions that threaten to rob you of good health and vitality. The action plans you create must be tailored to the cues that trigger the behavior that results in the consequence—even when a particular consequence appears positive in the short-run. This process, which starts with self-watching and self-awareness, ultimately leads to self-intervention.

The overall goal of behavior modification is to strengthen and reinforce self-control and enjoy the rewards inherent in overcoming destructive behavior. As former addicts of all kinds know, the joy of getting through the withdrawal and experiencing life without the destructive behavior is itself a great reward. The same is true for those who are able to overcome habits which, while not as destructive as a drug addiction, for example, still detract from one's quality of

Table 5.2: Action Plans to Change Adverse Lifestyle.

Below are some components of plans to change adverse lifestyles, with examples of the activities in an action plan.

Component of Changing Behavior	Comments
Self-identification (self-watching)	The individual has to catch himself or herself in the act. A diary of events helps unravel the ABCs.
Attacking antecedent cues	The individual understands the circumstances that precipitate the behavior or adverse lifestyle and takes evasive action; *e.g.*, the overeater stays out of fast food restaurants.
Substituting alternative rewarding behavior	Early in the withdrawal phase, a prop can be used; *e.g.*, nicotine gum instead of smoking. The obese individual could join Weight Watchers, etc.
Prevent relapse	The individual must anticipate temptation and develop coping techniques.
Exposure to the temptation	A dangerous but effective activity where the individual tempts fate but applies resistance.

life. For all the talk we hear today about the concept of self-esteem, nothing builds your healthy self-concept more than correcting behavior that you know is detrimental to your health.

Five key recommendations for changing behavior and exerting self-control are summarized in Table 5.2. You will also find the components of a potential action plan. Of course, this entire discussion is based on the premise that you *want* to change detrimental habits and addictions. Education and self-watching help provide the motivation to enact positive change. While a detailed discussion of all the possible ways to correct lifestyle issues is beyond the scope of this book, use the information that follows as a guide to replacing destructive behaviors with those that improve your health.

Smoking

Cigarette smoking is a cardiovascular risk factor that stands out above the rest. This probably comes as no surprise, and your health-care providers have no doubt delivered all the possible sermons about the dangers of smoking. Public service television commercials reinforce the well-known facts about the dangers of smoking, and each year brings more restrictions on smoking in public places—it is not as easy to smoke as it used to be! There are dozens of good reasons to quit smoking, from saving hundreds of dollars each year to having cleaner teeth to developing increased stamina for exercise. In fact, the only incentive to keep smoking is the power of the addiction itself. And it is now apparent that smokers may be doing as much harm to the health of other people in the environment as they are to their own health. This provides additional motivation to protect public spaces and eventually rid our society of cigarette smoking. Regardless of how "high-minded" some individuals sound, though, cigarette smoking is not a moral issue but remains as it always was—a serious health concern.

Today's challenge is finding the right method for individual smokers, many of whom have attempted to let go of the smoking habit numerous times before becoming successful over the long haul. The strength of the smoking addiction is enormous. During my work with heroin addicts, I became aware that their addiction to cigarette smoking was most often stronger than their addiction to heroin. If I had asked these addicts which substance they would prefer to take on a trip to the moon, their hands-down choice would have been cigarettes! And just like those who are recovering from drug and alcohol addiction, most former smokers accept the fact that they are always at risk for relapse.

That said, there is reason for hope. Millions of men and women have quit smoking and have enjoyed the benefits of the nonsmoking lifestyle. Most will tell you that quitting smoking required intense willpower and behavior modification. Many also report that the toolbox of aids for smoking cessation may be of significant help, but in the end they are Band-Aids, just as weight-loss drugs are short-term crutches for the dieter. This is not to say that these crutches are worthless to the struggling nonsmoker. While nothing is more important than a commitment to quit, a plan of action is also a must, and this plan may include one or more of the common smoking cessation methods and tools.

Quitting "cold turkey." Is the "cold turkey" method better than gradual withdrawal? It is certainly the method used by most people who have quit smoking. Until recently, there were almost no effective alternative methods. I must say that my preference is for the abrupt withdrawal method. I have advised many others (and myself) to go through the discomfort and be done with it, rather than prolong the agony. Gradual withdrawal by cutting back on the number of cigarettes smoked per day represents a situation where one is still giving in to the strong, enduring habit of reaching for a cigarette. So, when it comes to giving up the habit and the rituals involved in smoking cigarettes, cold turkey is preferable in many ways.

Nicotine replacement. Within the last decade, nicotine replacement products have gained in popularity, particularly after becoming available without a prescription. Popularly known as "the patch," this method offers the advantage of slow, gradual withdrawal from nicotine, but without actually picking up a cigarette. (Nicotine may also be delivered in the form of gum and, more recently, through an inhaler.) The steady release of nicotine into the body allows the quitter to adjust his or her lifestyle without the discomfort (some really do call it agony) of physical symptoms. Because smoking involves both psychological and physical dependency, the patch allows for a gradual adjustment to life without the act of smoking, but with nicotine present in the body. Many former smokers maintain that they could work, sleep, talk on the phone, drive, go out with friends, and so forth, without discomfort because of the nicotine dose they received through the patch. The gradual withdrawal and adjustment is no doubt a lifesaver for many people because they can live normally.

For those who are unable to face withdrawal from both the smoking rituals and nicotine, the patch or gum is a good choice. More recently, nicotine inhalers have been developed. They are alleged to have the advantage of more closely resembling the act of smoking than other methods of nicotine substitution. Although you can easily buy nicotine replacement products, I recommend talking with your health-care provider about individualizing the plan to suit your needs. For example, some people benefit from staying on nicotine replacement for up to six months. This is three to four months longer than the average regimen and should be supervised by a physician.

Homeopathic techniques. Homeopathic medicine appears to be rapidly increasing in popularity. It is based on the idea that "like will cure like." Some individuals see this as contrarian thinking, but homeopathy assists in garnering the strength of the body's own innate ability to heal itself or create altered functions. Dr. Samuel Hahnemann, the father of modern homeopathy, proposed that if a substance that creates a symptom or sign (expression of disease) is administered in minute dilution, then it can be used to treat the condition that caused the symptom. In a very skeptical scientific climate, homeopathic physicians have struggled to explain how homeopathy works, but evidence in recent, peer-reviewed medical literature implies that it does work in a wide variety of conditions.

Homeopathic remedies have been administered in a variety of ways, including creams, lotions, tinctures, and tablets. I have developed a homeopathic patch in which the homeopathic agents that assist in smoking cessation are incorporated into liposomes (little "fatty" envelopes) in a gel that is placed in a special patch with a window. This technology has proven quite valuable in open-label experiences in weight control, and it deserves further research for smoking cessation. This patch system could help in smoking cessation in many different ways.

Bupropion hydrochloride (Zyban). This drug works by increasing the availability of serotonin, a neurotransmitter—chemical messenger—in the brain that influences mood. Some believe that one group of addicted cigarette smokers unconsciously uses nicotine as an "antidepressant," and bupropion hydrochloride acts to correct the balance of neurotransmitters in the brain, thereby ending the need for constant "self-medicating." The drug is marketed under the trade name Zyban, and while it has some potential side effects, including insomnia, nervousness, and weight loss, it does show promise for some people, particularly those who have been unable to quit smoking after several attempts. Zyban is available by prescription only. Overall, my advice is to avoid drug therapy for this problem, but Zyban may be useful for a specific group of recalcitrant smokers, especially those who have major emotional responses to smoking cessation.

Hypnosis/relaxation tapes. Hypnosis is a clinical tool that is used to plant suggestions in the subconscious mind. As a tool that has been used to control pain in dentistry, for example, it has shown variable results. There are no doubt individuals who have quit smoking, lost weight, or changed some other habit with the help of hypnosis, but some people find it of little or no help. A school of thought exists that believes in "aversion" suggestion; that is, planting the idea that cigarettes will taste or smell like burning rubber or some other noxious substance. But an ex-smoker once told me, "I just learned to like the taste of burning rubber!" I guess this is an example of the "law of unintended consequences." If you choose to use hypnosis, I recommend those techniques that emphasize relaxation and visualization of positive images and ideas.

Relaxation tapes can be valuable for reducing stress, which any person trying to break an addiction will need to do. Relaxation tapes are often the first step in learning meditation practices, so they have value beyond being a smoking-cessation tool. Both relaxation and self-hypnosis tapes are available in bookstores and in some specialty stores, but I would ask your health-care providers for their suggestions.

Support groups. Hospitals and clinics regularly run smoking-cessation clinics, often in cooperation with organizations such as the American Lung Association. There is also a program based on the twelve steps of Alcoholics Anonymous that offers ongoing support to maintain abstinence from cigarette smoking.

Reluctantly, I add the following: if cessation is not possible, a reduction in cigarette consumption to about five cigarettes per day is desirable. At least at this level there is not much statistical evidence of a major health risk. Remember, though, statistics can lie!

Alcohol and Heart Disease

There are many medical reasons to avoid excessive drinking, not the least of which is that it is strongly correlated with excessive smoking and smoking "relapses." In addition, alcohol is toxic to the muscle tissue of the heart. Elegantly designed clinical experiments show that alcohol can have profound effects on cardiovascular responses by dilating blood vessels and depressing myocardial (heart muscle) performance. On occasion, alcohol can trigger abnormal heart rhythm. Beyond the direct physical effects, there are psychological ramifications. Alcohol can unleash behavior that places a susceptible individual at acute risk of a heart attack.

Much has been made of the potentially beneficial effects of moderate alcohol intake on cardiac function and cholesterol levels. Unfortunately, these benefits are often outweighed by the negative effects of alcohol on cardiovascular well-being. Reports that red wine contains chemical components that promote a healthy heart do not serve as an excuse to gulp a bottle of wine with dinner. Clinical studies in the medical literature, including my own, have shown that modest alcohol intake raises HDL, but overall it does not normalize blood fats. Given these results, evidence of cardiac benefits is arguable. Less arguable, in my opinion, is the benefit of grapeseed extract used as a dietary supplement to promote cardiovascular health.

What I am talking about here is the tendency to interpret evidence about red wine or other effects of alcohol as reason enough to encourage a daily alcoholic drink or two—almost as if a bit of alcohol is now medicinal. While I have no objection on health grounds to light social drinking, I do not think it is necessary to drink any alcohol in order to have a healthy heart. Given the amount of alcohol abuse among people of all ages in our society, it is clear that excessive drinking is a problem with far-reaching implications, not the least of which is the risk factor for heart disease when drinking occurs above safe levels of alcohol consumption. Unfortunately, safe levels of alcohol ingestion have defied accurate definition!

When drinking is out of hand. Most people assume that they would know if they are drinking hazardous amounts of alcohol. However, this is a big misconception. As with all forms of adverse lifestyle, drinking occurs in degrees of severity. Chronic alcoholics are at one end of the drinking spectrum, and abstainers or "teetotalers" are at the other. One cannot use the all-or-nothing approach when considering drinking. There is a spectrum of drinking habits—and shades of gray prevail. Dr. Harvey Skinner of the University of Toronto and I have published several articles on the early identification of problem drinking and methods for intervention to correct this adverse lifestyle.

The vast majority of drinkers use alcohol in moderation. About five to ten percent of the population are frank—overt—alcohol abusers, and they are experiencing some of the medical, psychological, or social consequences of excessive drinking. Alcoholic individuals often reveal their disease by their behavior or by organic illness—or both. However, many problem drinkers often are hidden from society. Medical literature is full of descriptions of "closet alcoholics" who are unrecognized in the workplace, social circles, and even during hospital stays. Recent evidence suggests that about 20 percent of the population may be problem drinkers. This means that at least twice as many problem drinkers exist for every overt alcoholic.

Studies of young males between the ages of eighteen and thirty-five indicate that excessive drinking is occurring in epidemic proportions. It has been estimated that 30 or 40 percent of all young males are problem drinkers. Many of these young problem drinkers may go on to develop true alcoholism, or they will continue to be problem drinkers and—unfortunately—cause an array of difficulties for their families and associates.

What is sensible drinking? Light drinking is unlikely to be harmful, but because drinking problems develop over time, it is advisable to take a close look at your drinking habits. Because tolerance to alcohol varies among individuals, it is not possible to set rigid guidelines about what constitutes "sensible" drinking versus "risk" drinking. However, women may be more vulnerable to developing some alcohol-related illnesses, such as liver disease, when compared with men whose intake of alcohol is identical. Women are also strongly advised not to drink during pregnancy because of the risk of fetal alcohol syndrome, which causes potentially devastating birth defects in the fetus. In addition, some increased risk of breast cancer has been associated with alcohol consumption, but the amounts of alcohol necessary to increase the risk is not yet clear. In both sexes, there is wide variability in the tendency to develop drinking-related illnesses.

The following information can serve as useful guidelines against which you can assess your drinking habits. For men of about average weight and height, sensible drinking would be no more than four average drinks at a time—one sitting—and no more than twelve drinks in a week, with an attempt to be inconsistent. Recommendations for women are lower. Women of average height and weight should consume no more than two drinks at a time or no more than ten drinks a week. As you can see, these guidelines are not particularly restrictive, and those who enjoy an occasional glass of wine or beer with their dinner should never feel deprived.

Using generally accepted standards, one drink refers to one 12-ounce bottle of beer, a 1½-ounce shot of liquor, a 5-ounce glass of wine, or a 3-ounce glass of fortified wine, such as sherry, port, or vermouth. Remember that safety is always an issue. One drink is too many if you are driving or operating machinery. I believe it is also sensible and healthful not to drink alcohol every day; some days should be alcohol-free.

Finally, adverse interactions between alcohol and a wide range of medications, drugs, nutrients, herbs, or botanicals are not only possible, but more common than many people believe. Since these interactions can endanger your health or well-being, be sure that you ask your physician or pharmacist about any potential consequences of mixing alcohol and your medications.

Using alcohol is an adult decision and should always be made with the knowledge that alcoholism is a serious disease, which often leads to premature death, not to mention the social consequences, which are vast. Most of us know a person whose life has been touched by alcoholism. Therefore, alcohol is not a substance anyone can treat lightly.

Other Substance Abuse

Everybody has the potential to become addicted to a drug. Frankly, questions about the legal status of any drug matter less than the lethal potential of a drug or its ability to impair functioning. Ultimately, addictions of any kind are self-defeating and dangerous to well-being and happiness. Unfortunately, drug addiction is one of the biggest problems facing humankind.

In recent years, the term "addiction" has been superseded in many settings by the kinder term "dependence." However, addiction is actually a better word because it reinforces the reality that something nefarious has gained a strong, habitual, and enduring hold. These three words are important: the hold is *strong*, it is a *habit*, and it is *enduring*. Obviously, the words are applicable to nicotine and alcohol addiction, but also to other substances, too. The activity that *counters* the addiction must be as strong as the habit if the "cure" is to endure. If an individual has a strong commitment to stop the substance abuse, support groups, medical advice, and psychological support are generally needed.

In our highly "medicalized" society, the amount of abuse and misuse of prescription drugs is alarming. Both the person taking the medication and the prescribing physician may have difficulty identifying this problem. Both parties may be blind to the developing condition because the symptoms are not obvious. Too many people believe that a drug must be relatively safe if a physician prescribes it! Classifying certain drugs as controlled substances has helped, but the abuse continues. Remember, dietary supplements are not all innocent.

The prescription drugs that are most likely to be abused are those that have mind-altering effects (psychoactive properties) such as sleeping tablets (hypnotics) and tranquilizers. The so-called minor tranquilizers are among the most abused of all drugs. Such drugs include a group referred to as benzodiazepines, which include diazepam (Valium), chlordiazepoxide (Librium), and lorezepam (Ativan). Although these tranquilizers are safe and effective for short-term treatment, they have a propensity to be addicting.

Dependence—addiction—probably has at least two components. The first is the psychological component, in which the individual becomes addicted to the complex effect of the drug on the mind. The sensation experienced as a consequence of the active tranquilizing effect is obvious, but a more nebulous example includes the dependence that develops from the mere act of taking the drug! The second component of addiction is the physical (or pharmacological) component, which is a result of chemical changes that occur in body tissue, such that the body seems to *need* the drug to function (this is experienced by the person who has become addicted.) Scientists are only beginning to understand the complex components of addiction.

If you are taking prescribed mind-altering medications, please discuss the risk of dependency with your physician. It is never a good idea to stop taking these drugs abruptly, nor should you attempt to adjust your dosage without the supervision of a physician. That said, this is an issue that you ignore at your own peril. When you begin a self-watching program, do not overlook the possibility that you have become addicted to prescription or over-the-counter drugs.

Some readers may be puzzled by the way drug addiction crept into a book on heart disease. In my opinion, polysubstance abuse—abuse of many substances—is a major underestimated risk for heart disease. Over-the-counter quick fixes (such as antiacids) can facilitate an individual's continuing adverse lifestyle—popping an antiacid, H_2 receptor antagonist, before drinking excessively. It is difficult to understand how so many people have been duped into believing that marijuana is safe. These individuals need to learn more about its ability to affect cardiac function and even precipitate heart attack or angina. My colleagues and I described the possibility of these events in the 1970s. Finally, a common problem for intravenous drug users is cardiovascular disease from infection or embolism.

Exercise

Among the behaviors that can easily be self-monitored, exercise is at the top of the list. Either you engage in regular exercise activities, or you do not. Very few of us spend much time performing hard physical labor these days, and the person who walks to and from work or the supermarket is rare indeed. For most of us, exercise comes in the form of deliberate activity, from brisk walking or running to aerobic dancing to swimming or tennis. For some, exercise is a joy; for others, it falls into the category of a chore. Attitude aside, there is no doubt that exercise can make important contributions to your physical and mental well-being.

I hope you will become motivated to get off your couch and into the pool or on the treadmill, but if you have been living a sedentary lifestyle, it is critical that you check with your health-care givers before you begin. Professional trainers and physicians will be able to provide advice about the type and amount of exercise that is ideal for you, given your current age and health status. It is a sad reflection on the medical profession that health club staff often know more about exercise physiology than do average physicians. If you undertake a program that is too arduous, you could risk injury or even cause damage to your heart and/or to your bones and joints.

The effects of exercise are direct. Exercise has a very beneficial and direct effect on the heart, lungs, muscles, joints, and bones. Exercise is a critical ingredient in a weight-loss program because calories are burned, the tendency to accumulate body fat is reduced, and, over time, the percentage of fat in the body diminishes. (This will happen more efficiently when the diet is carefully planned to use more calories than ingested.) In addition, if vigorous exercise is sustained for at least fifteen minutes, it results in improvements in cardiovascular and respiratory function of the body. Exercise also helps stabilize blood sugar, making a regular exercise program a must for men and women with diabetes. Of course, exercise also helps prevent diabetes from developing in the first place.

Without doubt, engaging in routine daily exercise or workouts is one of the most important actions you can take to prevent respiratory and circulatory diseases. Exercise increases circulation and improves muscle tone and strength. It is possible to benefit from exercise in many different forms, including walking, dancing, jogging, biking, gardening, housework, swimming, weight training, and stretching.

Obviously, your physical condition and limitations define the kind of exercise program you can undertake. However, people with a variety of disabilities can usually find an appropriate exercise regimen. For example, "jarming" (rapid arm exercise) can be used by wheelchair-bound individuals or those who have other conditions that limit the use of their legs. Jarming involves jogging with the arms alone. The motions involved in jarming often resemble the actions of an orchestra conductor. Some have even speculated that the longevity prevalent among the famous conductors can be attributed to the regular cardiovascular workout they achieve every time they work!

No "weekend warriors," please! The most noteworthy fact to remember about exercise is that in order to reap the benefits, it must be done regularly. A Saturday tennis match and a thirty-minute walk in the park on Sunday do not combine to form an adequate exercise program. The sporadic exerciser is at higher risk for becoming injured—or worse. Each year we hear local news reports that someone has had a fatal heart attack while shoveling heavy snow or while mowing the lawn in oppressive heat. These individuals are generally not physically fit in the first place, and the exertion proves too vigorous.

Exercise is much more beneficial when it is undertaken several times a week rather than only now and then, when the mood strikes.

Exercise requires patience, because the benefits it affords are not necessarily immediate. Stamina and strength increase over time, and change is incremental. Make unreasonable demands on your body, and you will be rewarded with sore muscles, injuries, and, most often, a sense of discouragement. Above all, do not push yourself to perform an exercise you loath. Enduring a stint on a treadmill day after day makes no sense if you enjoy aerobic dance classes or swimming. Most people will eventually stop engaging in activities they do not like.

Exercise and your weight. Even when not strenuous, exercise will help burn calories; therefore, it plays an important role in dieting. Unfortunately, there is a common misconception that a workout has to be strenuous in order to burn calories. With the advice of a qualified health-care provider who can guide you to an appropriate and supervised exercise program, you can build fitness safely over time. Many dieters find it helpful to keep a daily log of exercise activities, which enables them to track their progress toward goals they set. A daily activity diary is most useful when it contains the date and time of the exercise session, description of the activity, a notation on the number of times the exercise is repeated (*i.e.*, laps in the pool or miles walked), and duration of the activity (*i.e.*, minutes walked or cycled). Comments about the degree of difficulty are helpful, if only to make sure you are not pushing too hard or, perhaps, not hard enough.

If weight loss or maintenance is your goal, calculate the number of calories burned during exercise sessions. The activity chart (Table 5.3) provides guidelines. The chart indicates how many calories are being burned, based on a person weighing 160 to 170 pounds.

Fitness is the real fountain of youth. If you need any more reason to consider physical fitness a priority, consider that exercise promotes a sharp mind *and* a healthy body. One study showed that individuals who participated in a walking program performed better on memory tests after only *twenty-six days* of exercise. At any age, the physically fit perform better on tests of intellectual functioning. Exercise promotes increased oxygenation of the brain, which has a direct effect on mental acuity.

Table 5.3: Exercise Table.

Select a specific exercise and calculate how long you need to do the activity in order to burn off certain food items.

Activity	Calories Burned/Hr.	Activity	Calories Burned/Hr.
LIGHT	**50–199**	**VIGOROUS**	**Over 350**
Lying down or sleeping	80	Table tennis	360
Sitting	100	Wood chopping	400
Driving an automobile	120	Ice skating	400
Standing	140	Tennis (singles)	420
		Calisthenics	440
MODERATE	**200–350**	Bicycling (10 mph)	440
Walking, (2 mph)	200	Waterskiing	480
Walking, (3 mph)	320	Rope skipping	540
Bicycling, (5½ mph)	256	Skiing (10 mph)	600
Gardening	220	Squash or handball	600
Raking leaves	236	Bicycling (13 mph)	660
Golfing	250	Running (7 mph)	740
Housework, heavy	280	Running (10 mph)	900
Lawn mowing (power)	284		
Swimming	300		
Fishing (wading)	316		
Tennis (doubles)	316		
Square dancing	350		
Volleyball	350		
Rollerskating	350		
Badminton	350		

Duration of exercise required to burn off each food item.

Exercise/Time	Food item
16 minutes of jogging (10 mph)	1 piece of chocolate cake
5 minutes of jogging (10 mph)	1 medium apple
3 hours of sitting	a 3-ounce hamburger on a bun
48 minutes of sitting	1 hard-boiled egg
1 hour, 11 minutes of walking (3¾ mph)	a chocolate milk shake
17 minutes of walking (3¾ mph)	8 ounces of skim milk
31 minutes of bicycling (5½ mph)	10 french fries
9 minutes of bicycling (5½ mph)	1 cup of green beans
90 minutes of housework	1 cup of ice cream
38 minutes of housework	1 ounce of cheddar cheese

The same diseases that cause physical decline as we age, including cardiovascular diseases, contribute to mental decline as well. According to the National Institute on Aging, middle-age men and women with high blood pressure are more likely to experience problems with their memory as they grow older. A study that tracked close to four thousand men over a thirty-year period revealed that men who developed hypertension were two and a half times more likely to have problems with intellectual functions, including memory, than men with normal blood pressure. A study performed in Finland showed that exercise lowered death rates, even after considering genetic profiles and other lifestyle issues.

A harsh word for "muscle heads." I am puzzled why people who want to sculpt or build muscles do not want to build bones and concentrate on cardiovascular health. Exercise nuts should be more interested in becoming balanced, healthy nuts. If ever there was misinformation and witchcraft, it is to be found in the domain of sports nutrition fads. The use of dangerous dietary supplements and the propagation of fads and fallacies are rampant among self-declared sports nutrition experts. I know I sound negative here, but I believe that bad advice to bodybuilders is placing many people at risk, especially a cardiovascular risk. This is now a major public health concern.

For example, some athletes are advised to consume excessive amounts of animal protein, but this advice does not take into account the accompanying excess saturated fat and cholesterol load. Despite warnings from elite athletes such as Arnold Schwarzenegger on the dangers and inadvisability of excessive protein intake, many bodybuilders are preoccupied with "protein loading."

The use of hormone precursors such as DHEA and androstenedione, which are little more than the indirect use of anabolic steroids, is also a great concern. These steroids have been banned in some sports because of their potential danger. The unsupervised use of growth hormone is also a popular and dangerous tactic, reinforced by claims about its antiaging benefits. Excess growth hormone causes acromegaly (gigantism), and these unfortunate individuals die prematurely with agonizing arthritis and degenerative heart disease. In addition, certain hormones are potent carcinogens (cancer-causing agents). Hormonal agents have great advantages when used appropriately, especially in hormone-deficiency states, but playing with hormone balance is a form of Russian roulette.

Can you think of any more excuses? Given the variety of activities available to virtually everyone in our society, there are truly no excuses left not to exercise. Every public health agency and private health organization recognizes and promotes the value of exercise. This has resulted in a steady increase in accessibility of various activities. For example, shopping malls across the U.S. often open their doors early in the morning to accommodate mall walkers. Most communities have several private health clubs that offer a wide variety of exercise classes and equipment. Some offer yoga and t'ai chi classes which, beyond the well-known physical benefits, are also excellent stress management tools. An investment in a health club membership will pay rich dividends—provided it is used, of course!

Facilities such as a YMCA or a YWCA are valuable for adults as well as for children, and public swimming pools and exercise classes held in community centers are also accessible to many people. Even if you do not want to leave your home to exercise, there are exercycles, treadmills, and a vast array of exercise videos. Videos for men and women at every fitness level are plentiful, and specialized programs exist for pregnant women, the elderly, people with arthritis, and those with other disabilities. One need not leave home to buy them. The Internet offers numerous sites that discuss—in great detail—the content of a huge selection of exercise videos.

The value of walking endures. Author Andrew Weil, M.D., advocates regular walking, even if you engage in other exercise activities. He believes that the coordinated motions of your arms and legs provide beneficial conditioning in the brain. The rhythmic swing of your arms in opposition with your legs and feet are among the most natural motions the body uses—walking is one exercise we learn in infancy and do not forget how to do. In addition, it is entirely possible to build and maintain adequate fitness using nothing other than regular sustained walking. Dr. Weil also points out that walking can be done alone, with a partner, in groups, in silence, while carrying on a conversation, or while listening to music (or books or even foreign language programs) on tape. Barring physical disability, walking will be available to you for the rest of your life, and it is possible, but sometimes difficult, to do in the most urbanized centers or in the most remote rural town.

In the United States, where the "cult of the car" has all but taken over, making walking a part of your daily routine probably sounds impossible. However, I have read numerous suggestions from various health and fitness professionals about ways to increase walking, and I pass them on to you. For example, park a few blocks from your office and walk the rest of way to work; get off the bus or train a stop or two before the one that is closest to your office and walk the rest of the way; or park at the far end of the shopping center or mall. Walk to your neighborhood bank or library, or just take a walk around the block. Some communities are pressing for more sidewalks and bike paths in an effort to curb automobile traffic, but an additional benefit is that walking may make a comeback. It is ironic that several states in the U.S. that are recreational centers or holiday locations have few sidewalks. Try walking in Florida and Southern California without dodging automobiles! Even access to restaurants can involve a perilous negotiation past the drive-through lanes.

Before I close this section on exercise, let me remind you that far too many children are developing childhood obesity. Lack of exercise is one reason why so many children gain unwanted weight. For many children, physical activity—if any—is limited to an organized sport. Sure, playing soccer or basketball is terrific, but there is something odd about driving our kids to all these activities. Walking to school when possible or riding a bike around the neighborhood should be encouraged. Charles Attwood, M.D., author of *Dr. Attwood's Low-Fat Prescription For Kids,* recommends that children who are overweight should be well-established in an exercise program before parents try to reduce the amount of fat in their diets. Dr. Attwood is also one of the leading voices warning parents about the dangers of high cholesterol levels in children.

Let your children complain and carry on, but do them the favor of pushing them into physical activity. Show them by example that exercise is a regular—and normal—part of life. Years from now, their healthy hearts will thank you.

THE TEN LIFESTYLE COMMANDMENTS

As you can see, a wide variety of behaviors and addictions—or, in the case of exercise, a lack of activity—are involved in causing chronic degenerative diseases including, of course, heart disease. An enormous amount of epidemiological research (research that studies illness—and wellness—in population groups) confirms this crucial link. This underscores the importance of work in experimental and clinical psychology that promotes changes in lifestyle behavior by providing practical help. Attempts to change ingrained destructive habits require great motivation, commitment, and a clear plan of action.

I have prepared a list of lifestyle guidelines—I call them commandments—based on lifestyle issues. (See Table 5.4) They are meant to be reminders of adverse behaviors that you may need to work on to achieve optimal health. These commandments have no religious connotation, but you may notice that these lifestyle commandments look like general recommendations for health. The well-kept secret is that general health recommendations crossover completely to cardiovascular wellness.

Table 5.4: The Ten Lifestyle Commandments.

1. Control your intake of alcohol, or completely abstain if you have recognized a problem.
2. Avoid substance abuse; *e.g.*, excesses of caffeine-containing beverages, unnecessary use of over-the-counter or prescription medications, etc.
3. Stop smoking.
4. Exercise regularly and consistently.
5. Be in touch with your moods and stress levels. Simplify your life if you can.
6. Eat because you are hungry, and eat only to satisfy your appetite.
7. Eat a healthy balanced diet; *e.g.*, high fiber, low sodium, and low cholesterol.
8. Have periodic health examinations, such as an annual physical.
9. Practice monogamy or safe sex.
10. Never use illegal or recreational drugs.

SUMMARY

Remember that cardiovascular wellness does not happen by accident; it results from the choices you make day after day. The best way to handle lifestyle issues is to assess them yourself and, if necessary, seek help to correct them. Do not wait until you have a medical emergency to "wake up."

Adopting a heart-healthy lifestyle should be a positive addition to your life, and it is also an intensely personal process. You must ask yourself what habits and behaviors continue to hurt your chances for a long and vital life.

What You Can Do

- Use the "Ten Lifestyle Commandments" to guide positive change.
- Excessive drinking and illegal drug use cause untold harm to individuals and families—and society as a whole. I urge you to seek professional help and perhaps support groups, too, if your life is out of control because of substance abuse.
- Smoking is not illegal, but it is a primary risk factor for cardiovascular and pulmonary diseases. True enough, this is "old news," but the good news is the fact that there are numerous methods to help you leave the smoking habit behind. Review the methods listed in this chapter and take steps to quit smoking today. It is one of the most important things you can do to improve your health.
- Exercise is an essential element of a "heart-smart" lifestyle. In addition, there is evidence that exercise increases psychological well-being and may even help keep the mind sharp as we age. Join a health club or your local YMCA or YWCA, walk in your neighborhood or on a treadmill, slip an aerobics tape in the VCR. Dance, ride a bike, swim, or take up tennis—just start moving.
- If you have not been physically active for a long time,

check with your health-care provider before you begin a vigorous exercise program.

• Keep a journal detailing your efforts to improve your lifestyle and track your progress as you enhance your well-being.

CHAPTER SIX

YOUR EMOTIONAL AND SPIRITUAL HEALTH

In Chapter 5, we examined some key lifestyle issues that are largely under your control. They are tangible areas, in that you can measure how much you drink or smoke or exercise. Other lifestyle issues—ones that have a direct effect on your heart—are less easily measured. Over the last few decades personality types, emotional well-being, and stress have received increasing attention. No thorough discussion of heart disease would be complete without addressing them, which is why I decided that they deserved a chapter of their own.

You have probably read that stress can make you ill—and perhaps even lead to premature death. Yet, if I asked you to define stress, you might have some difficulty being specific. Most likely, you would answer the question by talking about everyday events that you label as stressful: preparing for a job interview, juggling your children's daily schedules, fretting about delays in traffic, arguing with your spouse over money, and so forth. In fact, you might tell me that stress is a daily experience, and that just about any of the important circumstances in your life are potentially stressful. You are correct, and because of what you have heard about stress, you may be worried—and worry is stressful!

In actuality, stress is a serious issue and you are right to think about what you can do to reduce the stress in your life—or, at the very least, to lessen its effects. Along with lack of exercise, stress is frequently underestimated as a cardiovascular risk factor. One of the most interesting—and important—effects of stress is its negative consequence for blood cholesterol levels. For example, studies of students undergoing prolonged periods of stress during examinations showed elevated blood lipids, and research in groups of accountants revealed elevated cholesterol levels with a rise in blood pressure during their busy tax season. The proof of the stress-related rise in cholesterol levels is the tendency of the blood lipids to return to normal after the periods of stress are over. This information should lead everyone to consider stress as more than just a vague concept, but one with serious physical repercussions. No one can afford to ignore stress as a health issue.

Most people are aware that stress encompasses unpleasant or painful emotions such as anxiety, worry, frustration, hostility, anger, and the like. In addition, it is associated with the exhaustion of overwork or unrelenting pressure. Day-to-day life is filled with stressful situations. To one degree or another, this is inevitable and even necessary. The person who is *completely* free from anxiety, worry, and periodic blues is not a model for perfect health—that person would be dead!

To be truly alive, we must experience the full range of our emotions and be mentally available to handle events as they arise. As much as we would like to rid ourselves of unnecessary stress, our real challenge is to learn to manage ourselves, our emotions, and the choices we make. Perhaps most importantly, we also must recognize that stress does not descend upon us from "out there," but rather is a self-generated, internal response. In other words, it is not the size of the traffic jam that causes our frustration, and in some cases, even rage. Our response to the traffic jam is the issue. In simple terms, stress is produced by the person who experiences it.

One of the central questions of modern life is: How do we manage ourselves and our lives? Will we cope better with traffic or our teenagers by relaxing more, thinking positive thoughts, and by exercising every day? This is good advice as far as it goes, and as you have seen, starting or continuing an exercise program is a concrete action you can take without delay. The other two pieces of advice are a bit more complex, however, and require in-depth examination.

TYPE A BEHAVIOR

In the 1970s, two cardiologists and researchers, Meyer Friedman, M.D., and Ray Rosenman, M.D., described the negative effects of an assertive, time-dependent personality, to which they assigned the label Type A personality. These physicians asserted that the Type A individual is prone to coronary artery disease, hypertension, heart attacks, and even strokes. The description put forth by Dr. Friedman and Dr. Rosenman fits the image of a high-powered, aggressive executive or a harried air traffic controller or a career-driven salesman. Usually fiery fast-talkers, these individuals were also described as quick to anger and perhaps even to become hostile. For the most part, Type A personalities were linked with men rather than women.

In contrast, these doctors also identified a Type B personality. These individuals are "laid back" and more in control of their emotions. The doctors hypothesized that the Type B individuals have less tendency to develop cardiovascular disease than their Type A brothers—and a few sisters.

Dr. Friedman and Dr. Rosenman were convinced that cardiovascular disease had its roots in aggressive, impatient temperaments. In their book, *Type A Behavior and Your Heart*, they write: "In the absence of Type A Behavior Pattern, coronary heart disease almost never occurs before seventy years of age, regardless of the fatty foods eaten, the cigarettes smoked, or the lack of exercise. But when this behavior pattern is present, coronary heart disease can easily erupt in one's thirties or forties." Perhaps these physicians did not take enough account of the fact that "balanced people" also may tend to smoke or gorge themselves with junk food. The statements of Dr. Friedman and his colleagues are not completely accurate, of course, but undeniably, the incidence of cardiovascular disease is higher among older individuals of all descriptions.

The main features of Type A behavior are summarized in Table 6.1. As you can see from this table, Type A behavior is very complex, and Dr. Friedman and Dr. Rosenman describe the Type A pattern as an action-emotion complex. In simple terms, this means that a minor event or challenge may provoke an explosive reaction. Therefore,

Table 6.1: Main Features of Type A Behavior.

Modified from Friedman and Rosenman (1974). The comments provide examples of the behavior.

FEATURE	COMMENT
Time urgency	This is regarded as the key aspect of Type A behavior—not enough seconds in a minute!
Accentuation of words in speaking	Type As typically hurry to finish a sentence.
Rapid eating, walking, and movement	Easy to spot in the Type A.
Overt impatience	Type As want people to get on with what they are saying or doing.
Doing or thinking more than one thing at once	The Type A individual contaminates leisure time with thoughts of work or problems.
Conversation focusing	The Type A individual steers the theme of a conversation to egocentric topics.
Inappropriate guilt	Type As cannot rest without discomfort.
Can't stop and smell the roses	The Type A individual must have things here and now.
Creates tight schedules	Type As fit more appointments in less time.
Has a face that makes people feel like punching it!	The Type A person is confrontational and does not engender sympathy for his or her own affliction.
Numerous tics and gestures	Finger pointing, table thumping, and jaw protrusion are examples of Type A aggression.
Belief that speed gives an edge	The Type A person has to move quicker than everyone else.
Measuring others' deeds or actions	The Type A person may apply numbers to activities, thoughts, or deeds.
Type A plus Type A makes sparks	The Type A is rapidly engaged by a fellow Type A.

attempts to change the Type A pattern must focus on increasing self-awareness in order to change the internal responses to outside events.

Studying Type B behavior may be a good way of identifying and correcting potentially adverse traits (see Table 6.2). It has been recognized that a Type B personality is much less likely to get coronary heart disease than the Type A individual even in the face of similar risk factors.

Type B individuals are not necessarily outwardly docile; indeed, they can have greater ambition than their Type A counterparts. However, they are not so obsessed with doing ever-increasing numbers of things in ever-decreasing amounts of time.

Switching from Type A to Type B behavior may be ideal, but it can be extremely stressful to attempt to change one's basic personality type. After all, some people thrive on the pressure of "taking the last shot," for example, and their competitive personality type helps them excel in their professions. That said, it is probably wise to take the edge off the Type A tendencies, just as it is equally important for the extremely passive person to become more assertive. Balance is probably all that is required. The concept of "balance" is at the root of religious philosophy, ancient medical disciplines, and a happy life—ask any Buddhist monk how he's lived so long.

Dr. Friedman and Dr. Rosenman have provided help in understanding personality types, and it is a useful exercise to identify which description more closely resembles you. Bear in mind, however, that 10 to 20 percent of the population are a complex mixture of Type A and Type B tendencies, and neither pattern may entirely and accurately describe any individual.

Table 6.2: The Type B Behavior Pattern as Modified from Friedman and Rosenman (1974).

The Type B trait is free of Type A habits and activities:
• No sense of time urgency
• No experience of free-floating hostility
• No need to keep discussing victories or topics of self-interest
• No need to portray self as superior
• Relaxes without guilt
• Works efficiently but steadily
• Not necessarily docile or "brain dead"

The link between personality traits and heart disease cannot be viewed as absolute. For example, it has been shown that the Type A person may recover *better* from a heart attack. Other studies suggest that the Type A personality is a risk factor in younger men, but does not operate to the same degree in the older male.

Too much emphasis on personality typing could lead to a false sense of complacency among those who view themselves as resembling Type B. For example, until recently, Type A traits were generally associated with males, but heart disease among mature women has been substantially underestimated. Furthermore, the importance placed on prevention programs for males and females of all ages and personality description diminishes if a general belief exists that heart disease primarily affects the powerful, aggressive males who fill our executive suites. This is obviously a mistake.

Most people who fit the Type A personality can identify themselves, and they probably are well aware that their behavior leaves them tense and stressed. Depending on other risk factors, the increased cardiovascular risk among these individuals may probably be related more to cigarette smoking, uncontrolled hypertension, and high blood cholesterol rather than to their behavioral traits. I realize, of course, that some behavioral scientists may not agree with me, but I feel that the mind and the body function together, and are heavily influenced by each other.

MIND AND BODY

When Dr. Friedman and Dr. Rosenman discussed personality type and heart disease, they opened the way to a wider examination of the mind-body connection in relation to heart disease. Not so long ago, many physicians looked at the proposed mind-body connection with a degree of scorn. However, the mind can make the body do almost anything! Now that this notion is widely recognized, your health-care givers are more likely than ever before to assess your psychological well-being. So close is the link that scientists now talk about the "mind-body" and present evidence that there are complex interactions involving "molecules of emotion," which happens to be the title of a new book by Dr. Candace Pert.

The Heart as Our Emotional Center

The negative effects of anxiety, stress, and even depression may be more deeply understood by using the metaphor of the "broken heart." Our language is filled with descriptive expressions that link the heart with emotional life. We may say that our heart "aches" over a sad event. A love affair gone wrong may be "heartbreaking" to those involved. On the other hand, we may say we have a "glad" heart when we are content. We may describe a person we love as having a "generous" heart or as being "goodhearted." And romantic love is considered an "affair of the heart."

In his book *Heartbreak and Heart Disease*, cardiologist Stephen Sinatra, M.D., has examined the metaphor of heartbreak as a risk factor for heart disease. It is not possible for me to do justice to Dr. Sinatra's book or his concepts here, but I recommend the book to those interested in deepening their understanding of the mind-body connection and holistic health philosophies. Dr. Sinatra has asked and addressed the following questions:

- To what extent do emotional factors and one's own intrinsic personality play a part in heart disease?
- Are suppressed feelings and emotions significant?
- Do negative feelings such as abandonment, heartbreak, betrayal, or humiliation create conditions that invite death?
- What part do positive emotions such as love, faith, and good humor play in the process of healing and staying well?
- What is the significance of the way we breathe?

In a sense, Dr. Sinatra has taken the personality type information provided by Dr. Friedman and Dr. Rosenman and expanded it to include a wider discussion of emotional health. As a young cardiologist, Dr. Sinatra was trained in the "nuts and bolts" of medicine. He notes that heart disease was viewed and treated as a biological disease process. However, experiences with his patients led him to examine his own emotional wounds. His journey has led him to explore the bridge between emotions and health. For example, Dr. Sinatra speculates that the person labeled Type A may be compensating for a sense of feeling unloved as a child. The need to control and the aggressive behavior may be the way in which such a person defends the wounded heart. The conscious mind may forget hurtful incidents, bereavements, and other emotional wounds, but *the heart remembers*.

To be certain that you understand the comprehensive nature of his work, I stress that Dr. Sinatra does not reject traditional cardiac care, including surgery when required, nor does he discount in any way the preventive benefits of nutrition and exercise. As a matter of fact, he is the author of a book on coenzyme Q10, which is discussed later on in this book. However, as valuable as these therapies may be, he believes that medical and lifestyle interventions alone may not be enough to achieve true healing. Therefore, Dr. Sinatra recommends examining the underlying emotional issues that may be involved in heart disease. The heartbreak about which Dr. Sinatra speaks may include loneliness, which is, quite frankly, rampant in our individualistic, impersonal, and "rushed" culture. Dr. Sinatra's work is important in our attempts to understand the many ways in which mind, body, and spirit work together to prevent or promote coronary heart disease.

Dr. Sinatra's approach is truly holistic. It does not deny the role of organic factors in promoting heart disease, and equally important, it takes account of the need to place mind, body, and spirit in harmony. In the most practical terms, Dr. Sinatra's work is another contribution to the efficacy of the expanding field of mind-body medicine. On a personal level, his work may provide an additional reason to examine your life and remove the psychological barriers to achieving optimal health. In some situations, medical intervention is required to treat psychological problems. Clinical depression is an example of such a situation, and depression has reached epidemic proportions in modern society.

Taking Depression Seriously

Although depression has been regarded as the "common cold" of psychiatry, it can never be taken as a casual event simply because it is seen so frequently. Depression is often vicious in its effects and can cause untold human suffering. Because depression manifests in various ways, some of them quite subtle, many people may not realize that they are afflicted. Depression does not have one easily identifiable set of symptoms, but instead may cause a spectrum of problems from mild unhappiness to complete immobilization associated with an overwhelming sense of despair. I have been there!

Understanding depression is the first step in fighting it. Likewise, understanding what depression *is not* is important, too. Depression is not the same as experiencing stress or feeling sad, even over a serious loss. For example, grieving the death of a loved one is not synonymous with depression. Although the metaphoric "broken heart" Dr. Sinatra describes may be present with depression, the heart that is wounded by a tragic event does not present the same condition as clinical depression. Unfortunately, the word depression is used rather loosely, and people might say they are depressed when they feel out of sorts for a day or two or are sad because they did not receive a promotion! Unlike the reaction to stressful and upsetting life experiences such as the loss of a relationship or a job opportunity, depression is always miserable, persistent, and frequently incapacitating. True depression may involve sleep disturbances, erratic eating patterns, and an inability to concentrate that is severe enough to interfere with job performance.

I believe that depression is a clear risk factor in cardiovascular disease and must be addressed by a health-care professional. Depression is a common event in people who have sustained a heart attack, and I believe that it compounds their risk for further cardiac events. Psychotherapy is often recommended, but depression sometimes requires medical intervention as well, either with antidepressant medications or, if less severe, the skilled use of herbal remedies such as St. John's wort. However, I do not believe anyone should self-medicate with herbal remedies for significant depression. To be fully effective, medications or herbal treatments must be accompanied by self-help efforts with skilled medical care.

In order to change their thoughts and, therefore, their feelings, some individuals may have to change their environment in a radical manner, which may not be easy to do. Along with medical treatment, self-discipline is needed and positive action is a must. *Taking action always elevates mood.* You can test this for yourself with a relatively trivial matter. Think of a recent time when you had a mild case of the blues. If you had continued to sit around feeling sorry for yourself, your mood would have deteriorated even more. But because you got up and took a walk or talked with a friend, you began to feel better. You may not improve 100 percent, but taking action on your own behalf is essential for a person suffering from depression. Indeed, it is part of a treatment plan.

Concern over having "enough time" is a modern phenomenon and is a cause of great stress. At times it seems that the world can be divided into two groups. The first expresses time by statements such as, "It's almost noon," or "It's around six o'clock." The second group anxiously peers at their watches and thinks—or says, "It's 11:51," or "It's two minutes after six." The advent of digital watches has made it easy for the time-obsessed to feel very normal! But a preoccupation with time can exacerbate conditions such as depression. Individuals who "live" by the clock should try leaving their wristwatch at home once in a while.

The Mind Tends the Heart

Conventional medicine has largely failed to acknowledge the role of the mind in cardiovascular wellness, yet it clearly recognizes the phenomenon of psychosomatic illness. For example, as many as twenty million Americans are troubled by irritable bowel syndrome (IBS). This is a common gastrointestinal disorder that is amenable to lifestyle change and behavioral interventions. This disorder is difficult to manage with synthetic pharmaceuticals, and conventional therapy frequently fails. It is well-recognized that there is a psychological component to this condition, and few would deny the mind-body connection in relation to IBS. I propose that we look at cardiovascular disease in a similar manner.

Does an entity we can call "irritable heart syndrome" exist? We can say with authority that the heart has an autonomic nervous system that is at least as intricate as that supplying the digestive system. In other words, the biological mechanisms for the physical response to stress—and other psychological conflicts—are capable of producing cardiac symptoms. These cardiac symptoms can occur in the absence of diagnosed organic heart disease. I propose that we recognize psychosomatic illness as a way to highlight the importance of the mind-body connection and behavioral interventions in promoting cardiovascular wellness. I believe in the concept of the "iritable heart syndrome" (IHS).

Several individuals have made significant contributions to changing the narrow perceptions of heart disease as just a matter of plaque in the arteries or as a list of risk factors, as important as these issues are. With their different yet compatible approaches, they offer mind-body concepts that you can use to improve your health.

Deepak Chopra, M.D., has popularized Ayurvedic medicine, a healing philosophy and system that developed in India over many centuries. Ayurvedic philosophy stresses the importance of emotional factors, thoughts, and awareness in promoting overall health. Dr. Chopra's book, *Ageless Body, Timeless Mind*, has become a classic in the field of longevity and in mind-body medicine. Perhaps more than any other modern physician, Dr. Chopra has been able to explain the way in which a thought influences the biochemical environment of every cell in the body. If you have ever heard Dr. Chopra speak on television or on audiotape, you know that he is passionate in his attempts to help you appreciate that talking about the "mind-body connection" is only a semantic necessity. In reality, the mind and the body cannot be separated, nor can the body be easily compartmentalized, with each organ or system viewed as separate from all others.

As a way of gaining a mental picture of this unity, Dr. Chopra emphasizes that every cell in the body knows if you are happy, sad, angry, or pleasantly excited. Our language limits us in that we say that thoughts originating in the brain ultimately affect the body, but while it is difficult to grasp, all our cells "think." Expanding our awareness of the "thinking body" (as well as the larger concept of the "thinking universe") is one of Dr. Chopra's important contributions to bridging the mind-body dichotomy. It should be recognized that these concepts are neither novel nor new. They form the basis of several ancient medical systems, including Ayurvedic medicine and North American Indian medicine.

We use the hyphenated "mind-body" term to express the notion that our systems have a generalized reaction to even simple stimuli, such as exercising. Whereas exercising creates both mentally and physically beneficial results, lack of exercise or even simple and minimal mobility can have a devastating effect on the body. If an individual sits in a chair with no stimuli, he or she will gradually experience decreasing mental awareness and a deterioration of physical health. This is a clear example of "disuse syndrome," a term coined by several leading gerontologists. (Dr. Chopra credits Dr. Walter Boritz with creating the concept.) In this context, "disuse" means that the physical needs of the body are given inadequate attention, which in turn leads to poor health and premature death. Men and women of any age with cardiovascular disease and the older person who is at risk of heart disease may rapidly go downhill if they stop engaging in physical activity. A sedentary lifestyle produces several predictable consequences, including obesity, a decrease in psychological well-being, musculoskeletal disorders, and premature aging.

Social contact among the elderly is at least as important an issue as physical activity to overall well-being. The elderly, as much as everyone else, require mental stimulation to maintain a sharp mind, just as they require social contacts to nourish their emotional health. Without physical and mental stimulation, depression and a decline in cognitive functioning may result. In the face of this knowledge, the modern family seems willing to abandon grandma or grandpa in the emergency rooms of our hospitals.

Ultimately, this information is elegantly circular—as you recall, the principal antidote to depression is activity. Perhaps the most important concept you can take away from this chapter is this: above all, the mind minds the body and the body can mind the mind.

The Body's Innate Ability to Heal

For more than two decades, Andrew Weil, M.D., and others have guided contemporary thought on holistic methods to enhance the body's intrinsic ability to maintain health and heal disease. This concept occurred to Hippocrates but has been lost in modern medicine, which concentrates on fighting disease rather than healing the whole being and promoting health. In his book *Spontaneous Healing*, Dr. Weil draws from several ancient health philosophies to define healing as restoring integrity or balance, and he points out that the word healing means "making whole." Ultimately, the goal of any remedy or treatment is to foster the body's innate powers of self-correction or regeneration.

Dr. Weil does not reject the value of conventional medical intervention, and he highlights the importance of pluralistic medical approaches in preventing and treating disease. He talks about "integrated" medicine, but I believe that this term exaggerates the already damaging dichotomy that exists between conventional and "alternative" medicine. As I have said, I prefer the term "pluralistic medicine," and since that term has not yet come into wide use, I tolerate the term complementary medicine (popularized by Robert C. Atkins, M.D.).

Like most of his contemporaries, Dr. Weil believes that individuals must take responsibility for seeking and evaluating treatments that will promote self-healing. He offers the following seven suggestions—he calls them strategies—that successful patients work with in their quest for healing. He believes that incidents of "spontaneous healing" would increase if these strategies were more widely employed. (The strategies themselves are stated in Dr. Weil's actual words as they appear in *Spontaneous Healing*. I have paraphrased and interpreted Dr. Weil in the following descriptive information.)

1. "Do not take no for an answer." In essence, this strategy means that we must reject a statement that our condition is "hopeless" and that "nothing can be done." These statements discourage individuals from taking actions on their own behalf. The words of physicians are powerful, but they must never be more powerful than your belief in your ability to improve your condition.

2. "Actively search for help." Successful patients take diagnostic and treatment information they receive from their health-care givers as a starting place. These men and women look for additional information and answers to their problem from a variety of sources. If you are reading this book and choose additional material from books I cite, you are promoting self-healing by increasing your own personal database. (Remember, too, that actively seeking information promotes your emotional health as well as your physical well-being.)

3. "Seek out others who have been healed." Without doubt, success is motivating. Do you know someone who appears robust and full of vitality, but has been diagnosed with heart disease? What has this person done to bring about the improvement? Role models for healing exist everywhere—find them, and use what they offer. It is no accident that we enjoy being with others in exercise classes, on walking trails, or in meditation groups. A self-care attitude can be contagious!

4. "Form constructive partnerships with health professionals." Your greatest allies are health-care providers who believe in your efforts to heal. These individuals are knowledgeable and competent, but they also recognize that their role is to support your healing process. These professionals know their limitations and encourage you to seek others who can help you heal yourself.

5. "Do not hesitate to make radical life changes." Illness can be a great catalyst for change. You probably know men and women who were diagnosed with serious diseases and, as a result, quit their jobs, changed careers, enriched their family relationships, or conversely, left bad relationships and dead-end careers behind. Sometimes patients view a diagnosis as a "wake-up" call, a call to change risky lifestyle habits and a push to do the things they have been putting off for too long.

6. "Regard illness as a gift." This is a hard recommendation for me to accept because it involves "turning the other cheek" to disease. Everyone knows that it is not easy to imagine illness as a gift. However, because illness often stimulates positive life change, individuals later say that the personal growth they achieved made the dark days worth it. While it may be tempting to feel "picked on" by the fates, constructively using illness is the healthier path.

7. "Cultivate self-acceptance." This is a corollary of the previous strategy. Accepting the reality of the circumstances we find ourselves in is a first step to change. Too often, we may struggle against our circumstances, but once we surrender to the reality of the illness our true healing work can begin.

MIND-BODY PRESCRIPTIONS FOR THE HEART

Although the recognition of the mind-body connection is centuries old, systematic approaches to healing that involve bioenergetic techniques have gained increasing popularity in recent times. Supported by scientific studies, psychotherapy, meditation, prayer, and spirituality have a role in promoting healing of the body and the mind.

In the final analysis, the overall goal is to use psychotherapy, relaxation, breathing exercises, lifestyle counseling, intimacy and sharing, visualization, meditation, prayer, and other spiritually oriented methods to protect and "mind" the heart by releasing repressed emotions and resolving conflict. These techniques vary in sophistication, but in essence they are extensions of stress-reduction training and behavioral therapy.

One of the perceived revolutionary aspects of the Dean Ornish program is its use of meditation, a support group, and yoga as integral to the therapy. It is interesting to note that Dr. Ornish anticipated the benefits of the yoga and meditation he included in his program. However, group meetings were initially considered necessary to convey information about the program, scheduling, and so forth. Within a short time, Dr. Ornish realized that the time participants were together in the group became part of the healing. For example, in his book, *Dr. Dean Ornish's Program for Reversing Heart Disease*, he explains that many of the men who entered his program had quite literally never opened up emotionally to others, particularly to other men. The group became a supportive setting for emotional issues to emerge. The so-called "broken heart" had a safe place to heal. The lesson here is clear. Emotional isolation can be as destructive to our health as too much "busyness" and a hectic lifestyle.

One of the most complete discussions of meditation as a therapeutic tool is found in *Full Catastrophe Living: Using the Wisdom of Your Body and Mind to Face Stress, Pain, and Illness,* by Jon Kabat-Zinn, Ph.D. First published in 1990, this book initially received attention from the public because of the provocative title. The phrase "full catastrophe" is taken from the play *Zorba the Greek,* and refers to a scene in which Zorba describes his life as a man, with all its richness, as the "full catastrophe." He means that his life runs the gamut from joy to sorrow; failure to success.

Perhaps the most important contribution Kabat-Zinn has made to mind-body medicine is that he has brought mindfulness meditation into the mainstream. An awareness of this type of meditation brings about the realization that most of us engage in a nearly constant inner dialogue that involves a kind of "judging": "This is good, that is better, this is uncomfortable, that is maddening, this is stupid, that is stimulating . . ." and so it goes. This inner prattle is actually the source of our stress.

Full Catastrophe Living explains the program offered by the Stress Reduction Clinic at the University of Massachusetts Medical Center, in which participants are trained in mindful meditation. Put in its most simple terms, mindfulness simply means "paying attention." We could look at it as "self-watching" at its most sophisticated and focused level. Mindfulness is a component—or practice—of many ancient healing philosophies and arts. It is at the root of Buddhism, and now it is practiced among individuals in many religious sects; thanks to people like Kabat-Zinn, its acceptance as a tool to deepen self-understanding and manage stress is making its way into health-care settings, against some stalwart resistance.

Mindfulness involves a specific way of paying attention to one's thoughts and thought processes. Few people doubt the power of this approach to healing. More than anything else, this program helps participants understand that mindfulness meditation involves learning what Kabat-Zinn calls "artful" ways to cope with life's problems. Rather than fighting our stress and the difficulties that come as part of living, we can use the difficulties, much the way sailors use the wind to move through the water. Our challenge is to learn new ways to live with the realities of life, and mindfulness meditation is a path to greater peace.

Kabat-Zinn's work is compatible with the programs set forth by Dr. Ornish, Dr. Sinatra, Dr. Weil, and Dr. Chopra, and also the work of Dr. Larry Dossey (see "Spiritual Connections," page 128). Although *Full Catastrophe Living* offers so much information that it is difficult to do it justice here, Kabat-Zinn describes the attitudes that are advantageous when approaching meditation and embracing the "full catastrophe":

1. "Non-judging." In brief, this is the process of "self-watching" that helps us identify the stream of judgments we make every day. Awareness of the thought patterns must precede attempts to change.

2. "Patience." Kabat-Zinn tells us that cultivating patience is a form of wisdom, and it results in an acceptance in the truth that many things unfold in their own time and cannot be hurried along. Furthermore, avoid rushing through some increments of time so that we can get to others means missing what each moment can teach us.

3. "Beginner's mind." This is simply the ability to put aside all that we think we know and open up to what actually is, or to the possibilities we cannot even conceive of. As experienced meditators will tell you, they try never to lose their beginner's mind. Medicine these days would benefit from the beginner's mind.

4. "Trust." When we develop trust in ourselves and our own intuition, we experience less distress, even if we make "mistakes." Trusting ourselves also means that we are less likely to put misplaced trust in others, including spiritual teachers. Consumers may have misplaced trust in both conventional and alternative medicine.

5. "Non-striving." Many people begin any kind of program by setting a goal. In many situations this is admirable and even necessary. However, in mindfulness meditation, goals and a focus on achievement interfere with the state of "non-doing." Paradoxically, if you enter a meditation practice with the goal of improving health, the best way to achieve that is to put the goal aside, rather than strive to reach it.

6. "Acceptance." This simply means focusing on "what is" at the present time. If you have diagnosed heart disease or have been told that you must improve your blood lipid profile, these are "what is." Kabat-Zinn uses being overweight as an example where acceptance is needed. The point is to accept the weight as it is now and love yourself the way you are in this moment. Typically, an overweight person will defer many things in life, including self-love, "until I lose weight." Adopting acceptance can alter this self-defeating attitude.

7. "Letting go." This is a form of nonattachment. A meditator will notice that we want to hang on to certain thoughts, but when we are able to suspend judgment, we can detach from the thinking patterns which, in some sense, keep us in our own form of bondage.

There are numerous ways to learn meditation. Taking classes, reading books, listening to tapes, or just sitting quietly and following your own breath will offer benefits. Meditation requires practice and discipline, although the rewards are great.

SPIRITUAL CONNECTIONS

Some decades ago, if I had inserted a section about spirituality or prayer into a book about improving health, the book would have been considered religiously motivated. Times have changed, however. Spirituality—as distinct from religious beliefs—has gone mainstream. Currently, the role of love and prayer in healing and wellness is a developing science. According to Larry Dossey, M.D., "Love makes it possible for the mind to transcend the limitations of the body." Dr. Dossey is the author of *Healing Words: The Power of Prayer and the Practice of Medicine* and many other books, some of which also discuss prayer. He has also served as the chairman of the National Institutes of Health Panel on Mind-Body Interventions. He is probably best known for bringing research information about the power of prayer and love to the general public through his books and lectures. For example, he drew attention to the finding that in a study of ten thousand males with cardiac disease, there was a 50-percent observed reduction in the frequency of anginal chest pain in men who recognized their spouses as loving and supportive. (The importance of this observation is well-illustrated in Levin's book *Heartmates*, discussed in Chapter 1.)

Several contemporary studies have drawn attention to the ability of prayer to influence health and healing. It is interesting to note that in some of these studies, patients were not aware that individuals they did not know were praying for them. In fact, in order to remove subjectivity from the process, some experiments with prayer have involved praying for bacteria in a petri dish. And yes, the bacteria that were "prayed for" grew faster than bacteria that were not! How did this happen? I do not know, but it shows us that not everything is explained by our current level of scientific knowledge. Other, unexplained forces operate in our lives.

For some, prayer may conjure up images of religion, and those without religious beliefs may dismiss these concepts as irrelevant or even superstitious. It is true that the research about prayer reinforces religious belief. However, atheists may take comfort if they explain these phenomena by using the language of quantum physics, which explains these changes at the material level in terms of energy and tells us that thoughts are powerful entities—things. So, what some people call God or Spirit or Allah or Krishna, others call energy. Still, one of the most interesting trends of our time is the bridge that steadily builds between science and spirituality in the West. Just as our society is understanding that we cannot separate the body from the mind, so are we respecting the power of spiritual belief and practice. (In the Eastern world, the material and the spiritual traditionally are not viewed as separate realities.) The attitude of "modern" medicine has been to donate the body and its physical needs to the physician and leave the spirit or emotion for the priest.

LOVE, SEX, AND THE HEART

While we appear to live in a society that seems overly preoccupied with sex, many people in the United States have grown up in a sexually repressive atmosphere. Because of this Puritanical climate, many men and women do not easily discuss sexual matters. But for those fortunate enough to have a loving relationship with a life partner, the warmth of love and sex can play a powerful—and natural—role in healing. In my book *The Sexual Revolution*, which explores natural ways to enhance sexual life, I urge men and women to explore their sexual attitudes and take advantage of new information about maintaining and enhancing sexual health. Sexual health is necessary for cardiovascular health.

Dr. Ornish explores the role of love and emotional intimacy in his book *Love and Survival*. As you may know, loving relationships with a partner, children, parents, friends, and associates are probably your best stress management tools. *Love and Survival* explores many concepts, including techniques to improve communication and listening skills and other ways to strengthen intimate connections. There is no question that loneliness, isolation, and lack of intimacy with others contributes to heart disease. Developing and enriching relationships with others is at least as important as your morning exercise routine.

Your common sense can guide you in ways to simplify your life and reduce stress, but perhaps the larger goal is to live more fully, doing more of what you enjoy and gives you satisfaction, even if these activities are challenging.

SUMMARY

There is scientific evidence that stress raises blood pressure and changes blood lipid profiles. When excessive or mishandled, stress is considered a contributing factor in cardiovascular disease. However, stress is a part of life, and our challenge is to manage stress, rather than eliminate it. For some, the concept of the Type A personality (driven and aggressive) and Type B personality (easygoing and "laid back") can serve as a way to define behavioral areas that need examination. There is some evidence that the Type A personality type may be a risk factor for cardiovascular disease in younger men. While we can learn from examining the characteristics of these personality types, applying a label to any individual cannot provide an accurate and complete description of risk for cardiac disease.

Balance is probably the most important concept to consider when evaluating your psychological and spiritual health. Fortunately, we live during an era when the body-mind connection is no longer a "way out" notion. More than ever before, your health-care providers are more likely to see you—and treat you—as a whole person.

I believe that depression is a clear risk factor for heart disease, and it—and other psychological issues—should be evaluated and treated. And as cardiologist Stephen Sinatra reminds us in his work, the heart is the emotional center. Another cardiologist, Dean Ornish, has added to a growing body of work about the power of the emotional centers to heal the heart, which is so vulnerable to disease.

Other health-care professionals have added to our knowledge about the mind-body connection and the philosophies involved in the development of integrative medicine. I prefer the word "pluralistic." While there is no single pathway to stress management, the benefits of meditation and other mind-centering techniques are receiving increased attention.

What You Can Do

- The quality of your relationships with others is as important as the medical treatments you choose. Focus attention on strengthening and enriching your relationships with your spouse, other family members, and friends and associates in your community.

- Read the work of the mind-body pioneers, such as Stephen Sinatra, M.D., Dean Ornish, M.D., Andrew Weil, M.D., and Deepak Chopra, M.D. These individuals—and many others—have made significant contributions to the integrative (pluralistic) medicine movement.

- If you believe you may be suffering from depression, do not delay. Do not simply hope that your depression will resolve on its own. Seek help immediately.

- Just as exercise is important to maintain a fit body, exercises that quiet and center the mind have great value as well. In his book, *Full Catastrophe Living*, Jon Kabat-Zinn, Ph.D., discusses the benefits of mindfulness meditation. Meditation and other methods such as visualization and deep relaxation techniques may have a positive influence on your health. Consider beginning a regular meditation practice, or just relax!

CHAPTER SEVEN

WEIGHT CONTROL

For individuals faced with what often is a lifelong battle to achieve a healthy weight, weight control is rarely an easy or pleasant issue. It is a difficult issue for health-care providers, too, because there are no simple answers and no quick remedies. Yet both patients and health-care professionals know that obesity is a risk factor for heart disease, hypertension, and diabetes. Obese individuals place more mechanical stress on their heart than a person of normal body weight, and I have never known a very obese patient who did not show up one day with arthritis or pain in weight-bearing joints. Obesity as a key factor in heart disease is such an important issue that I have written a book (*The Weight Control Revolution*) focused on that subject.

It goes without saying that anyone who has obesity dating back to childhood or has adverse medical consequences of obesity should seek supervision and advice from a well-informed health-care giver. Unfortunately, few physicians or pluralistic health-care providers have great experience or knowledge about treating severe obesity, so choose your physician carefully. The best help for the severely obese is often available at medical institutions that run special weight-control centers.

It is important to understand that, clinically speaking, overweight and obesity are two different things. One could say that anyone who is above their ideal weight is overweight, but to be considered obese, one must be about 20 percent or more above one's ideal weight. It is estimated that at least 25 percent of the U.S. population is obese by these conventional definitions. Some authorities have stated that the actual percentage is higher, and the number of people who are between ideal weight and 20 percent overweight includes many millions. Overall, at least 33 percent of Americans have a degree of being overweight that puts them at a medical risk.

One of the most problematic forms of obesity is termed morbid obesity, which has been defined as body weight that is 50 to 100 percent above desirable body weight. Medically, the term malignant obesity is used with individuals who have advanced complications of obesity, with very limited survival prospects. Few people realize that severe obesity can be a death sentence.

Given these figures, it is not surprising that weight control and obesity management are among the largest industries in North America. About one-quarter of the population annually spends about *thirty billion dollars* on weight control programs and aids. However, more money is spent on high-calorie junk food and "supersized" fast food meals. Approximately 15 percent of the population are on some form of diet continuously, and 75 percent of all midteen girls try to lose weight.

EATING DISORDERS

I have included a list and description of the four main eating disorders because they run the gamut from the person who is unable eat to one who cannot stop eating and/or purging (see Table 7.1). It is no accident that many young women today believe they are fat when their weight is, in fact, normal. Waif-like fashion models are terrible role models for our adolescent girls and young women. It is ironic, but the emphasis on body image has not led to a slimmer population, but to exactly the opposite; the U.S. population is heavier than ever.

Eating disorders are more prevalent among adolescents and young women, fifteen to thirty years old. Estimates about the prevalence of eating disorders in this age group may sound shocking, with some going as high as one-third of females in this age group. Of course, exact numbers are difficult to find because binge/purge eaters, for example, do not readily disclose their problem and will not respond to common survey methods. Unfortunately, the commercial diet programs and others who offer advice about weight loss may forget the importance of spotting the "inappropriate dieter." Obviously, assisting the bulimic or anorexic to lose weight can be a catastrophic situation. Eating disorders can pose a more immediate threat to life than cardiovascular disabilities. I urge you to look at Table 7.1 and assess your eating behaviors.

As you may know, a variety of diets are advertised and discussed— it seems as if there is unending talk about the latest diets. We should

Table 7.1: Characteristics of the Main Types of Eating Disorders.

Recognition of features in an individual should prompt seeking medical advice. Eating disorders are potentially life-threatening. I believe that they are all risks for cardiovascular disease.

DISORDER	MAIN CHARACTERISTICS
Anorexia nervosa	• Morbid fear of becoming fat • Marked loss of weight • Amenorrhoea (no menses) • Not caused by organic or psychiatric disease, but may be accompanied by such disease • BMI fifteen or less, 75 percent of ABW • Unusual weight-loss habits
Bulimia nervosa	• Compulsive binge eating • Many features in common with anorexia nervosa • Binge more than twice per week, for at least three months • Lack of control or severe dependence on eating • Regularly engages in strict weight-loss regimens • Persistent concern with body shape and weight
Atypical eating disorders	• Eating disorders otherwise not specified • Chaotic eating patterns • May have many but not all of the diagnostic criteria of anorexia or bulimia nervosa • May be recovering from or transitioning toward anorexia and bulimia
Obesity	• May or may not be an eating disorder per se • Very heterogeneous components • Has genetic, organic, psychological, and nutritional potential of origin • Severe obesity usually has a well-developed psychological component

examine the popular diets, however, in order to compare their strengths and weaknesses. Some emphasize "traditional" balanced eating, but others have special theories about the fastest ways to lose weight. Of course theories are not necessarily based on sound premises.

DISPELLING THE FADS: LOOKING AT DIETS

The very fact that there are so many different diets for weight control is sure proof that none are entirely satisfactory or effective. We also could conclude that although for many people permanent weight loss is very difficult to achieve, millions of people do not give up their quest to reach a healthy and attractive weight. Some health-care professionals recommend particular weight loss plans because health problems are appearing and the "bouquet" of risk factors is ominous. Diets are usually planned for a reason, be it to lose weight, lower cholesterol, control diabetes, or otherwise correct nutritional status, but for cardiovascular health, the ideal diet addresses all the risk factors and attempts to prevent diseases from developing. I am a great supporter of the concept of one diet for health *and* weight control. However, diets often need to be tailored to individual needs, especially if one disorder predominates (*e.g.*, diabetes) in an individual.

Some weight-loss plans include very specific meal recommendations and may supply the recommended or "allowed" food. This degree of regimentation is preferred by some, but over the long term it is complied with by few. It is difficult to live a normal life, especially in our hectic times, while trying to stick to a strict, regimented diet. If you do not choose a diet that matches your lifestyle—at least to some degree—failure is inevitable.

Certain diets are recommended by institutions or organizations and therefore have an aura of authority around them. However, just because a diet is promoted by a government or institution of high standing, it does not mean that the dietary recommendations are ideal. Some organizations have axes to grind or receive support from certain industries, which may color their recommendations. Table 7.2 summarizes two of these dietary proposals, both of which come from respected bodies. However, as you can see, these diets have some disadvantages or limitations.

Some of the more popular diets are summarized in Table 7.3. In some cases, both conventional and alternative health-care practitioners have rejected these diets for one reason or another. Like most things in life, danger is found in extremes. Claims that you can eat what you like and lose weight are misleading and often frankly untrue.

THE COMPLEX CAUSES OF OBESITY

The causes of obesity are often complex but usually involve overeating combined with some type of emotional factors in individuals who are prone to obesity. In addition to overeating, several causes have been identified and include: genetic tendency and family history, lack of activity and exercise, eating patterns, emotional issues, and various medically related causes, including side effects from certain drugs, endocrine disorders, specific brain diseases, and abnormal body metab-

---

Table 7.2: Some Potential Drawbacks of Well-Accepted, Health-Giving Diets.

The American Heart Association Diet
(less saturated fat, low salt, more complex carbohydrates)

- Easy to follow
- Widespread medical use
- Evidence it may prevent heart disease
    - But . . .
        - Omits the importance of essential fats in cardiovascular disease prevention or treatment
        - Some choices of polyunsaturated fat sources are suspect
        - Forgets the role of soy and vegetable protein

The U.S. Department of Agriculture Dietary Recommendations
("Pyramid of Foods")

- Aimed at general health promotion
    - But . . .
        - Does not consider importance of essential fatty acids
        - Too accepting of processed foods
        - No real focus of the health benefit
        - Pictorally promotes "junk food," inadvertently

Table 7.3: Popular Diets.

This table contains subjective comments based on a study of the diets by the author and consultations with medical practitioners and patients who have experiences with the diet(s). Some of the commonly used diet programs are listed with putative or actual concerns about their application. With exception of the well-accepted Ornish Program, the other dietary methodologies have been somewhat lacking in careful clinical study. Assessments of their safety and efficacy have been anecdotal. This situation may make criticisms of the diet plans appear anecdotal, so the author has focused on generally accepted medical interpretations of the basis, if any, for the dietary interventions. The "reviews" are not necessarily the opinions of Dr. Holt.

DIET/DESCRIPTION	THE REVIEWS
Dr. Atkins Diet Revolution (high fat, high protein, low carbohydrates)	• Not a revolution; used by Banting in the 1800s • Accelerated early weight loss is water loss • May result in abnormal blood lipids • Yo-yo regain of weight can occur • Ketosis induced with potential negative metabolic consequences • Cannot be recommended for the person with cardiovascular disease, except short-term.
Dr. Stillman's Quick Inches Off Diet (low protein, high carbohydrates)	• Few merits • Modification of 1950s rice diet • Accelerated early weight loss is water loss • Yo-yo regain of weight can occur • Nutritionally deficient
The Zen Macrobiotic Diet and other macrobiotic diets (grain-based vegetarian diet)	• Nutritionally incomplete • Not recommended long-term because of dangers • Beyond the average reach of compliance • Lack of certain essential fatty acids • Very variable dietary formulations that are complex, with questionable basis
The Living Foods Diet (based on uncooked organic vegetables)	• Ecological basis • Stresses inclusion of vegetables over grains in contrast to many macrobiotic diets • More to do with food preparation • Only for the very committed • Probably very healthy; a good dietary regimen

(Continued on page 138)

DIET/DESCRIPTION	THE REVIEWS
Weight Watchers (well-established plan for weight reduction)	• Quite successful • Shortcomings in the control of blood cholesterol and hypertension • Expensive • Forgets essential fats and soy
The New American Diet (a mostly vegetarian diet high in complex carbohydrates and low in saturated fats)	• Much to commend in this diet, which is a variation of AHA and USDA diets • Well-balanced and flexible • Good accompanying manual • Recognizes omega-3 benefits; underestimates omega-6 benefits • Forgets to emphasize soy
The Beverly Hills Diet or **The Fit for Life Diet** (fruit diet)	• The notion that fruit melts fat is not valid • Causes diarrhea • May cause weight gain
The Pritikin Program (quite severe diet restrictions; low fat, low cholesterol)	• Compliance problems • Nutritionally incomplete • Despite this, a major contribution • Cardiovascular wellness potential
The Dolly Parton Diet ("prescribed" diet; on/off eating)	• Little, if any, scientific basis • Food-juggling regimen is too complex
The Dean Ornish Program (a complete lifestyle program with low cholesterol objective)	• Very sound program that has been subjected to objective research • Designed specifically for cardiovascular wellness • Compliance problems
The Scarsdale Diet (short-term ketosis induction plan)	• Dangerous without medical supervision • Use for only two weeks advised • Loss of protein tissue (muscle) occurs • Rejected by many as a fad
The Last Chance Diet (liquid protein diet)	• Short-term • Risk of sudden death • Thrown out by many

(Continued on page 139)

DIET/DESCRIPTION	THE REVIEWS
Fasting Is a Way of Life (essentially, just don't eat)	• Prolonged fasts are decidedly dangerous • Boring • Stimulates overeating
The Cambridge Diet or **The Slim-Fast Plan** (beverage-assisted weight loss)	• Monotonous • No education on eating properly • Not nutritionally complete meal replacements • Compliance problems • Short-term success only
The Set Point Diet (theorizes that everyone has a set weight that the body tries to maintain)	• Balanced with natural foods • Similar to AHA and USDA diets • No emphasis on essential fatty acids • Principal aim is weight loss

olism. Obesity does not always indicate a failure of self-discipline with diet. Often it is not clear what the fundamental problem is. Although psychological problems figure high in the cause of obesity, few obese people want to recognize this component of their problem.

While overweight and obesity can be complex problems, the simple answer for many people is as follows: it is generally accepted that individuals who eat too much will tend to be overweight, and those who do not eat enough will tend to be underweight. That sounds logical enough, and most of us know it is true, but it is often forgotten in attempts to make various diets look attractive to potential consumers. Taking in more calories than the body uses for energy is, as it always has been, the surest way to add extra pounds. Obviously, overeating and a sedentary lifestyle usually go hand in hand to tip the balance toward being overweight.

One popular theory of obesity is the so-called "body weight set point." This theory implies that the body adjusts to a certain weight, and it defends itself from change, making the extra pounds resistant to weight-loss efforts. This theory promotes the notion that obese individuals have a high set point and will tend to resist weight loss when placed on a low-calorie diet. Clearly, this notion is simplistic and probably only partially correct. It might make overweight individuals feel better, but its acceptance does not help those who must lose weight to take on the challenge.

Table 7.4: Metropolitan Life Insurance Company's Height and Weight Tables (1996).

Crude guidelines only; revisions of BMI are perhaps better predictors of optimal weight.

Height (ft/in)*	Small Frame	Weight (lbs)* Medium Frame	Large Frame
		Men	
5'2"	128-134	131-141	138-150
5'3"	130-136	133-143	140-153
5'4"	132-138	135-145	142-156
5'5"	134-140	137-148	144-160
5'6"	136-142	139-151	146-164
5'7"	138-145	142-154	149-168
5'8"	140-148	145-157	152-172
5'9"	142-151	148-160	155-176
5'10"	144-154	151-163	158-180
5'11"	146-157	154-166	161-184
6'0"	149-160	157-170	164-188
6'1"	152-164	160-174	168-192
6'2"	155-168	164-178	172-197
6'3"	158-172	167-182	176-202
6'4"	162-176	171-187	181-207
		Women	
4'10"	102-111	109-121	118-131
4'11"	103-113	111-123	120-134
5'0"	104-115	113-126	122-137
5'1"	106-118	115-129	125-140
5'2"	108-121	118-132	128-143
5'3"	111-124	121-135	131-147
5'4"	114-127	124-138	134-151
5'5"	117-130	127-141	137-155
5'6"	120-133	130-144	140-159
5'7"	123-136	133-147	143-163
5'8"	126-139	136-150	146-167
5'9"	129-142	139-153	149-170
5'10"	132-145	142-156	152-173
5'11"	135-148	145-159	155-176
6'0"	138-151	148-162	158-179

*Weights for adults age 25-59 years based on lowest mortality. Weight in pounds according to frame size wearing indoor clothing (5 pounds for men and 3 pounds for women) and shoes with one-inch heels.

What Should You Weigh?

No one can say in absolute terms what an ideal weight should be for each person. Ideal body weight *range* should always take into account differences in age, body type, and other variables. The many standard weight tables can provide guidelines, and it is important to identify a range of weight where risk of morbidity and mortality are at their lowest. The Metropolitan Height and Weight Tables (Table 7.4) are based on actuarial studies that look at health-risk factors. By now, most people are fed up with looking at ideal body weight tables, and their value has become the focus of much argument and contention.

The process of assessing desirable weight can be made even more complex by using formulas. One such measure is the body mass index (BMI), which is essentially the relationship between height and weight. The math gets a little tricky, because it was developed using the metric system (figure 1 pound ≈ .45 kilograms, and 1 inch ≈ .025 meters). Overweight is approximately defined as a BMI of 25 to 30 kg/m², and obesity is a BMI above 30 kg/m². A BMI of greater than 39 is an indication of morbid obesity. The BMI is calculated by dividing weight by the height of an individual squared. A 180-pound (80-kg.) person who is 79 inches (2 m.) tall has a BMI of 80 kg. ÷ 2 m. × 2 m., which equals 20. The normal range of weight in terms of a BMI is 19 to 24.9. This calculation was chosen because an average weight is about 70 kg. (155 lbs.) for a male, and a weight of 80 kg. may conjure

Table 7.5: Body Mass Index/Risk.

Four grades of being fat can be readily determined from Body Mass Index measures, calculated as weight divided by height squared. The formula for BMI can be used to define underweight. Some muscular individuals will be misclassified into grade 1 even though they may have no excessive body fat.

Body Mass Index	Grade of Weight	Description
40 or more	3	Severe or morbid obesity
30–39.9	2	Obese
25–29.9	1	Overweight
19–24.9	0	Normal range

up the idea that the person was chubby—however, height is important in this equation, because 2 meters (6 feet, 7 inches) is taller than average—so height allays a higher-than-normal weight.

The mathematical projections work in the opposite direction. By these criteria, a staggering number of individuals in the U.S. are morbidly obese—estimated at approximately two million adults. Of these individuals, there are five times more women than men. Table 7.5 describes the BMI and what the numbers mean in terms of risk. The BMI is a better way of looking at measures of health risks and obesity than simple height/weight tables.

Distribution of Body Fat

There are so many methods for assessing the amount, distribution, and location of body fat that even health-care professionals become confused. One method sometimes used is the waist-to-hip ratio (WHR). The WHR is measured as a ratio of the minimal circumference of the waist to the maximum circumference of the hips. There is some relationship between the WHR and general body fat distribution. The WHR has implications for the design of exercise programs aimed at selective weight loss from certain parts of the body.

Measures such as the WHR can assist in defining upper or lower types of body obesity, which may carry different health risks. Individuals with predominantly upper-body obesity—affecting the back of the neck, shoulder areas, and inner abdomen—seem to have a greater risk of developing metabolic complications of obesity than those with lower body obesity. A few years ago, these differences were clarified for women by describing them as "apple-shaped" or "pear-shaped." The same description applies to men.

Upper-body obesity, or the "apple" shape, is associated with diabetes mellitus, high cholesterol and triglycerides, and cardiovascular disease. It is believed that individuals with lower-body obesity—affecting the hips and buttocks, or the "pear" shape—may be more stable from the metabolic point of view, and they may not be at such a great risk of metabolic disease, such as diabetes mellitus. The distribution of obesity appears to be relevant in dictating medical needs for weight reduction.

Regardless of body shape, epidemiological evidence shows the pervasive nature of obesity in Western communities. The results of a seven-country comparative study of obesity are summarized in Table 7.6. The striking finding in this study was that the Japanese, with their high-fiber, low-calorie, soy-containing diets, are at the bottom of the table in being overweight. Obesity is uncommon in Asia. Overall the rate of obesity increases with age, with the peak prevalence occurring in Western countries between the ages of fifty-five and sixty-five, when about one-quarter of all women and one-fifth of all men are obese.

The amount and type of fat in the Western diet is a pivotal element in obesity. Many nutritional surveys have shown that Western populations have changed their diets over the past century to increase calorie intake from fat, while decreasing the dietary intake of calories derived from complex carbohydrates. It is significant that if calorie intake is kept the same, a diet rich in fat will produce enhanced gain of body fat. This finding is well-documented in animal experiments.

The risks and complications of obesity are shown in Table 7.7. Being overweight carries a risk of premature death, but obese individuals often have other risk factors for early death, including high blood cholesterol and triglycerides, hypertension, coronary artery disease, renal failure, and other serious disorders. In addition to an increased risk for disease, we cannot underestimate the social toll of obesity, which is key to understanding the sense of defeat experienced by many obese people. American and other Western societies exude constant messages about ideal body types, which can lead to exceptional and often extreme discrimination against the obese person. Such discrimination is inappropriate and totally unacceptable, but not likely to go away quickly.

Table 7.6: Prevalence of Overweight and Obesity in Men from Seven Countries, from Keys (1970).

Country	Overweight	Obese
Italy	33	28
United States	32	63
Yugoslavia	19	29
Finland	15	14
Netherlands	13	32
Greece	11	11
Japan	2	2

Percent of Sample

Table 7.7: Risks and Complications of Obesity.

Glucose intolerance*
Diabetes mellitus*
Hypertension*
Hypercholesterolemia*
Cardiac disease: atherosclerotic disease, congestive heart failure
Pulmonary disease: sleep apnea, chronic lung disease
Cerebrovascular disease, stroke*
Cancer: breast, uterus, colon, prostate*
Gallbladder: stones*
Pregnancy risks
Surgery risks
Renal failure
Gout
Infertility
Degenerative arthritis*
Early death
Psychological problems: poor self-image
Social problems: discrimination in jobs, education, and marriage

* Complications of obesity that are amenable to partial correction by soy-based diets.

SOY FOODS ARE HELPFUL

Because of the complications associated with obesity, it is necessary to tailor weight-loss diets to make sure that they serve the overall health needs of the obese person. Soy protein and other soy-based products are ideal foods to include in the diet of the motivated person who is trying to lose weight and promote health. Soy, particularly soy protein, can help counteract some of the complications of obesity. Soy helps smooth out blood glucose levels, lowers cholesterol, and plays a role in helping to regulate blood pressure. In addition, soy foods are beneficial for people with arthritis and kidney disease, and they can help prevent the formation of gallstones, which are common in the obese person.

Soy foods are losing their reputation for being dull—and even a bit odd. The commercial diet program, Weight Watchers, is now including information about plant-based protein sources, including soy, in its literature. Soy foods and other legumes and beans fit well into a healthy diet that emphasizes complex carbohydrates and reduced fat. The fats in soybeans also tend to be the more healthful types of fat, unless they are hydrogenated and used in commercial products, in which case their health benefits are removed. My previous book, *The Soy Revolution,* discusses in detail the benefits of soy for a variety of conditions, many of which are part of both the causes and the effects of obesity. You will also notice that on the reading list found at the end of this book, some of the books I list include recipes for soy foods. There is much to be gained from taking soy in dietary supplement format, especially if soy foods cannot fit a person's taste preference. Soy protein containing isoflavones (such as in the brand Genista) can make a delicious smoothie drink loaded with health-giving nutrients.

Can My Wish Come True?

The fast food industry may frown at my recommendations, but they have woken up to the public's increasing demand for a more healthy diet. Salads have appeared in fast food restaurants as a token gesture to balance out our fat taste preference for the greasy hamburger, deep-fried chicken, and ever-present french fries. As the penny drops, the fast food industry will have to move toward vegetable sources of protein such as soy. Modern processing can make a soy-burger that is indistinguishable from the flame-broiled slab of ground meat that is the staple of many Americans' diets.

I am not engaging all of the fast food industry with criticism. Great things are happening. Health-conscious food chains like Smoothie King have appeared where soy drinks are served as a healthy alternative to fat-laden milkshakes. Smoothie King has taken the lead in promoting soy as a healthy alternative to dairy products.

If ever there was a clear health benefit for soy it is in the domain of cardiovascular wellness. Fractions of soy can lower cholesterol, lower blood pressure, assist in healthy weight reduction, and improve renal function. At present, the soy grown in America is mostly fed to the cows that provide our hamburgers and milkshakes. This does not make ecological sense. My wish is to see soy as the principal substrate for fast food. This step could help change the health of our nation.

AVOIDING THE EXTREMES

Sometimes an overweight person begins to believe that losing weight is all that matters and will set out to accomplish this at all costs. However, in doing so you disregard the principle that you must promote health at your own peril. Crash diets or long-term caloric restriction can sometimes be more of a risk than the obesity itself. I believe they are a risk for cardiovascular disease.

When all is said and done, the critical elements in any weight-loss program include: a diet designed to reduce calorie and fat intake, nutrition education, increased activity, and some form of behavioral modification. This is not what people like to hear, but it remains true. These elements appear to be the only reliable way to lose weight and keep it off. Weight loss should always be undertaken as a long-term strategy to build health, but also as a lifestyle change.

Routine medical treatment of obesity using diet alone has a failure rate of greater than 95 percent over a three-year period. The practice of drastic calorie reduction is known to be associated with a "yo-yo" pattern of weight loss and rebound weight gain. Yo-yo patterns of weight

Table 7.8: Commonly Used Types of Diet for Weight Loss.

DIET TYPE	DISADVANTAGES
Balanced, low-calorie diet*	Hunger; preoccupation with food and frequent failure
Formula diets	Discipline of the diet creates boredom and failure; formulas are expensive
Specific nutrient addition	Higher fiber is the frequent choice, but palatability is a problem; worthy of more study
Specific nutrient elimination	Specific nutrient deficiency syndromes; special preparation; poor compliance
Fad diets	Sometimes dangerous; often expensive; usually a variation of one or more of the above options

*Balanced low-calorie diets with fiber and soya addition presented creatively with other lifestyle adjustments are the best option.

loss can have serious health consequences and should be avoided at all costs. Reducing the calorie intake below 1,200 calories per day may result in weight loss, but an increase in calories will result in weight gain. This is the reason that so many dieters experience the cycle of losing weight, gaining it back—plus more—and then losing again, only to have the cycle start all over again. This is explained by looking at the fluctuations in body metabolism. Metabolism adjusts to accommodate a lower-calorie diet, and this adjustment does not rapidly reverse.

Almost every diet book describes this yo-yo syndrome. In her personal quest for permanent weight loss, television host Oprah Winfrey has described her own journey. She states that after she started dieting, the result was a seventy-pound weight *gain*, meaning that this is where calorie-restricted dieting led. She was not able to overcome her weight problems until she began exercising in earnest and stopped "dieting."

There are several different types of dietary approaches to weight loss (see Table 7.8). Each has disadvantages or limitations, underscoring the need for health-care professionals and patients to consider a more holistic approach to weight control. No matter what approach is undertaken, long-term changes in eating patterns are essential.

As an aside, drug therapies for obesity come and go in popularity and, as you know, some have been taken off the market. Amphetamines are still available and, although effective in the short-term, they are dangerous and should be avoided at all costs. Phenfluramine, or Phen-fen, has been taken off the market because of its serious cardiac side effects, including primary pulmonary hypertension, a direct cause of heart failure. A more recent drug, Meridia, is, at the very least, not suitable for individuals who have the very cardiac risk factors that are often associated with obesity. Treatment with any drug for obesity should be individualized, closely monitored, and stopped when efficacy is not achieved. In my opinion, if these drugs are used at all, it should be for the short-term in selected patients.

IT COMES DOWN TO BASICS

In the earlier chapters, I discussed the bouquet of risk factors that comprise the heart disease "time bomb." Excess weight is one of the most prevalent risk factors in Western societies and is especially widespread in the United States. There is obvious concern among the general population as well as in the medical community about the high rates of overweight and obesity. For this reason, advice about this or that diet is not hard to find. When all is said and done, the following guidelines appear to be among those that are found to work over the long term. Supervision by a health-care provider is essential, of course.

1. Eat a diet that is rich in complex carbohydrates, including soy food products. The new U.S. Food Pyramid, discussed in the final chapter, is a reasonably good guideline. Your physician may send you to a nutritionist who can help you plan your meals. In any case, your total calories should never fall below 1,200 per day. The days of the 800–1,000 calorie diets are over—they inevitably lead to the yo-yo syndrome.

2. Fat calories should comprise no more than 30 percent of total calories. Twenty to twenty-five percent is probably optimal. These fats should include the most healthful omega-3 and omega-6 fatty acids and only small portions of saturated fats.

3. Small quantities of low-fat animal protein are allowed, with an emphasis on fish and poultry. Move more to vegetable protein.

4. Work with your health-care provider to design an exercise program that suits your needs and abilities. If you are new to exercise, he or she may refer you to a facility in your community that has trainers or exercise counselors. If obesity is a long-standing problem that has resulted in joint pain and/or arthritis, water aerobics may be beneficial. For most people, walking is a safe exercise. The National Weight Loss Registry, a database that accumulates information about weight-control issues, reports that those who stick with their exercise program after weight is lost are likely to keep the weight off.

5. Work with a holistic health-care provider to determine the proper nutritional supplements that will support your weight-loss efforts. It may not be easy to find such a person, but I urge you to try. Eating a balanced diet—one that supplies all the vitamins and minerals in adequate amounts—is nearly impossible. Overweight is sometimes described as a disease of undernourishment, because the foods consumed, sometimes in large quantities, may have come from "nutritionally thin" refined foods.

6. Through stress management and/or counseling, begin to unravel the emotional issues that have led to overeating. Sometimes overeating is a habit—a response to a hectic lifestyle. No matter what the cause, you must become responsible for your eating behavior and work to change destructive patterns.

7. Accept that losing weight slowly, a half-pound to a pound or possibly two pounds a week, has been found to be the most realistic. At the beginning of a weight-loss diet, some individuals will initially lose some weight more quickly. Eventually, however, the rate of weight loss will level off. While this may be hard to cope with, slow weight loss helps you adjust to a new way of eating.

8. Track your diet and your progress. A diet diary is recommended, and research has shown that individuals who write down their food intake during the holiday season lose more weight than those who do not. Exercise should be tracked in a similar way. Some people also find that keeping a journal about the process of weight loss helps them understand and cope with the emotional issues.

9. The key to sustained weight loss is behavior modification. Regaining the weight is inevitable unless adverse lifestyle and habits are corrected through a process of self-identification and intervention. In the end, permanent change depends on you.

SUMMARY

Obesity is a risk factor for heart disease, diabetes mellitus, high blood pressure, and premature death. In addition, overweight men and women are prone to joint pain and arthritis. Remember that to be considered significantly obese, one must be 20 percent or more above one's ideal weight. Using this conventional definition, more than 25 percent of the U.S. population is obese. The point, of course, is to prevent those "few extra pounds" from developing into obesity.

As you may know, the consequences of obesity go well beyond the physical, and the emotional and social toll of living with chronic obesity is serious. In addition, the pervasive preoccupation—even obsession—with attaining an "ideal" weight and a "perfect" body has led to an increase in the incidence of eating disorders. Rather than focusing on one "magic number," it is best to think of an appropriate weight range. The body mass index—the BMI—provides an additional method to calculate degree of overweight.

The causes of obesity may be complex, but any eating and lifestyle plan that does not include reducing total calories and fat while increasing exercise is probably doomed to failure. Most people need education about proper nutrition and behavior modification techniques.

What You Can Do

- Ignore a chronic or developing weight problem at your own peril. Obesity is a significant cause of cardiovascular disease and other conditions that also contribute to heart disease.
- Avoid crash diets—in fact, it is best to avoid the word "diet" at all. Many make false promises or are unhealthy even for short periods of time. Focus on developing better eating habits while reducing total calories. A weight-loss quest requires a willingness to examine and change many lifestyle issues over the long-term, not just until the excess weight is lost. The best approach to weight loss is a balanced diet with calorie restriction and real efforts to change behavior. Yo-yo dieting is dangerous.
- Seek support for your weight-loss effort. Others who have struggled with a weight problem understand what you are going through.
- This chapter lists nine important guidelines for weight loss. If you follow them carefully, your health is very likely to improve as you lose weight at a steady rate.

CHAPTER EIGHT

NUTRITION FOR A HEALTHY HEART

THE EVOLUTION OF THE LOW-FAT TREND

We have entered a new age; new evidence about reversing heart disease indicates that established atheroma and coronary artery disease may be amenable to variable degrees of reversal. Even if reversal is not possible in some individuals, halting progression and general enhancement of wellness are worthy—and achievable—goals. Information about reversing atheroma comes from a variety of sources. For example, studies in primates who are fed high-fat, cholesterol-rich diets show regression of atheroma when fat and cholesterol are removed from the diet. Several human studies show similar effects, such as the Framingham Study in Massachusetts. In addition, epidemiological studies of the prevalence of heart disease during World War II linked a lower incidence of heart attacks in the United States to a reduction in the intake of foods high in saturated fat and cholesterol.

The idea of the "low-fat way to a healthy heart" has its roots in the Framingham Study that started in 1948 and documented the link between cholesterol levels and heart disease. This low-fat emphasis became popularized as a result of work done by people such as the late Nathan Pritikin, M.D., who created a program and a center that focused on diet and lifestyle issues. Dr. Pritikin became known for his advocacy of a *very* low-fat diet, which called for no more than 10 percent of total calories from fat sources. Later, Dean Ornish adopted ideas from Dr. Pritikin's well-known program when he designed his own protocols. (As an aside, both the Pritikin and Ornish programs have a commercial arm and produce food products based on their nutritional guidelines.) The recognition of the work of Ornish and Pritikin has been so widespread that their methods deserve thoughtful consideration.

Nathan Pritikin's work arrived on the scene at the very beginning of the low-fat "revolution." Unfortunately, his general recommendations are incomplete in that they lack understanding of the beneficial role of essential fatty acids to promote cardiovascular health. Pritikin and his followers were certainly correct in recognizing the overwhelming advantages of switching from refined to complex carbohydrates in the diet, but this knowledge was neither novel or new, even in Pritikin's era.

The Pritikin diet takes a wrong turn when it claims that the diet is not only safe and healthy, but maintains an ideal weight, too. This misinformation created concern among health-care givers because some individuals took seriously Pritikin's claim that those on his diet did not need to worry about quantity of food consumed, as long as it was the right kind of food. To accept this is to deny the role of calories in weight control and to reject the fact that excess carbohydrate is stored as hard, unhealthy fat in the body. Furthermore, it overlooks the increasingly common problems that occur in eating disorders, which include binge eating. Those who are prone to emotional overeating can consume large amounts of calories, whether those calories come from brown rice and whole wheat bread or from donuts and sugar cookies. Calories are calories, regardless of their source, and the body's response to excess calories is to store them as fat. It has always surprised me that Pritikin would get behind this "eat as much as you want" notion, and Dr. Ornish also has balanced on the brink of this notion. Unfortunately, this notion is propagated in other modern-day diets, but it has little support in science.

As has been previously mentioned, Dr. Ornish and his colleagues showed in controlled clinical research that stress management training combined with a diet low in animal fat, cholesterol, and salt resulted in improvements among patients in the program. It is notable that Ornish's patients reported improvements in their symptoms; *i.e.*, they generally felt better, they were able to exercise for increasingly longer periods, and the ability of their hearts to pump blood in response to exercise was enhanced. These individuals also showed reduced total blood cholesterol and triglyceride levels and improved blood pressure readings. So, improvements were both sub-jective, in that the participants in the program reported a greater sense of well-being, and objective, in that medical testing document-ed physiologic changes.

These early results sound extremely promising, but before you jump on the Ornish bandwagon too fast, remember that the program is intense and the lifestyle changes that participating patients made were enormous. Furthermore, the patients first treated with the Ornish program were in a residential program in a rural setting, and their lives were essentially devoted to learning a new lifestyle. For example, stress management training, exercise, yoga, and meditation consumed several hours a day. The diet provided is, by many people's standards, quite restrictive and calls for:

- A 1,400 calorie vegan diet—no animal products.
- No sugar, alcohol, or caffeine, and salt restricted to 325 mg. per day.
- Well-prepared foods, consisting of fruits, vegetables, and soy products, containing a total of 5.2 mg. of cholesterol.

Since I devoted two chapters of this book to lifestyle issues, I obvi-ously believe that addressing risk factors and engaging in exercise pro-grams, meditation, or other stress management techniques are most beneficial. I believe that Dean Ornish's recognition that lifestyle issues have an important role in *reversing*, not just *preventing*, cardiovascular disease is one of his most significant contributions. Logically—and intuitively—you know that in order to improve your health and the way you feel on a day-to-day basis, it is essential that you adopt a heart-sen-sible lifestyle. These changes will involve self-discipline and a strong willingness to change. Unfortunately, few among us can devote five or six hours a day to manage stress—this is a stressful thought in itself! It should be noted, however, that out-patient programs have shown some of the same beneficial effects of the "Ornish interventions." Dr. Ornish says that individuals can spend only a few minutes a day on his sug-gested interventions and still reap some benefits.

WHAT *ARE* WE GOING TO DO ABOUT FAT?

The selection of the ideal fat composition of a diet is an extraordinarily complex subject. Here are some minimal—and very basic—definitions to help you make some sense of it all.

- **Fat:** This might seem *too* fundamental, but there is confusion about what fats are. As a compound, fat is a complex mixture of carbon, hydrogen, and oxygen. Fats are concentrated energy sources. A gram of fat contains nine calories. (Protein and carbohydrates contain approximately four and five calories per gram.)

- **Fatty acids:** These can be described as chemical units of which fats are made. There are three basic types:

  1. **Saturated fats**, which are generally solid fats primarily of animal origin, with the exception of a few plant sources, including palm and coconut.
  2. **Polyunsaturated and monounsaturated fats**, which are liquid at room temperature, and generally are associated with health benefits.
  3. **Hydrogenated and partially hydrogenated fats**, which are unsaturated vegetable fats that have been converted to solid—hydrogenated—fats, and resemble saturated fats in their physical appearance. Even though hydrogenated oils are made from polyunsaturated fats, they are not considered healthful by many nutritionists.

     Trans-fatty acids are compounds found in hydrogenated fats. They play a role in raising cholesterol levels and are decidedly the least desirable of the "unhealthy" fats.

In general, saturated fats will tend to promote atheroma, whereas monounsaturated fats and polyunsaturated fats are not atherogenic. When healthful polyunsaturated fats are hydrogenated, as occurs during common food processing, to produce margarine, for example, it becomes an atherogenic substance.

Incorporating polyunsaturated or monounsaturated fats in your diet and decreasing saturated fats should be a primary goal in planning your diet. The problem in the typical diet in the West has not been just that it is high in fat, but that it is so high in saturated and hydrogenated fats. It is ironic that soybeans are largely used for animal feed and as a source of oil to use in commercial food processing (and for various industrial uses, such as an additive in paint and ink). So, this oil—which, in its unrefined form, offers health benefits—is turned into an unhealthful source of calories in foods that line the supermarket shelves. Few people realize that hydrogenated soybean oil is one of the principal sources of calories in the American diet. It is not healthy stuff!

What is the fuss about fat? Why not just do away with it? Some dietary programs come very close to doing just that. However, this is not a good idea, because there are beneficial effects of certain dietary fats and essential fatty acids. A diet grossly deficient in fat results in a low serum cholesterol and LDL, but HDL (good cholesterol) may also decrease. The implications of lowering HDL cholesterol are not entirely known and, to add to the confusion, polyunsaturated fats (good fats) in the diet may also lower HDL. This has led many experts to recommend using monounsaturated fat as the ideal source of fat— a commendable approach, at least in part.

A BAN ON CARBOHYDRATES: THE OTHER EXTREME

At the same time that the low-fat diets were gaining in popularity, there was corresponding interest in diets that were relatively high in fat and low in carbohydrates. When carbohydrate intake is significantly reduced—under 30 to 60 grams a day—weight loss may be rapid at first, which also causes the body to enter ketosis. Make no mistake, the early rapid weight loss results from loss of water in the body. When fat breaks down in the body, ketones are produced. Ketones need carbohydrates in order to be burned as a source of energy. In a very low carbohydrate diet, the body may stay in a state of ketosis as more and more fat is broken down. Ketones are then released from the body through the urine, the stool, or the breath. Some authorities believe that a state of ketosis is generally detrimental, while the low-carbohydrate diet advocates maintain that Type I diabetics are the only individuals who should always avoid such a restrictive dietary regimen.

Robert Atkins, M.D., has been one of the principal proponents of the low-carbohydrate diet. He is critical of the low-fat approach, and his dietary program has many proponents. While Dr. Pritikin failed to appreciate the intricacies of the effects of fatty acid metabolism on cardiac health, Dr. Atkins has addressed this issue to some degree. Both the Atkins diet and the Pritikin diet have some merits, but the ideal diet is achieved by neither in the long term, especially when it comes to promoting cardiovascular health.

In recent years, variations on the low-carbohydrate theme have developed. They could be called the moderate-carbohydrate plan, in that they modify both the fat and protein intake. For example, Barry Sears, M.D., the originator of "The Zone" approach to balanced eating, believes that the proper mix in an ideal diet is 40 percent carbohydrates, 30 percent fat, and 30 percent protein. Dr. Sears also believes that soy protein is a favorable source of protein in the diet, although The Zone approach also allows animal protein to supply the majority of the protein calories. The Atkins, Pritikin, Ornish, and Sears diets have one important component in common in that they all advocate complex carbohydrates and recommend avoiding refined carbohydrates. I have felt a sense of personal satisfaction because several of the modern "diet gurus" have, knowingly in some cases, endorsed my proposals for the role of soy in weight control.

In their book *Food Facts and Fallacies*, published in 1971, Dr. Carlton Fredericks and Dr. Herbert Bailey state that "there is no such thing as a calorie that confines itself to the production of energy. Excess calories will usually be stored—alas!—where they can be seen—usually as a belly bulge." I believe they were right to consider the notion that "calories don't count" as misdirected. Overall, this notion of "high or liberal fat" diets is partially invalid, perhaps dangerous. Unlike the balanced approach, these diets are examples of fads that come and go. Dr. Fredericks and Dr. Bailey recognized the importance of a diet balanced in protein, fat, and carbohydrate intake. I believe these authorities were right, even accepting the limitations of prevailing knowledge about health and weight reduction at the time they made their recommendations.

Dr. Ornish added an updated approach to dieting when he advocated a move toward vegetarian sources of protein. Early work had indicated that there was as much of a correlation between animal protein in the diet and mortality from coronary heart disease as there was between dietary fat and heart disease. A consensus has emerged from more objective studies, such as those of Ornish, that a movement toward vegetarian habits is both safe and efficacious in promoting health.

It is notable that in 1982 Dr. Ornish recognized the pivotal studies of Dr. K. K. Carroll in Canada and those of Dr. C. Sirtori in Italy, which showed that vegetable protein from soy protein lowers cholesterol. Unfortunately, Dr. Ornish indicated that these studies were controversial! Despite the apparent controversy, he incorporated soy foods into his cardiovascular health program. This "closet" approach to the use of soy may have been a function of his desire (or necessity) to float down the mainstream of medicine. Of course, many well-controlled clinical studies show an unequivocal benefit of soy protein containing isoflavones in reducing cholesterol and normalizing blood lipids. "The penny started to drop" as other proponents of cholesterol lowering began recommending fiber supplementation of the diet and recognized the health benefits of plant protein and essential fatty acids, such as those found in fish oil.

Acknowledging the value of vegetable sources of protein does not mean that one must become a total vegetarian to build health. However, over the last decade, it has become clear that animal protein is not superior to vegetable sources of protein. Despite the longstanding position of meat and dairy as the centerpiece of the Western diet, we now know that vegetable protein can, safely, partially replace meat and dairy products. When you plan dietary changes to promote cardiovascular wellness, I recommend thinking more about adding healthful foods and nutrients to your diet, rather than approaching the issue from what you must eliminate.

INSULIN: THE NEW WEIGHT CONTROL

In essence, new concepts about cardiovascular health and weight control center around the importance of *insulin*, a hormone that exerts very important and complex controls over body functions. Insulin is a hormone that is secreted by the body in response to carbohydrate intake. The way in which carbohydrates are consumed exerts major influences on the secretion of insulin by the endocrine portion of the pancreas. In simple terms, refined carbohydrates (simple sugars) are rapidly absorbed into the body and produce rapid responses in insulin secretion. Thus, excessive simple sugar consumption can flog the pancreas to death, and excessive insulin secretion occurs (hyperinsulinism). Furthermore, there is a stage where the body becomes resistant to effects of insulin (insulin resistance). This situation of hyperinsulinism/insulin resistance goes hand in hand with obesity and forms the basis of the modern epidemic of Type II diabetes mellitus.

By looking at the modern recommendations in the U.S. Food Pyramid, the issue is further illuminated. The food pyramid is perhaps promoting and supporting the massive consumption of junk food, albeit inadvertently. Let me put it this way: look at a picture of the U.S. Food Pyramid, and you will see photographs of supposedly health-building foods such as pasta and bread, which contain unhealthy amounts of refined flour and carbohydrates. In other words, while lip service is given to a preference for complex carbohydrates, typical consumers could buy "white" foods, such as white bread—even the more dense white bread found in gourmet bakeries, and even the finest white flour pastas—and believe they are eating by "pyramid" rules. At the same time, the issue of good fats in the diet— *e.g.*, fish oil—is played down.

We cannot ignore that our modern movement toward refined carbohydrates (by any name, this is junk food) is coincidental with the modern epidemic of maturity onset diabetes, which is characterized by insulin excess, insulin resistance, and obesity. Are the current widespread recommended dietary guidelines, such as those of the U.S. Food Pyramid, which inadvertently promotes consumption of excessive refined carbohydrates and flour, contributing to the common occurrence of cardiovascular disease in modern society? The answer is probably yes.

Diabetes Mellitus — A Cardiovascular Risk

Diabetes is now rampant and affects individuals of all ethnic origins in our society. Western society's alarming increase in the occurrence of diabetes mellitus is more notable in mature individuals, and it results in "maturity onset diabetes," which tends to be associated with obesity. Diabetes mellitus is inextricably bound up in the bouquet of risk factors that lead to cardiovascular disease. Like obesity, hypertension, and high blood cholesterol, diabetes is a common cause of cardiovascular diseases. Many people may die as a consequence of being in one of the stages of the evolution of diabetes without ever even knowing that they have diabetes. This is not a widely accepted opinion in conventional medicine. In order to understand this situation, we need to understand some controversial proposals about stages of diabetes and the evolution of frank diabetes, together with the inextricable link between diabetes and cardiovascular disease.

Most people do not know that consuming refined carbohydrates— junk food—results in "flogging" the pancreas to secrete insulin. Consuming the carbohydrates in junk food is probably the number one public health concern in modern society. Junk food tastes good because it is sweet with an abundance of refined carbohydrates. It has a pleasant sensation in the mouth because of saturated fats, hydrogenated fats, and sticky simple carbohydrates. In addition, it is often loaded with fat, which appeals to the modern fat taste preference that has enthralled our children and appealed to adults of all ages. Modern protagonists of revolutionary dietary concepts have described the evolution of diabetes in five phases. This hypothetical evolution of diabetes involves very interesting concepts that may not be embraced by conventional medicine. I emphasize that the following dialogue pertains to maturity onset (Type II) diabetes mellitus.

Frankly, many Western communities are inhabited increasingly by miniature blimps—our children are increasingly beleaguered by excessive weight, inactivity, and even high blood cholesterol. Against this background, *resistance to insulin*—the first stage in the development or evolution of diabetes—occurs. If people like junk food, they will take in more calories, satiate their learned food preferences, and become fat. Few would argue that people in Western society, especially the U.S., are "supersizing" their bodies and changing their body shape. Evidence for this phenomenon abounds. Recently, the international publication, *The Herald Tribune,* carried a tongue-in-cheek article about the changing body size and shape of Americans. The article focused on a new study costing millions of dollars that defines the needs for expanding the width of the seating for Americans in theaters, automobiles, airplanes, and in other public places. The findings may be amusing to some, but it should be perceived as tragic that average Americans cannot seat themselves anymore in regular-sized chairs.

Insulin is responsible for the efficient use of sugar by the body, and when resistance occurs, more insulin may be secreted, leading to hyperinsulinism—which, itself, has negative effects on body chemistry. *Hyperinsulinism* can be considered to be the second stage in the development of the diabetic diatheses. In fact, it may be easier to think about problems related to insulin controls in the body rather than think about diabetes alone.

As insulin resistance and hyperinsulinism progress, there is evidence of abnormalities in the way sugar is handled in the body. This cannot always be demonstrated by the simple glucose tolerance test that measures *increases in blood glucose* as a response to drinking a standard glucose solution. Measuring insulin release in response to meals may assist in detecting abnormalities. This constitutes the third stage of the diabetic diathesis.

We now have three stages of progression of diabetes; while frank disease is not yet present, cardiovascular risk is enhanced as a consequence of abnormal actions of insulin. These three early stages are associated with obesity, abnormal blood lipids, and increased risk of cardiac disease. Stages four and five of the evolution of diabetes involve the occurrence of Type II diabetes in stage four, where *insulin levels remain high.* Stage five of Type II diabetes occurs when insulin levels may tend to be low because *the endocrine portion of the pancreas finally gives up.*

The evolution of problems with insulin control is not quite as simple as presented, and much overlap occurs in this hypothetical progression of events. Coincidental with these changes, one sees the tendency toward elevated levels of bad cholesterol (LDL), lowered levels of good cholesterol (HDL), high blood triglycerides, and changes in lipoprotein status.

Modern cardiologists have talked about complicated variants of coronary artery disease; one catchy term involves the description of something called "Syndrome X." The hallmarks of Syndrome X are truncal obesity (fat belly; the apple-shaped body type), increased triglycerides level in the blood, low HDL, high blood pressure, insulin resistance and/or hyperinsulinism, and one or other of the stages of the evolution of problems with insulin control previously described. Whatever the situation or syndrome, problems with insulin actions and control are wrapped up with our modern epidemic of cardiovascular disease.

AN INTRODUCTION TO FIBER

In third world countries, there is a much lower prevalence of cardiovascular and other degenerative diseases that afflict more affluent Western societies. When fiber's modern-day champion, Dr. Dennis Burkitt, began to talk about fiber—and the lack of it in Western diets—he received considerable, and unjustified, criticism for his proposals. But he is another forward thinker who has achieved complete vindication in recent years.

There are many types of fiber in plant foods, but an all-purpose definition of fiber is that it is the nondigestible supporting structure of plants. Fiber has been called "unavailable carbohydrate," since it contains complex polysaccharides that are not a significant energy source because of their lack of assimilation by the body. Dietary fiber tends to fall into two broad categories: soluble and insoluble. Soluble fiber forms a gel with water, but it is not absorbed into the bloodstream. Insoluble fiber is "hydroscopic"; it holds water, but travels through the digestive tract virtually unchanged.

Plant fiber is delivered into the colon (large bowel), where it is metabolized and fermented by bacteria to produce volatile fatty acids, gas, and energy. The action of fiber in the colon is very important in understanding the effect of fiber on human physiology. First, most types of fiber absorb and retain water, which adds bulk to the stool. People who consume a high-fiber diet have softer, bulkier stool than those who consume a low-fiber diet. Fiber can alter the normal bacterial populations present in the large bowel, and it can promote the growth of more friendly types of bacteria. The idea of maintaining a healthy range of "friendly bacteria" in the gut is the basis of the popular concept of prebiotic and probiotic therapy. Fiber, like some nonabsorbable carbohydrates (*e.g.*, stachyose and raffinose in soy) is a useful prebiotic agent that will tend to promote the presence of friendly types of bacteria in the human colon and digestive tract.

Fiber and Longevity

In an earlier chapter I mentioned the Zutphen Study, performed in Holland. In addition to linking high cholesterol and adverse lifestyle issues with cardiovascular diseases, it showed that men with a low intake of dietary fiber had about three times greater risk of death from all causes than men who had a high intake of dietary fiber. The Zutphen Study indicates that a diet rich in fiber (of the order of about 35 g/day) is protective against death from several chronic diseases in Western societies. Though in the Zutphen Study other factors may have operated in addition to diet, such as exercise, cigarette smoking, environmental pollution, and psychological issues, of all disease-causing factors, appropriate diet seems to be pivotal in slowing the increase of degenerative diseases.

Soluble and Insoluble Fibers

The notion of differences between products in terms of soluble fiber and insoluble fiber content can be misleading or confusing. Soluble fibers, such as those found in apples (pectin) or beans (guar), are generally more effective at reducing blood cholesterol levels than insoluble fibers. The role of soluble fiber in decreasing cardiovascular risk has been grossly underestimated. Several controlled scientific studies indicate that oat bran or beans in the diet can reduce cholesterol by 19 percent, and guar, pectin, and psyllium supplements in the diet can lower cholesterol by 8 percent, 15 percent, and 16 percent, respectively. These findings imply that a diet that is high in fiber content is one way to promote cardiovascular wellness.

Beans, some fruits, carrots, and a variety of cereals have been shown to lower cholesterol. A few years ago, many people jumped on the oat bran bandwagon. In a 1988 study, 236 healthy volunteers followed the American Heart Association guidelines on diet and noted a reduction of blood cholesterol over a period of one month. After this initial period, the volunteers were split into two groups; one received oatmeal supplements, and one did not. The results then showed that oatmeal caused reductions in blood cholesterol. This and other studies show the beneficial effect of supplementing the diet with oatmeal, and offers an advantage because oatmeal is inexpensive as well as effective.

The efficacy of oat bran is impressive and, like soy protein, it has been proposed as a real option to avoid drug therapy in the control of blood cholesterol. An important study looked at the cost-effectiveness of oat bran versus two prescription cholesterol-lowering drugs (colestipol and cholestyramine), and concluded that oat bran could be considered more cost-effective than these drugs. While more potent lipid-lowering drugs have emerged since this study was performed in 1988, there is no reason to reject effective natural options to lower cholesterol, such as oat or soy fiber. I propose that soy protein containing even modest amounts of isoflavones (*e.g.*, Genista) and oat bran are first-line options to lower cholesterol and could be used in many circumstances before any cholesterol-lowering drugs are prescribed.

The Fiber in Complex Carbohydrates

A diet that has a relatively high content of complex carbohydrates usually means a diet that is high in fiber content. The Ireland-Boston Diet-Heart Study demonstrated the importance of choosing complex carbohydrates. In this prospective study, over a twenty-year period, the diets of three groups of individuals were analyzed and subsequent mortality was surveyed about twenty-three years later. The analysis showed that cholesterol intake and the ratio of saturated to unsaturated fats were higher in those with coronary artery disease, but the individuals who died of coronary disease tended to have much less total carbohydrate and fiber intake in their diet. The researchers concluded that the dietary difference that accounted for the increase in coronary heart disease was most likely more related to a decrease in the intake of complex carbohydrates rather than a change in the intake of dietary fat.

In practical terms, what does this mean for you? It is generally agreed that you should eliminate—or at least severely restrict—refined carbohydrates, a category that includes a vast array of foods: nutrient-stripped and bleached white flour products, white rice, sweets made with white flour, sugar, and, most often, saturated fats. This is especially important for overweight individuals, but applies across the board. Studies have shown a relationship, albeit inconsistent, between the metabolic changes induced by sugar and coronary artery disease and diabetes. The results of several studies indicate that a high intake of sugar (refined carbohydrates) in the diet tends to correlate with raised blood levels of triglycerides and cholesterol. It is known that long-term consumption of simple sugars, such as sucrose or fructose, enhances cardiovascular risk factors (though starches and complex carbohydrates in fruit and vegetables do not seem to share this negative effect.) Fruit and vegetables not only come with advantages of fiber, they also contain vitamins, flavanoids, and other compounds that fight chronic disease.

The Fiber Hypothesis

Neil Painter and Dennis Burkitt, who published their work in the 1970s, are regarded as the emblem-bearers of the fiber hypothesis. These scientists proposed that a deficiency of plant fiber in the diet may predispose individuals to many of the chronic degenerative diseases that afflict Western society. The fiber hypothesis, as first proposed, relied on a great deal of epidemiological data derived from population studies and clinical observations. They reached their conclusions from the profiles and occurrence of certain diseases in the West as compared with those in rural and less industrialized cultures, which were largely consuming vegetable-based diets.

On average, a vegetarian consumes more than twice the amount of fiber as an individual who consumes a recommended healthy Western diet (greater than 40 g/day versus less than 20 g/day). In nonurban societies, such as those of African natives, the daily dietary fiber intake ranges from 50 to 150 g/day, especially when maize is the dietary staple. It is interesting to note that the stool weight of many Westerners may be 100 g/day or less, whereas the African native eating maize diets may pass up to 1 kg. or more of stool per day. Comparisons of the diets of white and black South Africans have shown that as urbanization of the black population increases, the proportion of fat and protein in the diet increases, too. In addition, more refined carbohydrates are consumed, and the total dietary fiber intake falls dramatically. Coincidental with these dietary changes, the urban black develops a disease profile similar to that of the urban white. Disorders such as colon cancer, diverticular disease, varicose veins, and heart disease tend to become more prevalent as dietary fiber intake is reduced.

Dietary fiber, in a variety of forms, has been shown to reduce cholesterol, and it may play a major role in the prevention of colon cancer, gallstones, inflammatory bowel disease, diverticular disease, diabetes mellitus, varicose veins, and functional gastrointestinal disease (spastic colon; irritable bowel syndrome). Fiber has an established therapeutic role in the treatment of obesity, diverticular disease, colitis, constipation, and functional bowel disease.

Fiber is sometimes considered to be a laxative, but this may be misleading. Bran, when consumed with an adequate fluid intake, can cause a laxative effect, but certain gel-forming fibers, such as pectin, can be used for their balancing effect to control diarrhea. Therefore, it is more appropriate to consider fiber as a modulator of bowel and other gastrointestinal functions. The overall hypothesis of fiber for health has extended to the identification of compounds within dietary fiber that account for its health-giving potential. For example, lignans may have estrogen-like actions in the body, and much has been made about the potential versatile health benefits of phytates (phytic acid). Phytates are linked to the presence of inositol hexaphosphate, which has been labeled "IP6" by supplement purveyors. Inositol hexaphosphate has interesting anticancer properties, but it is not a health panacea, as it has been described. Phytates are abundant in soybeans.

Working Fiber into Your Diet

If you decide to add extra fiber to your diet, it is best to introduce it slowly. The production of fatty acids and gas from the colonic fermentation of fiber explains why there may be a temporary and often unpleasant period of time when the colon adapts to an extra fiber load. The fatty acids result from the metabolism of fiber by bacteria in the colon, and this may promote more frequent bowel action and excessive gaseousness. Many people believe they cannot "handle" a high-fiber diet because they are not prepared to withstand its early phase of gastrointestinal adaptation. For Westerners, increased fiber can be both a gastronomic and physiological shock because they are used to having contracted, constipated colons that produce small, hard stools.

There are several ways to increase fiber in the diet. First, you may choose to add—gradually—more foods that are rich in insoluble and soluble fibers. This is a difficult goal for the average person, and it often involves moving toward a vegetarian diet. You can also choose to use dietary supplements. Unprocessed wheat bran is desirable, but many people consider it unpalatable; hydrophilic preparations that contain predominantly gel fibers (*e.g.*, Metamucil, Citrucel) lack the overall combined benefits of soluble and insoluble fiber.

Soy contains both insoluble and soluble fiber, giving it advantages over many cereal sources of fiber. Relatively little research has been

Table 8.1: Fiber Supplement Ingredients.

Preparation	Description	Contact with water
Bran fiber	Fibrous outer layer of cereal grains, usually wheat	Poorly soluble with water holding dependent on particle size
Plantago sp. (Ispaghula) *ovata* P. *pysllium indica*	Small dried ripe seeds; cellulose-containing walls of endosperm and mucilage-containing epidermis	Colorless transparent mucilage forms around insoluble seed
Ispaghula husk	Epidermis and collapsed adjacent layer or Plantago species.	Swells rapidly with water to form a stiff mucilage
Sterculia gum	Gum obtained from *Sterculia* species	Forms a homogeneous adhesive gelatinous mass
Methylcellulose	Methyl ether of cellulose	Slowly soluble, giving a viscous, colloid solution
Soya fibers	Insoluble and soluble cotyledon and pulp	Universal beneficial properties Swell and hold water

performed on the health benefits of soy fiber in comparison with other sources of fiber, such as bran. There are several reasons to explain this disproportionate interest in bran fiber. The benefits of cereal fiber have received considerable support from the cereal industry, and this interest has led to the marketing and generation of the scientific support to promote several commercially available insoluble fiber products that are marketed as pharmaceuticals and over-the-counter medications. In other words, commercially isolated fiber products have been researched in the West for "treating" a condition largely caused by lack of natural fiber in the diet!

It is generally agreed that an intake of between 20 and 35 grams of dietary fiber in the diet is optimal, but there may be great differences in individual requirements. There is no magical dose of fiber, and certain people have a limited tolerance to dietary fiber as a consequence of altered frequency of bowel habit or flatus production. In general, science supports the use of combinations of soluble and insoluble fiber. Soluble fiber appears to be particularly effective at lowering blood cholesterol, and it has clear advantages when incorporated into a heart-smart diet. Insoluble fiber has more general effects as a modulator of bowel function and may help protect against cancer.

Fiber products are available in several modified forms. For example, bran is available in tablets and even gel-soft preparations, pea fiber can be added to flour, and psyllium has been incorporated into cereals. However, there is a lack of confidence that these modified fiber products have the same health-promoting benefits of the crude or natural sources of fiber.

The guideline of 20–35 g/day is recommended by the Federation of American Societies for Experimental Biology (FASEB), which matches recommendations made by the American Diabetes Association and the National Cancer Institute. The Reference Daily Intake (RDI) of dietary fiber proposed by the FDA for labeling purposes on nutritional products in the United States is 25 g/day, which matches recommendations in several European countries and those that have been made by the Department of Health in Australia. In contrast, the World Health Organization (WHO) has been more specific in defining dietary fiber requirements by expressing recommendations by using the term "non-starch polysaccharides." The WHO daily dietary recommendation for nonstarch polysaccharides is 16 to

24 g of dietary fiber per day. This is consistent with estimates of 27 to 40 g of total dietary fiber per day. The WHO has tended to recommend higher fiber intake than other agencies, but now the Department of Health in Australia is recommending 30 g/day of dietary fiber as a goal for the Australian public by the year 2000.

BUTTER VS. MAN-MADE SPREADS

Alternative thinking about the causes of cardiovascular disease points to the finding that beginning in the early twentieth century, there was a progressive move to include cheap sources of fat in Western diets as a substitute for expensive dairy products, such as butter. The margarine industry took healthy, fresh, vegetable oils and processed them by hydrogenation to produce solid margarine, which has gained increasing popularity over the past fifty years. This has led to margarine versus butter arguments. The reality is that both butter and margarine have disadvantages and limitations.

The notion that most types of margarine are protective against heart disease is probably fallacious. The debate about butter versus margarine is not particularly relevant when it comes to choosing a heart-smart diet, particularly one in which weight loss is also a goal. While it's true that butter contains cholesterol and many margarines do not, margarine is little more than a chemically processed food in which the potentially healthful fat has become an unhealthful one. Because of the hydrogenation process, I would choose a small amount of butter over highly processed margarine products.

It is quite easy, actually, to turn a health-giving fat into an unhealthy one. As explained, hydrogenating an unsaturated fat is one such way. Some studies have shown a link between hydrogenated fats and atherosclerosis, implying that vegetable shortenings, margarine, and other hardened fats are to be avoided. Indeed, several studies have shown that hydrogenated polyunsaturated fats may actually elevate blood cholesterol. This has been a big question that has been posed to the margarine industry when they reject butter as "unhealthy."

The cholesterol elevating effects of some hydrogenated vegetable oils is not completely understood but it may be related to the fact that hydrogenation produces the unhealthy type of fatty acid, *trans-fatty acids.* The most plausible explanation of this phenomenon is that the trans-fatty acids found in processed vegetable oils have an antagonistic effect on the action of essential fatty acids. Several scientists have studied the concentration of trans-fatty acids in the fat tissue of individuals who died from coronary artery disease, and they have found that the accumulation of trans-fatty acids appeared to be correlated with a risk of death.

We can also turn good fat into bad fats by frying and overheating unsaturated fats. Oxidation of fats tends to promote their atherogenic potential, and deep-fried foods are often notoriously high in cholesterol. The heating of cholesterol during frying results in the oxidation of cholesterol. Oxidized cholesterol is known to be toxic to arterial smooth muscle, and it may promote atherosclerosis. I recommend using a microwave oven over frying because this cooking method reduces the formation of oxidized cholesterol and fats in the diet.

You have probably heard about Olestra, which is essentially a fake fat developed to make some popular snack foods low fat, without losing their taste appeal. It is unfortunate that the market for these "empty" foods is so large; the fat-free rage has led to this. Apparently, these fake-fat products, which include chips, snack crackers, and so forth, are a marketer's dream. There is a big difference between removing fat from food products and adding a phony variety, whose safety may still be in question. Products made with Olestra are required to carry a warning that abdominal cramping and loose stools may be side effects of the products. In addition, Olestra inhibits absorption of some vitamins, and certain vitamins are added to the products. Overall, I recommend avoiding fake fats. Their long-term safety is not established and, particularly for your children, the better goal is to avoid developing the taste—or craving—for fat. A new development is the marketing of spreads that may help lower cholesterol (*e.g.*, Take Control and Benechol). These innovations are very valuable.

OLIVE OIL—ATHENA'S GIFT

When calories are not a big issue, many people find that best way to deal with the butter versus margarine dilemma is to use fresh vegetable oils in most cooking and olive oil as a spread. You may have noticed that many restaurants are "going Mediterranean" and using olive oil, along with various types of vinegars and herbs, to serve with their bread. This convenient substitution can be beneficial for those individuals at special risk for cardiovascular disease. Olive oil has very special benefits in preventing and perhaps treating common cardiovascular problems.

Studies of Mediterranean people who eat monounsaturated fat in the form of olive oil show that their rates of cardiovascular disease are as low as people who consume low-fat diets. The main issue here is that monounsaturated fats do not lower HDL, and this may be a key factor in promoting cardiovascular wellness. Olive oil in the diet is commended and recommended for the heart-smart person.

The olive has a long and rich history; in ancient religions, it is linked with maturity, fertility, and even longevity. In addition to being a monounsaturated fat, olive oil contains *phenolic* (anticancer) compounds, which have antioxidant properties. Olive oil contains beta-carotene (pre-vitamin A) and tocopherols (forms of vitamin E); it has its green tinge because it contains chlorophyll. Olive oil is also rich in magnesium, an essential nutrient that is important for maintaining a healthy heart. Finally, olive oil contains *triterpenic* compounds, which are believed to have anti-inflammatory effects on the body, which benefit the cardiovascular system. You can see why many people have referred to olive oil as a gift from Athena, the Greek goddess of wisdom.

The fatty-acid composition of olive oil is important in that it contains compounds that are believed to decrease the oxidation of LDL cholesterol, the so-called "bad" cholesterol. As you are aware, the process of oxidation of bad types of cholesterol is important in the cause of plaque formation in the arteries. A number of studies have indicated that olive oil may help reduce cholesterol levels, inhibit the formation of blood clots, and reduce blood pressure. In the 1950s, a study compared the diet and rates of heart disease in seven countries. This study showed that coronary heart disease was less common in two Greek islands than it was in urban populations. In the 1950s, the nonurbanized population of these Greek islands had a plant-based diet, with relatively small quantities of meat protein, but a strikingly high amount of fat—about 40 percent of total calories. Much of this fat was in the form of olive oil. A favorable reduction in coronary artery disease was noted in countries in which large amounts of olive oil were consumed, but where the diet also included a generous supply of vegetables. The vegetables added substantial quantities of antioxidants and were fiber-rich. Over the past decade, several studies have provided direct and indirect evidence that a traditional Greek diet, rich in olive oil, may tend to have a protective effect on the incidence of coronary artery disease.

It is important to note that several different compounds may combine to make olive oil a health-promoting food. One substance, DHPE (di-hydroxyphenyl-ethanol) is known to inhibit platelet aggregation (clumping), and several flavonoids in olive oil may have the same effect. The monounsaturated fat, *oleic acid*, may be one of the principal agents in olive oil that is responsible for lowering blood pressure.

Taken together, these beneficial properties of olive oil have led the expert panel of the National Cholesterol Education Program and some cardiac treatment centers to approve some inclusion of olive oil in the diet. This recommendation is based in part on some studies that seem to indicate that oleic acid, together with omega-3 fatty acids, may help prevent recurrent heart attacks. In addition, olive oil has been linked with a possible anticancer property, particularly breast cancer, and it may offer benefits for some who suffer from arthritis, digestive disorders, and diabetes.

Extra-virgin olive oil is the most pure and health-promoting type. The best olive oils are cold-pressed, rather than those subjected to heat, which can lead to their deterioration. Oils processed in this way also have the least amount of acidity and the best flavor. High-grade olive oils purchased from health food stores are probably the most predictable and reliable. The olive oil products sold in typical grocery stores tend be more refined and, therefore, less healthy. So, the olive oil of choice is extra virgin and cold processed, but it must be *fresh!* When stored, oils will spontaneously oxidize and decompose. They are best stored away from sunlight and in an opaque bottle.

A word of caution is in order, too. Telling people that olive oil is a health-building food can be risky if common sense is in question! Just as any potential health-benefits of red wine, for example, are eliminated when used excessively, the same is true for olive oil. In general, any oil should be used sparingly. A tablespoon or less on a fresh salad or with bread (wholemeal) should be considered a serving.

THE GOOD EGG

Not all saturated fatty acids are necessarily atherogenic. The main offenders have odd-sounding names: palmitic, myristic, and lauric acid, which are found in animal fats. However, some foods have been labeled unhealthy because they contain saturated fat. Coconut oil, cocoa butter, and eggs fall into this category. Eggs are rich in cholesterol, but as much as 50 percent of the fat in eggs is monounsaturated, and they are a rich source of lecithin, which can itself be considered an anti-atherogenic principle.

Eggs are an inexpensive source of enjoyable, dietary protein and I caution eliminating your omelets and scrambled eggs. Egg whites are a source of high-quality protein, and data on the negative effect of egg yolks on blood lipids are less than convincing. Some diet programs recommend using one egg in a dish, such as an omelet, along with two egg whites. This significantly reduces the calorie count of the dish, but supplies the protein. I do not believe that the odd egg in the diet causes harm, especially in view of the observations that blood cholesterol levels appear to be more responsive to saturated fat intake than they may be to dietary cholesterol intake.

THE FRENCH PARADOX AND THE "SLOW FOOD" MOVEMENT

The effect of alcohol consumption on cardiovascular risk factors, particularly blood cholesterol levels, has provoked much debate. Overall, as stated elsewhere in this book, I believe the evidence suggests that drinking in moderation is not overtly harmful. Some of the best evidence for a beneficial effect of moderate drinking on cardiovascular risk comes from a study by Dr. Rimm and his colleagues that was published in *Lancet* in 1991. In this study, the relationship between alcohol intake and coronary disease was examined in a prospective manner in 51,529 male health professionals. Increasing alcohol intake (to modest levels) was found to be inversely related to the incidence of coronary disease, after adjustment for other coronary risk factors were made. There are other beneficial effects of moderate drinking, which include a reduction in platelet aggregation and an increase in diameter of the coronary arteries. There may be a link between moderate drinking and moderate lifestyles in general, which in turn are linked to overall health and longevity.

The protective effects of alcohol consumption were the subject of considerable debate in the early 1990s when "The French Paradox" was defined by scientists. The term "The French Paradox" refers to the scientific evidence that showed that despite high-fat diets and a lifestyle often deficient in exercise, French people were less likely to suffer heart disease than several of their neighbors in Europe or their American counterparts.

The red wine consumption by the French was postulated to account for this paradox. This observation then led to the search for constituents other than alcohol in red wine that could account for this situation. Several compounds are present in grapes that are known to exert beneficial cardiovascular benefits. These include com-pounds known as OPCs, which is an easy abbreviation of the term oligomeric proanthocyanidins. Another interesting compound is resveratrol, which has been synthesized and, in very elegant scientif-ic experiments, has been shown to be cardioprotective.

As a result of these scientific findings, grapeseed extract has become a very popular dietary supplement in the U.S.; it is used pri-marily for its cardiac benefits. Not all scientists believe in these agents as the explanation for The French Paradox. Some people postulate that it is the mindset and habits of the French concerning food that are responsible. What does this mean? The best way to describe this is through a description of the "slow food" movement, which ascribes to the relative cardiovascular health of the French and their tendency to relax and enjoy their meals, rather than gulp them down. The slow food movement has become organized, and a few years ago it became a "society" in Italy. It has thousands of members worldwide who are engaged in philanthropic activities to help feed the poor. It probably comes as no surprise that individuals in the U.S. could greatly benefit from the slow food movement. Is it possible that the next millennium will see a battle between the slow food and the fast food movements?

Another consequence of our fast-paced society is massive caffeine consumption. Caffeine comes in many forms, most notably in coffee and cola drinks. A study performed in Norway indicated that coffee consumption is a predictor of coronary death, and it operates at a level higher than can be explained by its known effects on raising blood cholesterol. Unfortunately, decaffeinated coffee does not clearly afford protection, so the jury is still out on this issue. However, I believe that for a person with no known heart disease, it is probably safe in moderation. Individuals with established heart disease should avoid excessive caffeine intake because it can alter heart rate and rhythm, as well as increase platelet reactivity and raise blood pressure.

A SALT BY ANY OTHER NAME

The addition of salt (sodium chloride) to food is a learned habit that can be broken with effort. It has been described as a habit most people "can't shake." Recently, some evidence has emerged indicating that salt from more natural sources may have some benefits. However, the body recognizes salt as salt, and I find it difficult to believe that natural sources of salt have a great deal to offer in protecting the body from the well-known blood pressure elevating effects of salt in general. Several natural agents have been proposed in playing a role in lowering blood pressure; they are listed in Table 8.2.

Ordinary table salt may have started from a natural salt source, but the processing methods strip it of its natural mineral companions. Normal salt is usually prepared from a saline solution that is kiln-dried at very high temperatures. In this process, many trace minerals with health-giving potential are lost. After drying, table salt has many chemical additives, including potassium iodide, silico aluminate, tri-calcium phosphate, magnesium carbonate, sodium bicarbonate, and yellow prussiate of soda. With the exception of iodide addition, these other agents are added to provide an ideal physical appearance to salt, to prevent caking, and to ensure free flow of the material through a salt shaker. It is interesting that additions have nothing to do with health but more to do with aesthetics, which make it easier for a consumer to get hooked on the salt habit.

The best way to break the salt habit may be to replace salt in your cooking with tasty herbs and spices. A number of true "salt-substitute" products are available. However, you should be aware that many salt substitutes do contain salt in the form of sodium chloride. I think most professional cooks will agree that the most creative combinations of spices and herbs that can be used as salt substitutes include onions, garlic, peppers, citrus peel, carrots, oregano, celery seed, marjoram, thyme, cumin, coriander, mustard, and rosemary. The creative use of herbs as salt substitutes can offer a great deal for cardiovascular health. Do not forget that many of these alternatives to salt are beneficial as well to cardiovascular health, especially garlic, celery, cumin, and rosemary. I suggest you become adventurous and try your own combinations as well as the salt-free herb and spice combinations available in most supermarkets.

One way or another, you can kick the salt habit. You should focus on eliminating salt at the table as well as in cooking. If you often eat in restaurants you may need to ask about the salt content of the food. Once you begin to cut back your salt intake, heavily salted food will not be particularly pleasant. Oriental food seems healthy because of its preponderance of vegetables. Chinese fast food, however, is often loaded with salt, as is the popular Japanese dish, miso.

Table 8.2: Nutrients and Natural Agents Capable of Lowering Elevated Blood Pressure.

Individuals with high blood pressure are recommended to seek medical advice and attention. Do not self-medicate to lower your own blood pressure.

Decreased sodium intake
Optimal potassium intake
Optimal zinc intake
Niacin
Vitamin C
Essential fatty acids, especially omega-3, fish oil
Bioflavonoids
Mushrooms (shiitake)
Taurine
Coenzyme Q10
Mistletoe (*Viscum album*)—toxicity is a problem
Black cohosh (*Cimicifuga racemosa*)
Hawthorne—toxic in high doses
Calcium
Magnesium
Celery seeds (toxic at high doses)

Salt and Potassium

The importance of restricting sodium intake has overshadowed the importance of optimal potassium intake for patients with elevated blood pressure. If potassium intake is not sufficient, the body is not able to secrete sodium efficiently; then, sodium and water retention occurs, elevating blood pressure. Modern medicine has focused on the use of diuretics (water pills) to rid the body of excessive salt and reduce blood pressure. However, many water pills cause potassium loss, and potassium conservation is important for normal cellular function in the body.

Unfortunately, some physicians may often ignore the issue of potassium supplements. Be aware that self-medication with potassium supplements is quite dangerous, especially if an individual has poor kidney function. If potassium builds up in the blood, then it may cause abnormal heartbeat and even cardiac arrest. However, it is quite easy to obtain potassium in the normal diet by drinking fruit juices or eating fruit that has a high potassium content. Several fruits are notably high in potassium and relatively low in sodium content. An outstanding source of dietary potassium is the banana. An average size banana contains approximately 500 mg. of potassium and only approximately 2 mg. of sodium. There have been some scientific studies that have looked at populations of individuals who eat bananas and some evidence that, on average, their blood pressure tends to be lower than populations that do not consume this fruit. Other good sources of potassium, with relatively low sodium content, include oranges, lemons, peaches, melons, potatoes, and lima beans.

Remember, too, that in addition to potassium, adequate calcium and magnesium intake is required to have normal blood pressure. A deficiency of magnesium, which is frequently found in people who drink excessive amounts of alcohol, can result in high blood pressure. Also, individuals who have a low calcium intake are prone to hypertension. Calcium supplements are a good addition to the diet of all adults, and they may play a special role in promoting health by helping to reduce osteoporosis (thin, brittle bones) in later life. Calcium is not the whole answer; soy isoflavones exhibit remarkable benefits in preventing and perhaps treating osteoporosis and indirectly in lowering blood pressure.

SUMMARY

Nutrition is key to prevention, and it may also contribute to *reversing* established coronary artery disease. While adopting a low-fat diet is not a cure-all, it provides a place to begin because the typical Western diet is currently high in hydrogenated and saturated fat. In general, fat should comprise no more than 30 percent of total daily calories, although some programs recommend an even lower percentage. However, the type of fat is at least as important as the total fat.

Remember that hydrogenated fats (primarily animal fats and processed vegetable fats) tend to promote atheroma, and monounsaturated and polyunsaturated fats, which are generally of plant origin, are not atherogenic. However, avoid the unsaturated fats that been hydrogenated and are made into a solid food product such as margarine.

While some diets have restricted animal protein and others call for all but eliminating carbohydrates, they have one thing in common—these diets recommend emphasizing *complex carbohydrates* and limiting overly refined foods. As a rule, avoid the "white" foods— white sugar, white bread, white pasta. The U.S. Food Pyramid emphasizes carbohydrates, but mistakenly; it does not stress the importance of eliminating these "white" foods. The pyramid philosophy also partially ignores the importance of good fats; *e.g.*, fish oils and healthful polyunsaturated vegetable oils.

Complex carbohydrates provide fiber, which is essential in a "heart-smart" diet. Both oat bran and soy fiber are viable options to help lower cholesterol. In addition, a diet adequate in both soluble and insoluble fiber may be protective against developing a variety of gastrointestinal disorders, diabetes mellitus, and colon cancer. Vegetable protein containing isoflarones (Genista) can lower cholesterol.

What You Can Do

- Shift your diet away from heavily salted, saturated fat-laden refined foods, including the readily available "fast foods," to one that includes more complex carbohydrates and moderate amounts of unsaturated fats from vegetable sources. Use salt sparingly.

- Avoid deep-fried foods because the beneficial effects of the most healthy fats are reversed by the oxidation and dehydration that takes place when fats are heated.
- "Fake fats" are just that, fake. Avoid them. Some people experience unpleasant gastrointestinal symptoms, including cramping and diarrhea, when they consume these foods.
- Even the proposed health benefits of red wine and olive oil can be destroyed if used to excess. A tablespoon of extra-virgin olive oil that is *cold-pressed*, rather than processed using heat, is a serving. There is no need to drink *any* alcohol, but if you do, one glass of red wine is a serving.
- Egg whites are an inexpensive source of high-quality protein, so it is not necessary to entirely eliminate eggs from your diet. Just use them in moderation.
- *Slowly, gradually*, add fiber to your diet. Your goal should be to consume 20 to 30 grams of fiber per day. However, if your diet has been low in fiber, you will experience unpleasant gastrointestinal symptoms if you suddenly consume large amounts of fiber.
- Bring pleasure back to your meals by eating slowly and enjoying your food. Meals should be a time to relax and enjoy the companionship of your family and friends.

CHAPTER NINE

VITAMINS AND SUPPLEMENTS

THE ALL-IMPORTANT VITAMINS

A great deal of work exists on the role of vitamins in the prevention or treatment of cardiovascular disease. Unfortunately, much of the data is conflicting. This confounds opinions. Some things can be said with a degree of certainty, however. For example, few health-care givers would argue against the notion that antioxidant vitamins (vitamins A, C, E, and so forth) exert a beneficial role in allaying atherosclerosis and heart disease. Considerable emphasis has also been placed on a form of one of the B vitamins, niacin, because of its cholesterol-lowering ability.

Nicotinic acid is the form of niacin that has been shown to lower cholesterol, and it may reduce the risk of heart attack and death. However, nicotinic acid—when given in significant amounts—has unpleasant side effects, such as flushing of the skin and itching. These adverse effects limit its use in treatment. It is not possible to consume enough niacin in food to have a beneficial therapeutic effect in fighting cardiovascular disease. You might consume 15 to 35 mg. of niacin a day, but you would need 1.5 to 3 *grams* of nicotinic acid a day to lower cholesterol. Nicotinic acid is available over-the-counter, but it should always be used with medical supervision because it has potential complications for certain people. One serious limitation of niacin therapy involves its use with individuals who are under treatment for Type II diabetes mellitus. In this situation, niacin may cause poor blood sugar control and increases in serum uric acid. Niacin is still used as a cholesterol-lowering agent, but for this purpose alone, it is actually obsolete. One saving grace for niacin is its ability to raise HDL while lowering LDL.

The Arrival of the Nutriceuticals

Many people take a multivitamin each day, and this is probably a good idea, although it is not a substitute for a balanced diet. You may take a vitamin supplement to make sure that your nutrient intake is balanced because you cannot be certain about the nutrient content of your food. This is a common practice in Western societies and can be

---

Table 9.1: Nutrients That Are Used in Dietary Supplements Which Lower Blood Cholesterol.

Some nutrients can be used to lower cholesterol with variable success. The author proposes that these nutrients be taken in food or dietary supplement form as an adjunct to a low-cholesterol diet to lower blood cholesterol. The most effective dietary supplements to lower cholesterol are soya protein, containing isoflavones, and fish oil, containing omega-3 series fatty acids. Dietary supplementation with Fisol and Genista (fish oil and soy protein supplements, respectively) are highly effective adjuncts to a low-cholesterol diet in lowering blood lipids. The products Fisol and Genista were formulated by the author. Fiber is strongly recommended for general health.

Nutrient		Comment
Soy protein containing isoflavones		Highly effective, safe, inexpensive. Lowers blood lipids with many ancillary health benefits.
Omega-3 series fatty acids (fish oils)		Safe, effective, palatable in an enteric coated, delayed-release format. Must be taken with cofactors to be effective.
Others		
Fiber	Iodine	Fiber is highly effective and health-giving, but unpalatable. Overall, the cholesterol-lowering actions of several of these nutrients are not as well-defined as they are for soy protein containing isoflavones or fish oil.
Garlic	Zinc	
Orotic acid	Lecithin	
Carnitine	Chromium	
Niacin (B3)	Selenium	
Vitamin C	Magnesium	

---

considered a self-care tool for preventing disease. However, more is not necessarily better, and excessive vitamin intake, especially of fat-soluble vitamins (A, D, E, and K) can be dangerous to health.

We enter the world of nutriceuticals when we use specific vitamins, minerals, or fractions of foods (*i.e.*, soy isoflavones, green tea extracts) for therapeutic purposes. Using nicotinic acid to lower cholesterol could be considered an example of using a nutriceutical, but when a disease is treated, the term "drug" has to be used. When you move into the realm of using nutriceuticals, it becomes important to seek medical advice from a health-care provider who is familiar with their use. It makes no sense to go to a physician who may have vast knowledge of pharmaceuticals but little knowledge of or even belief in the therapeutic use of vitamins, minerals, herbal remedies, and so forth. My advice to be cautious is in no way meant to diminish the potential benefit of an array of vitamins. Several vitamins have been shown to have a positive effect on both prevention and treatment of atherosclerosis (see Tables 9.2, 9.3, and 9.4). Vitamins C and E may have a special role because of their antioxidant effects, which require special consideration.

ANTIOXIDANTS VS. FREE RADICALS

The heart is quite susceptible to damage by free radicals, which are unstable and destructive molecules. This type of damage is sometimes referred to as oxidative stress. However, it should be understood that free-radical formation is a natural process itself. Free radicals are produced by normal metabolic processes, and even your healthful exercise program causes free-radical activity. Free radicals also result from exposure to polluted air, radiation, or any number of environmental factors. We have a built-in mechanism to handle free radicals and oxidative stress. The antioxidant nutrients are a premiere part of this natural system, and these nutrients are often called free-radical scavengers. These compounds are on a constant "search and destroy" mission.

Vitamin C is one of the best-known of the antioxidant vitamins. Considerable research has shown that this important nutrient has the ability to prevent oxidation of LDL and help the body clear LDL from the liver by transporting it into the bile, where it then can be excreted. In addition, vitamin C may help raise HDL, the "good" cholesterol.

Low levels of vitamins C and E in the bloodstream have been documented in some studies of patients who have suffered a heart attack. It is not clear whether a low level of these nutrients is involved in the onset of the event, or is perhaps a consequence of the heart attack itself. Vitamin C also may have a mild effect on lowering blood pressure. When I say "mild," I mean that it is not dramatic and does not mean that you can take vitamin C instead of blood pressure medication. Any efforts to lower blood pressure should be undertaken only with the supervision of your health-care provider.

Vitamin C has a number of benefits, including a potential ability to prevent cancer and a protective effect against cataracts. Overall, vitamin C promotes a healthy immune system and is essential to build health and prevent disease. The Recommended Daily Allowance (RDA) for vitamin C is 60 mg. a day, but as you may know, the RDA for any nutrient is a minimum in the sense that it is the amount necessary to prevent a deficiency disease—a *known* deficiency disease. This amount of vitamin C will prevent scurvy! While the "father" of vitamin C research, Dr. Linus Pauling, took as much as 18,000 mg. a day, that is probably more than you need to maintain your health and certainly more than you should take on your own. Typical therapeutic dosages range from 200 mg. to 1000 or 2000 mg. a day, although higher doses may be beneficial in some cases. Although vitamin C is extremely health-giving, its optimal dose remains poorly defined and it varies, depending on the reason for using it in vitanutrient therapy.

Vitamin E and a Healthy Heart

Another antioxidant vitamin is finally garnering the respect it deserves: vitamin E is making its way into the conventional medical practice, but this was not always the case. Two Canadian physicians and brothers, Evan and Wilfred Shute, are responsible for alerting the health-care community about the benefits of vitamin E. The doctors used vitamin E treatment extensively in their practice, and later, researchers began to corroborate the beneficial observations that they made in their research. It is now known that low vitamin E levels are linked with elevated blood pressure and high cholesterol. Like vitamin C, this nutrient prevents oxidation of LDL. When LDL and vitamin E are present together, LDL is resistant to oxidation. Vitamin E also is a natural anticlotting agent, and the higher the serum level of vitamin E, the less sticky the platelets become. Given all the evidence about vitamin E as a natural blood thinner, one has to wonder why it is not used universally in the treatment of patients with cardiac disease. Since vitamin E prevents, or slows down, plaque buildup in the

---

Table 9.2: Vitamin Effects on Atherosclerosis.

A summary of the putative role of some vitamins in the prevention or treatment of atherosclerosis. Readers are referred to a medical practitioner because of the potential danger of adverse effects from some vitamins in the presence of established cardiac disease.

Niacin	Lowers LDL and total cholesterol, and raises HDL; has side effects.
Folic acid	Supplementation may reduce plasma levels of homocysteine, an atherogenic amino acid.
Vitamin B6	B6 deficiency in animals results in atherosclerosis. Blood B6 levels fall in myocardial infarction, and supplementation of B6 may inhibit platelet aggregation and prolong clotting time.
Vitamin C	Blood and leucocyte C levels are decreased in atherosclerosis. Cholesterol-7-alpha-hydroxylase is vitamin C dependent. Vitamin C stimulates lipoprotein lipase and is required to hydroxylate proline, the principal amino acid in collagen.
Vitamin B12	Deficiency of B12 raises homocysteine levels, which fall with B12 supplements.
Vitamin E	Plasma levels of E are often lower in heart disease. Supplementation may increase HDL, prevent oxidation of LDL, reduce the size of a myocardial infarct, inhibit platelet adhesiveness, and stimulate endothelial repair. High doses of E are not recommended except under close medical supervision.
Vitamin D	Animal studies show deleterious effects of high doses of Vitamin D on blood vessels. Vitamin D should be used with caution in the presence of cardiovascular disease.

arteries as well as possibly raises levels of HDL, it is one of the pre-miere heart-smart nutrients.

Vitamin E comes in many forms, the most complete of which is d-alpha-tocopherol, which is the most biologically active. Natural vita-min E is preferred to synthetic vitamin E, but it is more expensive. It is also the form of vitamin E that has been used in many modern studies. Dosages of vitamin E vary according to need, but the average therapeutic dose is about 800 IUs a day. However, vitamin E at this level can tend to alter and even increase blood pressure in an unpre-dictable way. Hypertensive patients may need to refrain from taking vitamin E supplements in doses higher than 200 IU per day. Again, seek guidance from your own health-care provider.

The Power of Beta-Carotene

Along with vitamins C and E, beta-carotene is a powerful antioxidant nutrient that helps prevent LDL from damaging the arteries, perhaps by acting to prevent it from attaching to the artery wall. There is also a suggestion that when serum levels of beta-carotene (along with vita-mins C and E) are high, there may be a tendency for fewer adverse cardiac events. Additional work with beta-carotene shows that it may have a protective effect against stroke, and it strengthens the immune system, which may ultimately have implications for pre-venting cancer and perhaps treating patients with HIV or AIDS.

Beta-carotene is converted to vitamin A in the body. As you may know, vitamin A can be toxic at very high levels. However, beta-carotene is converted to vitamin A on an "as-needed" basis, so it is not as toxic as vitamin A at higher levels of intake. Beta-carotene is one of the carotenoid family, of which there are many members. The carotenoids are found in varying amounts in a variety of fruits and vegetables. It is unwise to count on supplements of beta-carotene alone because the benefits of the other carotenoids are not fully known. What is known about them makes it clear that the whole fam-ily has important functions in the body.

Carotenoids form a group of several hundred different com-pounds. While there is no RDA for these other carotenoids, that does not mean they are less important, but rather, it tells us that we lack information about them.

From Selenium to Glutathione, and NAC

An essential trace mineral, selenium is needed to produce *glutathione peroxidase*, a powerful antioxidant enzyme. In recent years, gluta-thione has been identified as one of the most important protective antioxidant agents—in this case, an enzyme. Vitamin E and selenium work synergistically, and vitamin E protects against selenium toxicity. The exact heart-protective mechanism of this mineral is not known, but epidemiologic studies show a relationship between low selenium levels and higher risk of heart disease. Selenium intake is measured in micrograms, and the RDA is 70 mcg. for men and 55 mcg. for women. The National Research Council states an optimal range of intake of 50 to 200 mcg. It is best to take selenium along with the other antioxidant nutrients, rather than alone.

Table 9.3: Mineral Effects on Atherosclerosis.

A summary of some of the effects of minerals on atherosclerosis. Self-medication with minerals is not advised in the cardiac patient.

Calcium	Calcium can decrease total cholesterol and triglycerides; calcium deficiencies or excesses of calcium can promote atherosclerosis. It is believed that calcium within cells is involved in atheroma formation.
Copper	Copper deficiency is associated with high blood cholesterol and decreased HDL. Copper is toxic in high doses.
Iron	Iron may contribute to atheroma formation.
Chromium	Chromium supplements may raise HDL and lower total blood cholesterol and LDL. Deficiency of chromium is a risk factor for arteriosclerosis.
Magnesium	Magnesium deficiency is more common than recognized. It can result in an increased risk of coronary disease, sudden cardiac heath, heart attack, and abnormal heart rhythm.
Selenium	Low blood levels of selenium predispose to atheroma.
Zinc	Atherosclerosis may reduce zinc blood levels. Zinc may exert both beneficial and untoward effects on blood lipids.

It is important to note the potential cardiac benefits of an amino acid, N-aceytl-cysteine—NAC. There is some evidence that NAC has potential benefits in the treatment of angina, in that it may enhance the effectiveness of nitroglycerine. It also may reduce oxidative stress that occurs in patients undergoing cardiac surgery; specifically, bypass surgery. NAC is another of the substances that has potential cardiovascular benefits when used under medically supervised conditions. Because NAC may aggravate diabetes, as well as have other side effects, I stress again the importance of seeking the help of a knowledgeable health-care practitioner and remembering that NAC supplements should not be casually used.

L-Carnitine

If you are a bodybuilder, you may have heard that L-carnitine helps build muscle tissue, but it has implications for cardiovascular health. L-carnitine is sometimes thought to be an amino acid, but it is rather a compound formed by the two amino acids, lysine and methionine. It appears that L-carnitine may help "fuel" a weak or failing heart by transporting fatty acids to the cells, where they can be used for energy. There have been reports that L-carnitine, in combination with coenzyme Q10, can bring about significant improvement in patients with congestive heart failure. In addition, it may help protect the heart during heart attack, meaning that it may help contain or limit the damage. As a preventive nutriceutical, it appears to help raise HDL and lower LDL and help lower triglycerides. There is no known optimal dose of L-carnitine at this time, but under supervision, L-carnitine in doses starting at about 500 mg. per day have been used successfully in cardiovascular problems, with dosages going as high as 2,000 mg.

COENZYME Q10: A POWERFUL ANTIOXIDANT

As you can see, vitamins and minerals are not the only sources of antioxidants. Some powerful antioxidants are components of common plants (see Chapter 12). Isoflavones, found in soybeans, are also antioxidant substances. One of the most powerful known antioxidants comes in the form of coenzyme Q10, or coQ10, and otherwise known as *ubiquinone*. Coenzyme Q10 is grabbing increasing attention as a beneficial nutriceutical for cardiovascular wellness.

The discovery of coenzyme Q10 was an important scientific breakthrough and brought researcher Peter Mitchell, Ph.D., a Nobel prize in chemistry in 1957. Its value as a preventive and therapeutic agent has been recognized in Europe and Japan (where virtually all the coQ10 is produced), but the conventional medical community in the U.S. has given it scant attention or recognition. This situation is rapidly changing, however, because information about coQ10 is appear-

Table 9.4: Nutrient Effects on Atherosclerosis.

Miscellaneous nutrients that exert a potential benefit on atherosclerosis. In many cases the evidence to support their use is incomplete.

L-Arginine	Supplementation may assist endothelial function in blood vessels.
N-Acetylcysteine	Administration has been reported to reduce lipoprotein(a).
Aspartic acid	A nebulous role with Mg^+ and K^+ in cardiac disease.
Beta-carotene	May reduce heart attacks in established coronary heart disease.
Bioflavanoids	Reduces platelet adhesiveness; antithrombotic.
Carnitine	May improve lipid metabolism and has an effect on myocardial energy expenditure.
Coenzyme-A	Uncertain, beneficial effect on blood lipids.
Coenzyme-Q10	Lipid-soluble antioxidant with protective effect against atheroma; reduces blood viscosity; cardioprotective.
Glycosamino-glycans	Anticoagulant and lipid-lowering effects.
Lecithin	May normalize blood lipids and reduce platelet aggregation. Effect on lipids is limited and probably related to linoleic acid content.

ing in medical literature—and, perhaps even more important, in the popular press. As a result, health-conscious consumers are asking their health-care providers about its function in the body.

In simple terms, an enzyme is a protein that acts as a catalyst to bring about chemical changes in other substances. A coenzyme can be considered a "helper" chemical in that its job is to enhance the action of enzymes. Coenzyme Q10 is found in every type of cell in the body except red blood cells. Its function is to help the cells convert oxygen into energy.

Our cells have energy producers—or energy centers—called mitochondria, the plural of mitochondrion. The mitochondria in a cell are like little factories that produce energy to sustain life. The mitochondria are constantly at work producing energy from the fuel our food provides, and they need coQ10 to do it efficiently. Cells in different parts of the body have different numbers of mitochondria, depending on the cell's specific requirement for energy. The heart has more mitochondria than any other organ because its demand for oxygen and energy is so great. When the heart muscle is weak, *i.e.*, lacking energy, it has a difficult time doing its job of pumping blood. If coQ10 works to increase energy to all the cells, then the benefits to the heart are obvious.

CoQ10 is known to be a powerful antioxidant, thereby giving it an important role in protecting the arteries from damage by LDL, the so-called bad cholesterol. In fact, this coenzyme may do this important job even better than vitamin E, and, in addition, help vitamin E work more efficiently. CoQ10 can increase energy in the heart, giving it great potential, or treat congestive heart failure, arrhythmia, and even heart attacks.

While coQ10 is not widely recommended by conventional physicians in the U.S., Karl Folkers, a scientist from the University of Texas, has studied coQ10 for over twenty years. His results have consistently shown that this coenzyme has important implications for fundamental treatment for heart disease. One of Dr. Folkers' studies showed that 72 percent of men and women with cardiovascular diseases showed a deficiency of coQ10. It is also believed that cholesterol-lowering drugs may interfere with the body's ability to produce coQ10. A study in the 1980s showed that 100 mgs. of coQ10 improved heart function of patients being treated for congestive heart failure.

In addition, there is increasing evidence that coQ10 can reduce the frequency of episodes of angina.

Other studies have shown that coQ10 is also useful for treating high blood pressure, diabetes, and lung diseases such as emphysema. In the course of research about coQ10, a positive side effect appeared in that it appears to play a role in preventing and treating gingivitis, the common gum disease that affects millions of people. Incidentally, poor dental hygiene and gum disease have been unequivocally associated with heart disease. The effect of coQ10 on gingival health may be one of many mechanisms of the positive cardiac benefits of this agent. The energizing effect of coQ10 in the body also helps enhance athletic performance. In general, coQ10 is reported to increase energy levels and decrease the fatigue that results from taking some medications, including the beta-blocker drugs that are commonly prescribed for heart disease and hypertension.

Because of its powerful ability as an antioxidant, coQ10 may play a role in protecting the body against cancer. The converse may be true as well, in that a deficiency of coQ10 has been associated with the occurrence of cancer. A study performed by Dr. Folkers revealed *deficiencies* in levels of coQ10 among a group of cancer patients with diverse types of cancers. As a group, breast cancer patients had the greatest deficiencies. CoQ10 has amazing versatility in cancer management. For example, it has been observed that coQ10 may reduce the toxic effects of certain chemotherapy drugs used in cancer treatment.

Dr. Stephen Sinatra, author of *The Coenzyme Q10 Phenomenon*, has treated thousands of cardiac patients with this coenzyme and has seen no significant adverse reactions. In fact, he describes some patients who needed to cut back on their dosage of the nutrient because they had *too* much energy! In some people, CoQ10 can cause symptoms of excessive stimulation, similar to caffeine, in which case, the dosage will need adjustment. On occasion, individuals report some indigestion or nausea, but this is usually corrected by changing the time of day the supplement is taken in relationship with meals. Dr. Sinatra believes that coQ10 will one day be recognized as an anti-aging nutrient, because of its ability to neutralize free radicals, its positive effect on the heart, and its neuroprotective function, meaning that it has a role in protecting tissue in the central nervous system from damage.

You may wonder where coQ10 comes from and how we ingested sufficient amounts of this nutrient before we even knew it existed! It is found in many foods, including eggs, red meat, organ meats, fish, some nuts, spinach, and broccoli. When coQ10 is used as a preventive or therapeutic agent, it is taken in supplement form in varying dosages, depending on the reason for using it.

Many experts believe we need 30 to 60 mgs. a day to maintain health, and therapeutic doses increase from that base point. However, I cannot with authority tell you how much coQ10 to take either to maintain health or treat any condition. It is important to note that there may be no benefit in supplementing with coQ10 when there is no deficiency. In medical literature, 120–180 mgs. a day are commonly mentioned for treating congestive heart failure and angina. To date, no dosage can be considered standard because this is not yet a standard treatment and a consensus about optimal dosages, even minimal amounts to maintain health, does not exist. Although I believe coQ10 is safe, and many millions of Japanese people take this supplement without harm, do not self-medicate, particularly if you are taking medications for heart conditions or other disorders. The prudent road is to seek the advice of a health-care provider who will monitor your condition and track your progress.

BEYOND ANTIOXIDANTS: THE ANTI-HOMOCYSTEINE NUTRIENTS

In a previous chapter I discussed the "homocysteine theory" of heart disease; as you learned, vitamins B6 and B12, together with folic acid, are critical in maintaining low levels of homocysteine, an amino acid that is a byproduct of protein metabolism. The amino acid methionine is the indirect source of homocysteine. The research into homocysteine has shown that it is present in higher than optimal levels in individuals with coronary artery disease; further, homocysteine itself can damage the walls of the blood vessels and encourage clotting of the blood.

The presence of high levels of homocysteine may result from a genetic flaw in the body system by which homocysteine is metabolized. With further research, we may learn if this genetic anomaly plays a role in premature heart disease, especially when no other cause can be identified; *i.e.*, high cholesterol levels, plaque formation, and so forth. Based on past research, this is a reasonable hypothesis. In 1992, a study published in *JAMA* stated that high homocysteine levels represented an independent risk factor for cardiovascular disease.

Equally important, however, is the knowledge that the essential micronutrients—folic acid, B6, and B12—have the ability to lower homocysteine levels. B vitamins are found in variable amounts in most standard daily vitamin pills. Vitamin formulations found in health food stores tend to have higher amounts of all the nutrients, including the B complex. In order to use them therapeutically, as nutriceuticals, regulated and consistent doses are required. The B vitamins are found in many foods, but if you are attempting to regulate homocysteine levels, supplements are required. In his book *Healthy Heart, Longer Life*, Joe Goldstrich, M.D., recommends a daily B vitamin supplement that includes 50–100 mg. of B6, 400–800 mcg. of folic acid, and 50–500 mcg. of B12. The other B vitamins are taken in 50 mg. doses, which exceeds the RDA. The use of B vitamins at these dosage levels is presumed to be safe. (These are guidelines only—check with your own health-care provider before self-medicating with these vitamins.) At very high levels, in the area of 1,000–2,000 mg. a day, B6 can be toxic.

Using B vitamins therapeutically is a sound practice, but it can be a difficult feat as well. It is one thing to take B vitamins at levels exceeding the RDA for prevention purposes, and quite another to attempt to lower homocysteine levels on your own. It is probably wise to have homocysteine levels checked and B vitamin and folic acid dosages then recommended based on the results. Periodic testing then establishes if the vitamin therapy is working.

The discovery of the link between elevated homocysteine and cardiovascular disease represents an exciting development in preventive medicine. You will no doubt hear more about the role of B vitamins in lowering homocysteine, and I urge you to discuss this issue with your health-care providers, whether you believe you are at risk for early heart disease or not. I also recommend that you eat a diet that favors unrefined and minimally processed foods. B vitamins are found in varying quantities in many foods, but they can be destroyed in processing. One forgotton area is the use of food that is biotransformed by fermentation. The process of fermentation with yeasts tends to load food with available vitamins, especially B-class. I believe that part of the health benefit of soy described in population studies in Eastern Asia is due to the use of fermented foods, especially soybeans.

TMG: ANOTHER IMPORTANT COMPOUND

The B vitamins just discussed, along with the chemical trimethylglycine (TMG) represent a group of nutrients involved in methylation, a physiologic process that works to protect the body from disease. Through methylation the methyl groups—a particular type of molecule—adhere to certain chemicals in the body, thereby either protecting or changing them. Methyl groups are involved in converting potentially harmful homocysteine to the more beneficial amino acid methionine. One of its benefits is that it produces a chemical that is a natural antidepressant. TMG, which is found in broccoli, spinach, and beets, enhances methylation, making these foods important additions to a health-building diet.

THE MAGNESIUM BALANCE

Magnesium is necessary for energy production in every cell. In addition, it has the important job of balancing the physiological activity of potassium and calcium in the body. There is evidence that magnesium can help the heart withstand heart attack, and some studies have shown that magnesium, if given at the time of the initial cardiac event, results in a reduced death rate several weeks after the event. Scandinavian and Israeli studies showed the beneficial outcome of administering magnesium during heart attacks in double-blind, controlled clinical studies.

Magnesium may have a role in normalizing blood lipid levels, and animal studies have shown that supplementing the diet with magnesium can assist in reducing the severity of atherosclerosis. A most important feature of magnesium is its role in maintaining normal heart rhythm. Magnesium deficiencies are associated with cardiac arrhythmias, which are life-threatening situations. However, excessive magnesium can also alter heart function, so the amount used is critical. Magnesium supplementation has also shown some benefit for patients with peripheral vascular disease and in patients with congestive heart failure.

The RDA of magnesium is 350 mg. per day for men (280mg./day for women), and it is likely that a typical Western diet may be deficient in this mineral. This is especially true among people using diuretics. With the exception of an individual with kidney disease, including kidney failure, magnesium supplements are generally considered safe. However, magnesium intake must be balanced with adequate calcium intake in the diet.

Calcium is important for, among other things, regulating blood pressure (as is magnesium). It also may play a role in raising HDL and lowering LDL. Calcium, magnesium, potassium, and sodium are of critical importance, but they must be used in balanced amounts. There is an ongoing fluctuation and "balancing act" in the body that regulates these minerals. For this reason, supplementation with these minerals should be supervised.

DR. STEPHEN LEVINE, PH.D., AND HIS COLLEAGUES ON THE "COMPLETE HEART"

Dr. Stephen Levine is a biochemist par excellence and a pioneer of nutriceutical therapies. He has made many major contributions to the field of antioxidant research and has applied his expertise in formulating several valuable biopharmaceutical preparations. Many of his products are the mainstay of dispensation in professional practices in the U.S. that focus on nutritional medicine and remedies of natural origin. It is apparent in this chapter that there are many different cardiovascular functions that can be supported by a complex array of biopharmaceuticals and nutrients. Of all combination products available in dietary supplement format, I have been impressed by the systematic approach to the formulation of Dr. Levine's "Complete Heart" formula that is produced by NutriCology of

Hayward, California. This product is for use by physicians engaged in preventing or treating heart problems.

The Levine formula teaches us a great deal about the power of combined nutrients in the promotion of cardiovascular health. The areas of concern that are addressed by Dr. Levine in the nutritional support of cardiovascular function include: general nutrition, energy production (ATP), homocysteine metabolism, antioxidant function, maintenance of serum viscosity, and vascular health. Dr. Levine recommends a wide range of supplements to provide general nutritional support for cardiovascular function and specific agents to promote certain physiological functions.

Many people, including physicians, are concerned about the balance of nutrients that are available in a consistent manner in the average diet. "Complete Heart" is almost a "one-stop shop" for many essential vitanutrients to support cardiovascular function. The formula contains vitamins, minerals, amino acids (largely from soy), essential fatty acids, and other agents that should be used only under medical supervision.

My residual concern about this and other "complete" formulas is the need to monitor this therapy because of its content of a number of agents that are not entirely suitable for self-medication. In this regard, my concerns about "Complete Heart" for self-medication exist because of its content of hawthorn berry, DHEA, and pregnenolone. I am not a supporter of self-medication with hormones or hormone precursors, and I refer the reader back to Chapter 2 as to the reasons why. I express strong antagonistic opinions about self-medication with hormones in my book *The Sexual Revolution,* but I accept that they may be valuable when used under medical supervision.

SUMMARY

Vitamin and mineral supplements are not a substitute for a healthy, balanced diet. However, certain nutrients are recognized as having a role in preventing and treating heart disease. Nicotinic acid, a form of niacin, one of the B vitamins, has the ability to lower cholesterol, but to be effective, it must be used in fairly large doses. Therefore, it should be taken only under medical supervision.

In recent decades a group of vitamins, minerals, and other substances have been identified as antioxidant nutrients. This means that they can prevent damage done by unstable molecules called *free radicals*. Antioxidant nutrients, which include vitamins C and E, beta-carotene, the trace mineral selenium, coenzyme Q10, and many other substances, are nature's "search and destroy" forces. They aid in the natural process of "scavenging" for free radicals and preventing oxidative stress on the body. In addition, vitamin C may help raise HDL, the "good" cholesterol, and lower LDL, the "bad" cholesterol. Vitamin E may help regulate blood pressure and work as a kind of natural blood thinner.

Low levels of magnesium, calcium, and the B vitamins folic acid, B6, and B12 are also linked to heart disease, and optimal levels of these nutrients may help prevent—and may help treat—heart disease.

What You Can Do

- Nutrients tend to work synergistically in the body. Do not favor one antioxidant or one B vitamin at the expense of other important vitamins and minerals.
- Take nutrients in doses that greatly exceed the Recommended Daily Allowance only under supervision of a knowledgeable health-care provider. Excessive doses of vitamins and minerals can be as harmful as nutritional deficiencies.
- Educate yourself about the role of individual nutrients, including those that are emerging as important for cardiovascular health. In the coming years, you are likely to hear more about the value of coQ10, the enzyme glutathione, and one of its relatives, NAC (N-aceytl-cysteine). L-carnitine and the chemical trimethylglycine have value as cardioprotective agents. These substances have various positive effects on the cardiovascular system.

CHAPTER TEN

THE OMEGA FACTORS

Essential fatty acids—the omega factors—are essential for health. Scientists are struggling to precisely define and describe the health benefits of specific types of fatty acids. Studies of fatty acid metabolism have led to Nobel prizes, and more await the scientists who clarify these issues. A Pulitzer prize probably awaits the person who can explain the facts about these valuable fats in a language that everyone can understand! In actuality, understanding the importance of omega-3 and -6 essential fatty acids (EFA) in the diet is hard work, even for health-care professionals. But before you decide to skip this chapter, pause a moment and consider that essential fatty acid deficiency is probably one of the most important—but overlooked—influences on cardiovascular and general health. It is estimated that 80 percent of the population of Western countries consume insufficient quantities of certain types of EFA in their diet. EFA deficiencies may be more important than vitamin deficiencies. Obviously, since fat intake is generally thought to be too high in our society, it is clear that the solution to the fat dilemma is more complex than just "going low fat."

The medical world has yet to tip its cap to the pioneers of lateral thought in the field of essential fatty acid research, but the list of these individuals is distinguished and includes: Udo Erasmus, Dr. Edward N. Siguel, Dr. Caroline Shreeve, Dr. David Horrobin, Dr. Michael Schmidt, and Dr. Michael T. Murray. The layperson's knowledge about the so-called "good fats" has been greatly expanded because of their work.

NOT ALL FATS ARE BAD

First, remember that fat is not a dirty word, although it has been regarded as such by many health-conscious individuals. This unfortunate assumption overlooks the importance of essential fats as health-giving nutrients, and it has helped to lead us to a modern dietary deficiency state of EFA. In fact, essential fatty acids are called *essential* because they are necessary for health, must be obtained from dietary sources, and cannot be synthesized by the body. It was determined in the 1930s that the omega-6 and omega-3 fatty acids were essential, so this is not recent news.

In our quest to reduce overall fat in the diet, we have overlooked EFAs. So, while it is quite clear that saturated fat has a role in the cause of a variety of common killer diseases, the role of certain fats in the promotion of health is still clouded. Fats are as important as carbohydrates and protein in maintaining health and preventing disease. As Dr. Michael Schmidt points out in his book *Smart Fats*, 60 percent of the structure of the brain—the most complex organ in the body—is fatty material. The notion of "feeding your head" with EFA (especially docosahexaenoic acid, DHA) is well-founded.

The conventional wisdom is that the person who wants to prevent cardiovascular disease or certain types of cancer should avoid fat in the diet. While saturated fat of animal origin is associated with cardiovascular disease and some cancers—colon and breast cancers, in particular—certain types of unsaturated fats are associated with the prevention or treatment of cardiovascular disease and cancer. This is the nature of the confusing situation we currently face.

The omega-6 and omega-3 series fatty acids are the two most important categories of EFAs. Omega-6 series fatty acids are ubiquitous in the diet and are found in vegetables, whereas omega-3 fatty acids are found largely in fish and marine mammals. Certain legumes, such as soybeans, also contain significant amounts of the precursors of omega-3 fatty acids. Flax seeds are also sources of omega-3 fatty acid precursors, and the coarsely ground seeds or prepared oils are increasing in availability as information about the health benefits of EFAs becomes more widely known. One of the biggest misconceptions that has been propagated by the dietary industry is that flax (seed or oil) is a reliable source of omega-3 fatty acids. It contains precursors of omega-3 that cannot always be made readily available for use by the body. Please consider dropping flax for fish oil. The science favors fish oil use.

Within these omega-3 and -6 series, there are several varieties or types of fatty acids. The two most important omega-3 fatty acids with health-giving benefits are eicosapentaenoic acid (EPA) and docosahexaenoic acid (DHA). These are the major active components of fish oil. (Fatty acids have such complex names that a virtual "alphabet soup" of abbreviations has developed.)

A BRIEF CHEMISTRY LESSON

Fats may be solid or liquid, and the key chemical structure of a fat includes one molecule of glycerol, with three fatty acid molecules attached. Fatty acids come in various sizes, and their chemical nature determines their overall structure. Neutral fat, or *triglycerides*, circulate in the bloodstream. These substances contain fatty acids and are found in fat stores throughout the body. Fatty acids are part of the principal structural components of cells. They help form the membranes of the cell walls and the intracellular walls that surround cellular components (organelles), such as mitochondria or lysosomes. These organelles within cells of the body are key sites that are responsible for body metabolism.

A saturated fatty acid is one in which the bonds between the carbon atoms in the molecule contain a shared pair of electrons to form a single bond. In contrast, unsaturated fatty acids contain double bonds. In broad general terms, saturated fatty acids are found within the less healthful types of fats, whereas unsaturated fatty acids are found within the more healthful types of fats. Saturated fatty acids occur mainly in food of animal origin, whereas unsaturated fats tend to be found in food of vegetable origin.

The presence of a double bond in the unsaturated type of fat is key to understanding fats. Unsaturated fatty acids tend to be more active chemically and capable of reacting with a variety of chemical substances that crop up in metabolic processes in the body. These metabolic processes, which involve reactive, unsaturated fatty acids, include reactions with oxygen, sulfur (to form sulfhydryl groups), or water (to form hydroxyl groups).

The term polyunsaturated fatty acid merely refers to unsaturated fatty acids that have two or more double bonds within the molecule. The general use of the term "polyunsaturated" fat applies to omega-6 fatty acids, which are found in vegetable oils that are used often in food and cooking. In contrast, omega-3 fatty acids are often referred to as "superunsaturated" fatty acids to distinguish them from the garden-variety omega-6 type fatty acids. There is a general belief that increasing the dietary intake of polyunsaturated fatty acids in the diet is an ideal goal. Overall, however, this is not beneficial, because it has led to the consumption of polyunsaturated fats, generally of the omega-6 type, at the expense of the omega-3 factors (EPA and DHA). If anything, the Western diet is overabundant in omega-6 type fats, and we shall learn that the ratio of intake in the diet of omega-6 and omega-3 fatty acids is important. The omega-3 fatty acids EPA and DHA play a pivotal role in protecting the body against cardiovascular disease.

WHAT FATTY ACIDS DO

Fatty acids are very efficient sources of energy for the body. One gram of fat contains more energy than one gram of carbohydrates or protein. About nine calories of energy are derived from the body burning one gram of fat, whereas only five calories come from burning one gram of carbohydrate. Fats may be the most efficient source of energy, but excess fat intake can readily lead to excess pounds of body weight. This is why it is so important to avoid the wrong kind of fats, which are easy to find, and eat sensibly the healthier varieties, which are conspicuous by their absence in refined foods. Snack foods taste good because of their unhealthy fat content, most notably saturated fats and hydrogenated oils. Junk food is often a "sinful delight" for body function.

Fatty acids are described in terms of "chains of atoms," which relates to their chemical complexity. Longer fatty chains require

Table 10.1: Effects of Essential Fatty Acids and Prostaglandins on Body Function.

- The normal function of the immune system
- Formation of substrates for hormone production and effector properties
- Regulation of blood pressure by involvement in vascular tone and collateral circulations
- Regulation of responses to pain, inflammation, infection, and cancer
- Control of glandular secretions and their composition
- Regulation of smooth muscle and neural function
- Cell membrane structure and mitosis of cells
- Regulation of cell oxygenation and nutrient intake
- Provision of energy substrates for key organs

more complex mechanisms of digestion and metabolism than do shorter length fatty acid chains. Saturated fatty acids containing less than sixteen carbon atoms are used more preferentially as an energy source by the body than fatty acids of a length between sixteen and eighteen carbon atoms. These longer-length fatty acids are used most often to construct cell membranes or to provide a substrate—a foundation, of sorts—for the body to convert to unsaturated fatty acids of different types.

One of the most important functions of omega-3 and omega-6 essential fatty acids is that they are the precursors for hormonal compounds, especially prostaglandins. (A precursor is a substance that is needed for another substance to form or to be used.) Prostaglandins are a type of hormone-like substances that play a major role in maintaining body structure, function, and homeostasis. In Table 10.1, I have summarized the roles of essential fatty acids and prostaglandins in body metabolism.

THE ESSENTIAL NATURE OF THE ESSENTIAL FATTY ACIDS

If an essential fatty acid is not consumed in the diet, a deficiency will result in exactly the same way that other nutritional deficiencies result as a consequence of an unbalanced diet. The most common

Table 10.2: The Role of Omega-3 and Omega-6 Fatty Acids as Precursors of Compounds That Are Necessary for Healthy Body Functions.

Obviously, this is a simplified version, but I present it to help you more easily understand this complex issue.

Family	Omega-3 Fatty Acids	Omega-6 Fatty Acids
Principal precursors found mainly in vegetables	Linolenic acid (omega-3)	Linoleic acid (omega-6)
Fatty acid derivatives found mainly in animals (6) or fish (3)	DHA, EPA	GLA, DGLA, and arachidonic acid
Prostaglandins	Type 3 and less inflammatory leukotrienes	Type 2 and leukotrienes

health-building types of polyunsaturated fats in the Western diet are of vegetable origin, and these fats often contain omega-6 fatty acids. In contrast, only a relatively small quantity of the Western diet contains omega-3 fatty acids. Omega-3 fatty acids, in their most biologically active form, are found predominately in fish and marine mammals; *i.e.*, saltwater fish and shellfish of cold-water origin. In Table 10.2, I have summarized the importance of omega-3 and omega-6 types of fatty acids as precursor molecules. For cardiovascular health, we need to think omega-3 more than omega-6 in broad, general terms.

Sources of Essential Fatty Acids

Remember that the "omegas" are families, and just like any other family, they have members with individual names, which brings us back to the "alphabet soup." The omega-3 family of fatty acids includes:

- alpha-linolenic acid (LNA)
- stearidonic acid (SDA)
- eicosopentaenoic acid (EPA)
- docosahexaenoic acid (DHA)

Although omega-3 fatty acids are primarily found in marine sources, some (mainly precursors) are found in plants, especially seeds. LNA is found in oils derived from flax, hemp seed, soybean, canola, walnut, pumpkin seed, candlenut, and other plants with dark-green leaves. In common with LNA, SDA is found in several seeds of wild plants, and SDA is a significant constituent of black currant oil. In contrast, EPA and DHA are found only in oils of marine origin, such as those found in cold-water fish and marine mammals. In general, EPA and DHA are the "active or "reactive" types of omega-3 fatty acids required for health.

Some mammals are minor sources of EPA and DHA, too, and include foods that are normally termed "offal." These are animal organs, such as the pancreas, adrenal glands, brain tissue, and gonadal tissue. In some cultures, offal is considered a delicacy. Unfortunately, offal is loaded with cholesterol and unwanted hormones and should be avoided as a regular part of the diet. The sources of different types of essential fatty acids and their derivatives in the diet are shown in Table 10.3.

Table 10.3: Dietary Sources of Essential Fatty Acids and Their Derivatives.

Essential Fat & Derivatives	Type of EFA	Food	Source
Linoleic	Omega-6	Vegetable oils, seeds, and nuts	Sunflower Walnut Soybean
Linolenic	Omega-3	Vegetable oils, seeds, and nuts	Linseed Walnut Soybean
Arachidonic	Omega-6	Mainly meat	Liver, muscle (steak)
GLA	Omega-6	Dietary supplements	Evening primrose, borage oil, black-currant oil, and pumpkin seed oil
EPA, DHA	Omega-3	Fish oil	Cold-water fish

Tracing the Origin of the Health Benefit of Fish Oils

The health benefit of fish oils has been recognized for a long time. Many children in the past two centuries have choked after swallowing a teaspoon of cod liver oil! Why did parents of the past think that this oil was a healthy tonic for a child?

At least in part, we can trace the answer to studies of the disease profile of populations that ingest large quantities of omega-3 fatty acids in fish oil. For example, Eskimo populations living under traditional conditions have a very high consumption of fat and protein in the diet, but a remarkably low incidence of cardiovascular disease. In fact, the Inuit language contains many words to describe snow, but no word to describe heart disease! It is of interest that the term "Eskimo" means "eaters of raw meat." Inuits, or Eskimos (natives of Greenland), in their natural habitat live largely upon both raw and cooked flesh and fat derived from fish or marine mammals, such as seals. Marine mammals and fish of cold-water origin are the most abundant source of the EPA and DHA members of omega-3 fatty acid family. I must stress that fish oil is a much better source of omega-3 fatty acids than plant or vegetable oils derived from flax, soybeans, and hemp. I believe it to be superior also to algae, as a source of omega 3 fatty acids.

Much of the current research interest in the health benefits of omega-3 fatty acids resulted from these epidemiological investigations. Eskimos rarely die of cardiovascular disease, despite the high fat, high cholesterol, low carbohydrate diet that typifies their existence—at least in their native habitat. Other differences appear when we compare the disease profiles of the Eskimo and members of Western society. These differences include a relatively low prevalence among the Inuit population of inflammatory bowel disease, arthritis, and other degenerative disorders.

Unfortunately, contemporary data on the epidemiology of disease in the Inuit population shows a shift away from the lower incidence of such disease states. This change has happened as these populations have moved toward a Westernized diet, along with the general introduction of some less desirable Western lifestyle habits.

Recent Studies on the Health Benefits of Fish Oil

If there was a single dietary supplement to consider for cardiovascular health, it would be fish oil—but contemporary accounts of its benefits have received far less attention and application than they deserve. Many studies published in leading medical journals have demonstrated that fish oils are effective in preventing arteriosclerosis, favorably altering blood lipids, and reducing blood pressure. In addition, several recent studies have convinced me that fish oil offers safe and effective treatment for several "untreatable" disorders such as rheumatoid disease and inflammatory bowel disease (*e.g.*, Crohn's disease).

In his book *The New Super Nutrition*, Richard Passwater has drawn attention to the ability of fish oil to lower blood pressure. Passwater cites a study at Brompton Hospital in London where sixteen patients with mild hypertension were shown to have lowered blood pressure over a six-week period in a placebo-controlled crossover study. Fifty milligrams of fish oil taken daily—a relatively modest dose—was found to produce modest reductions in systolic blood pressure. This research indicated that fish oil supplementation of the diet could provide a safe, acceptable therapy for patients with mild hypertension, where systolic (the higher, first number expressed in a blood pressure reading) hypertension was preponderant. Studies at Vanderbilt University in Tennessee also have found similar results, and many other observations of the hypotensive effects of fish oil exist.

One of the most complete descriptions of the health benefits of EFAs is found in the book *Fats That Heal, Fats That Kill,* by Udo Erasmus. Erasmus indicates the importance of EFAs, especially for promoting cardiovascular wellness and healthy neurological functioning. He reports that the omega-3 fatty acids (EPA and DHA) can be synthesized in humans relatively slowly from linolenic acid (LNA). Linolenic acid is a polyunsaturated fatty acid that is found predominantly in safflower, sunflower, corn, sesame, soybeans, walnuts, flax seeds, and pumpkin seeds. Seeds are abundant sources of omega-3 and omega-6 acids; I have summarized these in Table 10.4. It should be recognized that vegetable sources of omega-3 factors are not as reliable as fish oil. Fish oil contains EPA and DHA, and plant sources of omega-3 EFAs are largely precursor molecules of omega-3 factors.

The Importance of EPA and DHA

The omega-3 fatty acids (EPA and DHA) are *superunsaturated* fatty acids that help disperse aggregations of saturated fatty acids, which form plaque deposits in arterial blood vessels. In other words, these fatty acids can reduce the effects of harmful fats and help prevent

Table 10.4: Seeds and Fatty Acids.

This information is modified from the book by Udo Erasmus, *Fats That Heal, Fats That Kill*. While I have not undertaken a formal cost-effective analysis on the health benefits of seed oils, I believe that fresh soybean oil may be very cost-effective as a source of essential oils because it is cheap and ubiquitous.

Name	Fat Content (%)	18:3ω3*	18:2ω6*	18:1ω9*	18:0*	16:0*
Hemp	35.0	20	60	12	2	6
Flax	35.0	58	14	19	4	5
Pumpkin	46.7	0–15	42–57	34	0	9
Soybean	17.7	7	50	26	6	9
Walnut	60.0	5	51	28	5	11
Wheat germ	10.9	5	50	25	18	
Evening primrose	17.0		81	11	2	6
Safflower	59.5		75	13	12	
Sunflower	47.3		65	23	12	
Grape	20.0		71	17	12	
Corn	4.0		59	24	17	
Sesame	49.1		45	42	13	
Rice bran	10.0	1	35	48	17	
Rape (canola)	30.0	7	30	54	7	
Peanut	47.5		29	47	18	
Almond	54.2		17	78	5	
Olive	30.0		8	76	16	
Avocado	12.0		10	70	20	
Coconut	35.3		3	6		91
Palm kernel	35.3		2	13		85
Beech	50.0		32	54	8	
Brazil	66.9		24	48	24	
Pecan	71.2		20	63	7	
Pistachio	53.7		19	65	9	
Hickory	68.7		17	68	9	

*These notations are chemical shorthand—18:2ω6 means 18 carbon atoms, 2 double bonds methylene interrupted, where the first double bond starts at the ω6 carbon atom, which is the sixth carbon from the methyl (ω) end of the molecule.

the build-up of plaque in the arterial walls.

One of the most important functions of EPA is that it is the precursor of the type of prostaglandins (largely the type-3 family) that have beneficial cardiovascular effects, including potent anticlotting activity. The omega-3 fatty acids found in fish oil are very important in terms of their function as a substrate for the production of prostaglandins. Since prostaglandins play a variety of important roles in the modulation of acute and chronic disease, you can logically see why it is important to have a supply of the substance that is needed to produce them.

In addition to promoting cardiovascular health, several authorities have described beneficial effects of fish oils for treating inflammatory bowel disease, rheumatoid arthritis, psoriasis, migraine headaches, visual disturbance, cancer prevention, and even yeast infections. The potential health benefits of omega-3 fatty acids are legion, and you can understand them better when you have a grasp of the biochemical functions of essential fatty acids in general.

A BRIEF OVERVIEW OF ESSENTIAL FATTY ACIDS

The most important EFAs to consider are *linoleic acid* (LA), *alpha-linolenic acid* (LNA), and the two classic fish oil fatty acids, EPA and DHA, previously discussed. Linoleic acid is an omega-6 polyunsaturated fatty acid found in many vegetable seeds. Omega-6 fatty acids, like omega-3 fatty acids, can promote cardiovascular and general health.

The health benefits of linoleic acid are the focus of intense research, but their effects and potential benefits for health are still underexplored. However, we do know that the manifestations of linoleic acid deficiency are protean and include: skin disorders, such as eczema or hair loss; liver dysfunction; kidney disorders; central nervous system disorders, including behavioral problems; failure of certain immune function with susceptibility to infections; potent adverse effects on reproductive functions, including sterility in males and miscarriage in females; bone and joint disorders; cardiovascular disease; retarded growth; and failing glandular functions. Some of these disorders have been encountered in patients who have been placed on long-term parenteral feeding (feeding via the intravenous route), where LA was deficient in the administered solutions.

As I stated, LA research is ongoing and, to date, is still somewhat poorly defined, but it is likely that a spectrum of disorders of varying severity may occur as a consequence of varying degrees of LA deficiency. In Table 10.5, I have summarized the many signs, symptoms, and disorders that can be attributed to essential fatty acid deficiency.

Alpha-linolenic acid (LNA) is an example of a superunsaturated fatty acid of the omega-3 type. The term superunsaturated is used to distinguish LNA from LA. Keep in mind that LNA is an omega-3 fatty acid, whereas LA is an omega-6 fatty acid. This distinction is important because the health implications of omega-6 and omega-3 fatty acids and their effects may be quite different in many circumstances.

The results of a deficiency of LNA are as complex as those of LA. LNA has been associated with cardiovascular disease, central nervous system changes, behavioral problems, paraesthesia ("pins and needles" in the arms and legs), motor incoordination, muscle weakness, impaired learning ability, loss of visual acuity, and retarded growth.

When you look at these potential problems resulting from deficiencies of these essential fatty acids, you may see that they influence an amazing array of functions in the body, not the least of which are neurologic in nature. While EFA deficiencies can affect all age groups, it is striking that they are linked to conditions that affect the

---

Table 10.5: Signs, Symptoms, and Disorders Attributed to Essential Fatty Acid Deficiency (LA and LNA variably).

The reader is cautioned that these problems are not specific to fatty acid deficiency and may occur due to other reasons.

Chronic fatigue—all symptoms encountered in chronic fatigue syndrome
Mental changes—depression, poor motivation, poor higher central nervous system function, and, perhaps, dementia
Reduced function of the immune system
Cancer and neurological disease
Cardiovascular disease, angina, high blood pressure, poor exercise tolerance
Frequent infections; *e.g.*, colds and flu
Bone and joint problems; *e.g.*, arthritis
Gastrointestinal upset—flatulence, constipation, and bloating
Dry skin, dry hair, cracked nails, and dry mucous membranes, *e.g.*, eyes, mouth, and vagina

very young and may even influence their intellectual and emotional functioning. These deficiencies are linked to the elderly population, too. So, Dr. Schmidt did not name his book *Smart Fats* for nothing!

It is reasonable to assume that a deficiency of LNA may resemble, to some degree, a deficiency of EPA and DHA. It should be noted that these deficiencies generally tend to occur together. Deficiencies of omega-3 fatty acids in general may tend to result in: hypertriglyc-eridemia, high blood pressure, a tendency to form blood clots due to platelet stickiness, inflammation in a variety of body tissues, skin disorders (especially dry skin), tissue swelling (edema), deterioration in mental function, and general disorders of immune or metabolic functions in the body.

You may wonder why you have not heard more about fatty acid deficiencies and why the lay public has not been made aware that such a deficiency is even possible. As you can see from the list of possible consequences these symptoms can be caused by many factors, and there are no easily identifiable, specific classic symptoms of omega-3 fatty acid deficiency. However, as the information about essential fatty acids continues to accumulate, many authorities now recognize that essential fatty acid deficiency, especially a deficiency of omega-3 fatty acids, is much more common than was hitherto suspected. Equally important, evidence has emerged that many of the negative effects of essential fatty acid deficiency (including omega-3 fatty acid deficiency) can be reversed merely by adding essential fatty acids from fish oil to the diet in supplemental form. I believe strongly that omega-3 fatty acid deficiency in Western diets is at the root of the cause of common diseases such as depression and atherosclerosis.

PUTTING ESSENTIAL FATTY ACIDS IN PATHWAYS

It is clear that essential fatty acids are needed for many metabolic functions—we could call this their metabolic fate, which they meet after traveling through pathways. (For those who are interested in more scientific explanations, I have summarized the metabolic pathways of omega-3 and omega-6 fatty acids in Table 10.6.) The end result of the pathways of metabolism is prostaglandin production. The

Table 10.6: Metabolic Pathways of Omega-3 and Omega-6 Fatty Acids and Their Role in the Production of Prostaglandins and Leukotrienes (Simplified).

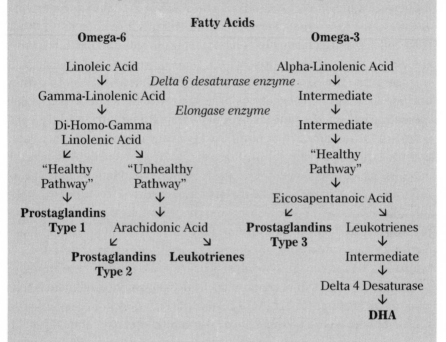

Table 10.7: Major Precursor Pathways of Type 1 (Healthy), Type 2 (Unhealthy), and Type 3 (Healthy) Prostaglandins.

The terms "healthy" and "unhealthy" are relative. There is no inter-changeability between the omega-6 and omega-3 pathways; this is the "family rule."

Cis-Linoleic acid omega-6	Type 1 prostaglandins (and indirectly type 2)
Arachidonic acid from omega-6	Type 2 prostaglandins and leukotrienes
Alpha-Linolenic acid omega-3	Type 3 prostaglandins and less inflammatory types of leukotrienes

types or families of prostaglandins and related compounds that are produced have an important bearing on health and disease.

Imagine the pathways as a complex series of roads where automobiles are merging into lines of traffic. One car can compete with another; one route may be blocked, but the other may be open. Each road must be driven on the "correct" side. Many factors determine the end product of the pathways.

The main feature of essential fatty acid metabolism is that they become active in body functions after their transformation into intermediates and prostaglandins or leukotrienes. Leukotrienes are compounds that are somewhat similar to prostaglandins. A "family rule" operates here, in that only omega-6 fatty acids will produce the omega-6 progeny of Type 1 or 2 prostaglandins and leukotrienes of an inflammatory nature. The best route for omega-6 precursors to take for health is the pathway towards the more health-giving Type 1 prostaglandins. These statements are oversimplifications, but are useful ways of unraveling the health benefits of certain types of EFA.

In the same way, only omega-3 precursors produce the omega-3 "daughter and cousin" compounds, most of which are favorable in their health benefits. Table 10.7 summarizes a simple sequence to remember in terms of the fate of the major omega-6 and -3 precursors. There is no interchangeability between the pathway of omega-6 and omega-3 fatty acids. This lack of "crossover" results in circumstances where the balance of omega-6 and omega-3 fatty acids in the diet is of major importance. I stress the notion of the balance between omega-6 and -3 EFA. This balance is very important for health.

The terms healthy and unhealthy are applied to *prostaglandin type*, which are expressed as numbers. These types are relative terms to describe the physiological or pathophysiological properties of each type of prostaglandins. Types 1 and 3 are generally regarded as the healthy types of prostaglandins, whereas Type 2 is a relatively unhealthy type.

Type 1 prostaglandins tend to reduce blood-clotting when compared with Type 2 prostaglandins. Furthermore, Type 2 prostaglandins are abundant in the presence of cardiovascular disease, hypertension, and cerebrovascular disease (strokes), whereas Type 3 prostaglandins work to block some of these unhealthy consequences. The effects of different types of prostaglandins are very complex in view of the number of different types and subtypes of these "hormone-like" substances.

GOOD AND BAD OILS FROM FISH

All fish oils are not created equal. While the omega-3 fatty acids contained within fish oil have unequivocal health benefits, some oils in
fish may be unhealthy. Cetoleic acid, a fatty acid containing twenty-two
carbon atoms, is found in herring, cod, and capelin in varying amounts.
Cetoleic acid resembles erucic acid, both chemically and functionally.
Erucic acid, which is found in mustard and rape seed, has been shown
to cause degenerative damage to the kidneys and hearts of rats
because it promotes fatty deposits in these organs. It is not clear, however, that these same effects are found in humans. The rat seems to
metabolize erucic acid in a manner different from humans, so we can
only surmise that similar damage may be possible, but not yet clarified.

Another potential problem with fish oils is that they may be easily
damaged by heat, light, or oxygen. Eating raw fish is common in certain
countries such as Japan, but much of the fish oil is contained within the
skin or subcutaneous area of the fish, and these parts are often exclud-
ed during the preparation of sushi or sashimi. One big concern with fish
oil is heavy metal contamination with mercury, lead, cadmium, and
organic chemicals (*e.g.*, pesticides, herbicides, and PCBs). Recent controls have helped to reduce this toxicological problem. Regarding the
safety of fish, there are suggestions that regulatory agencies are less
stringent in their inspection of fish than of meat. I believe that much of
the fish sold in stores in Western countries is not fit for consumption in
raw form. The notion that freezing fish at very low temperature is capable of removing toxins or parasites is quite misleading.

One of my major concerns is the contamination of northern
oceans with radioactivity following the irresponsible abandonment of
nuclear weapons and armory accumulated during the Cold War. We
still have very little idea about the degree of radioactive contamination of cold-water fish in northern seas, especially the waters adja-
cent to the northwest shores of the former USSR, where covert
dumping of radioactive waste may have occurred with alarming frequency. Many experts have indicated that fish caught away from
coastal waters may be safer, both in terms of less parasitosis and contamination by environmental waste. However, large metal containers
of radioactive waste have been dumped on the bottom of the ocean

bed far away from the coastal areas. It may be many years before we experience the negative effects of this environmental crime or even become aware of this modern-day disaster. I am not trying to make a case to avoid cold-water fish, but as an educated consumer you are wise to examine the origin of the foods you eat. In addition, you should be aware of the environmental factors that will continue to affect the safety of the food supply on a global level.

How Much Fish Oil Per Day?

Now we are again in Nobel prize territory because as yet, the precise required daily amounts and interactions of essential fatty acids in the human diet are not known. Several authorities have attempted to recommend certain dietary doses of various essential fatty acids, but this is hazarding a guess, at best. Even if an official recommended amount were established, that concept is quite misleading. You have a variable requirement for a variety of nutrients, and the requirement changes as circumstances change. Not only do individual needs exist, but factors such as environmental conditions, stress, physical activity, and your general health influence your requirements for all nutrients.

How much fish oil do we need to reap the benefits? Can we just eat more fish? Some estimates about optimal intake are surprisingly high. For example, the Council for Responsible Nutrition in the U.S. indicates that an individual may need to consume approximately a pound and a half *daily* of certain types of cold-water fish. It is alleged that this is the quantity of fish that contains enough omega-3 fatty acids to achieve a health benefit. Of course, fresh fish is quite expensive, and some find it difficult to prepare. Besides, many people do not find cold-water fish palatable in this quantity.

If you do like and eat fish often, the fish most likely to contain significant quantities of omega-3 fatty acids include yellowfin tuna, cod, rainbow trout, sea bass, herring, mackerel, salmon, shark, swordfish, grouper, and sardines. Several of these fish are rather uncommon in food shops in Western locations and, as mentioned, they tend to be quite expensive. Salmon has increased in popularity in the U.S., precisely because of media reports that it is a "heart-smart" food. Farm-raised salmon tends to be fattier, but has a lower concentration of the omega-3 fatty acids than wild salmon. Unfortunately, this information serves to confuse consumers even more. Still, both types of salmon are good sources of these vital oils and are available year-round. Because it is difficult to obtain a reliable amount of these oils, it may be more realistic for people to supplement their diet with omega-3 fatty acids from fish oil capsules.

Practically nothing of real clinical significance is known about differences in requirements of essential fatty acids between men and women, except that hormonal activity dominates in either sex at varying times, which probably determines changing requirements for essential fatty acids between genders. Other complex factors operate in omega-3 fatty acid requirements by the body. It has been estimated that up to as much as 18 grams per day of linoleic acid for either sex in the diet may be optimal (a staggering estimate!), but individuals who are obese, have blood lipid disorders, or ingest large quantities of *saturated* fatty acids may require more than this amount. About 5 grams per day of LA are required to prevent deficiencies of this fatty acid, but the optimal intake may be about twice this amount. Some studies in animals have attempted to define the optimal amount of essential fatty acid intake, but these studies may not be relevant to humans because of the significant differences in fatty acid metabolism among animal species.

In spite of the uncertainly about exact dosages, I strongly believe that it is necessary for the average person to supplement the diet with fish oil. It is necessary because of the widespread deficiency of omega-3 fatty acids, the general lack of dietary precursors of omega-3 fatty acids such as LNA, and the overriding health benfits of consuming adequate amounts of omega-3 fatty acids. Fish oils do not have an immediate effect on health, and it may require several weeks of supplementation to reach optimal biological effect. Remember, too, that the needed co-factors help these oils become processed and converted in the body.

Essential Fatty Acids and Their Co-Factors

In order to deliver their potential health benefits, essential fatty acids need to "hang out" with certain minerals and vitamins—hence the term "co-factor." In essence, co-factors need each other for their biological activity. These co-factors include vitamins B3, B6, C, E, A, and the minerals zinc, selenium, and magnesium. These co-factors are so important that it is not wise to take essential fatty acids supplements without the necessary co-factors. Consumers who seek the health benefits of essential fatty acids must recognize the importance of consuming adequate amounts of the important co-factors that permit the body to use EFAs.

ABOUT THE OTHER EFAs

The ideal amount of alpha-linolenic acid (LNA) in the diet is even more of a guess than the optimal amount of linoleic acid (LA). However, it is generally accepted that about one-quarter to one-half the amount of LNA is required in comparison to LA, which translates into approximately 5 to 9 grams of LA per day for a 155-pound human. (These figures, by the way, are only best guesses.)

Remember that when we discuss optimal amounts of EPA and DHA, the individual factors just mentioned must be considered. If an average human can transform LNA into EPA at a rate of about 2 to 3 percent per day of the LNA administered, then the body can make only limited amounts of EPA daily from LNA. Four to six grams of EPA is a projected, and, by some, an assumed, daily requirement of EPA and DHA that appears quite astonishingly large. If this is a required daily amount, it represents a need for several servings of fresh fish weekly—or, as an alternative, a combination of supplements containing EPA and DHA (fish oil), or oils containing LNA, assuming the conversion occurs optimally. The assumption that precursors (LNA) are valid sources of EPA and DHA has led to misguided advice to take flax seed or oil as a reliable source of omega-3 fatty acids.

Several dietary supplements have been made with fish oil, and an average fish oil capsule that contains between 500 and 1,000 mg. of fish oil with varying concentrations of omega-3 fatty acid (usually 18:12 ratio of EPA to DHA) may have to be taken in a dose of more than twelve capsules a day to meet the body's need if a deficiency of omega-3 fatty acids exist or if fish oil is used as a treatment (*e.g.*, for depression or inflammation). The whole situation is confusing because requirements vary, depending on stress, lack of other dietary co-factors, and many other influences on health status. Remember, too, that a therapeutic amount of omega-3 fatty acids may be much greater than what is needed to maintain health. Once the body is saturated with essential fatty acids in an attempt to reverse a deficiency state, then the subsequent amount of fish oil required to maintain adequate bioavailability of EPA and DHA is much lower. This reasoning assumes that the fish oil supplements are well-tolerated and absorbed and assimilated by the body.

DELAYED-RELEASE FISH OIL SUPPLEMENTS ARE DESIRABLE (PERHAPS MANDATORY!)

We are not finished with the complications! Not every individual can readily absorb large doses of fish oil, and few individuals can tolerate very high doses of fish oil that are not given in a special formulation, such as a delayed-release (enteric-coated) format. Individuals who have attempted to take several tablespoonfuls of any oils containing essential fatty acids will be aware of the problems of digestion and lack of palatability of crude preparations. (For many people, memories of cod liver oil come to mind.) This situation has led producers to develop special encapsulation techniques that deliver fish oils to their site of maximal absorption in the small intestines, where they are handled more efficiently. But there may be a significant portion of the population, perhaps as many as one in ten, who are unable to efficiently make EPA and DHA from LNA. Therefore, these individuals have an absolute requirement for fish oil supplementation in their diet. Edward N. Siguel, M.D., has suggested a supplementation regimen for individuals with omega-3 fatty acid deficiency. I have summarized this regimen in Table 10.8. But opinions on ideal dosage differ greatly.

Table 10.8: A Regimen of Diet Supplementation with Fresh Oils.

This regimen is suggested by Dr. Edward N. Siguel. I believe that these estimates are too conservative. Enteric coated fish oils are better tolerated and absorbed.

WEEKS	FISH OIL ω3 DERIVATIVE	FLAX OIL ω3 EFA	SOYBEAN OIL ω3 + ω6 EFA
1–4	1 teaspoon	½ tablespoon	1–2 tablespoons
4–10	Reduce	Same	Increase
10–20	Reduce	Same	Same/less
Over 20	Same/less	Less—more if ω3 different	Same/less

A Word of Caution

Most people are able to take regular fish oils without anything more serious than the common side effects of bad breath and abdominal upset. But at very high levels, fish oils can cause abnormal clotting function, with a bleeding tendency in some people. Always remember that nutrients, in all their forms, have a powerful influence in the body.

Based on the pathways of production of prostaglandins from omega-3 fatty acid, it is evident that linolenic acid can be converted to EPA (refer to Table 10.6). Although alpha-linolenic acid is found in fresh, green, leafy vegetables and a variety of vegetable oils, such as flax, soy, and linseed, supplementing the diet with these foods or nutrients will not result in an efficient production of EPA in everyone. The conversion of LNA to EPA is inefficient because converting enzyme systems are weak in their activity. Furthermore, the presence of relatively large amounts of the omega-6 fatty acid, linoleic acid, as is common in standard Western diets, tends to inhibit the activity of the conversion of alpha-linolenic acid to EPA. Excess saturated fat in the diet also inhibits the process of conversion of precursors to active omega-3 fatty acids. This reinforces my opinion that plant sources of omega-3 fatty acids are less reliable for health than fish oil.

HOW GOOD FATS CAN QUICKLY LOSE THEIR VIRTUES

The way fish is prepared is of critical importance. Unfortunately, much of the fish that is eaten in the West is prepared in a way that is not only deficient in essential fatty acids, but probably contains toxic byproducts of fats produced by frying. The British tradition of fish and chips has evolved—perhaps I should say devolved—into using low-fat containing fish (low in EFA and DHA) with potatoes deep-fried in damaged, saturated fat that contains carcinogens. Individuals from the north of Britain may love their fish-and-chips diet, but it may explain why areas in the north of England and the Scottish lowlands have among the highest incidence of heart disease and cancer in Europe. The deep-fried fish meals served "American-style" in restaurants all over the country are certainly no better, even though they are more often fried in vegetable oil.

Always remember that essential fatty acids and other unsaturated fats are heat-labile, which means that they are damaged at high temperatures. High temperatures decompose fats to produce oxidized, or denatured, products and change healthful "cis" fatty acid structures into unhealthy "trans" structures. Table 10.9 illustrates the average temperatures at which commonly used fats and oils can be decomposed by heating. The more unsaturated a fat, the more labile or fragile it becomes. Unsaturated fats "go bad" even with exposure to modest sunlight! The fact is that as soon as a bottle of fish oil is opened, it will rapidly deteriorate. There is no question that oil concentrates of omega-3 fatty acids, stabilized with vitamin E in enteric coated capsules (such as the brand Fisol) are the optimal way to take fish oil.

THE OMEGA-6 AND OMEGA-3 BALANCE

The ratio between omega-6 and omega-3 fatty acid intake in the diet is still another issue involving EFAs and has been the subject of much interest. The traditional Inuit diet has a ratio of omega-6 to omega-3 of approximately 1:3, whereas average Western diets have a ratio of omega-6 to omega-3 of anything ranging from 5:1 through 30:1. Based on dietary changes over the over the past 150 years, it is estimated that

Table 10.9: Average Temperatures at Which Common Fats and Oils Decompose.

Note that the healthy fats in olive oil are the easiest to decompose with heat.

Fat	Approximate Temperature of Decomposition °C
Corn oil	227
Butter	208
Lard	218
Margarine	225
Olive oil	175
Soy oil	210

the consumption of omega-3 fatty acids has dramatically fallen in the average Western diet. With this trend, there has been a corresponding rise in the consumption of omega-6 fatty acids, and this situation could be an underestimated cause of the modern-day epidemic of cardiovascular disease. I believe stongly that this is the case!

This modern change in diet is actually a striking trend, but it is almost forgotten by contemporary medicine. Such a fundamental change in fat content in diet, with a shift from omega-3 to omega-6 fatty acids, results in a completely different body composition of fat with important, but not very obvious, health implications.

There have been many other dietary adjustments over the past 100 years, and in addition to a switch in the ratio of omega-6 to omega-3 fatty acids in the diet, there has been an increase in foods high in saturated fat and cholesterol. Earlier, I mentioned that the presence of omega-3 fatty acids have protected Eskimo populations from heart disease. Clearly, however, other factors, including other dietary issues and lifestyle, influence disease profiles. Life expectancy of the modern Eskimo or Inuit population is not admirable. The prevalence of stroke is quite high among Inuits, presumably as a result of a high salt intake that may promote hypertension. In addition, Inuits living in traditional circumstances are deficient in water-soluble vitamins such as B complex vitamins and C. They can counter this tendency by eating raw food, but cooking is more common among the modern Eskimo. The Inuit diet also is relatively deficient in vitamin E. I mention this because it is important not to look at one type of nutrient and its effect on only one set of diseases and then draw overly broad conclusions.

The relative amounts of omega-6 and omega-3 fatty acids in the body varies dramatically, depending on the tissue in question. The omega-6 to omega-3 fatty acid ratio in nervous tissue is approximately 1:1, whereas the ratio in adipose (fat) tissue deposits is in the range of 3:1 to 7:1. On average, the ratio of omega-6 to omega-3 throughout most body tissue is about 4:1 or 5:1. The omega-6 to omega-3 ratio in populations with healthy types of diets ranges from 5:2 to 1:6, not the 20:1 that many Westerners take. I believe that an optimal ratio of omega-6 fatty acids to omega-3 fatty acids in the diet could be somewhere between 2:1 and 5:1. Remember, though, this ratio becomes unimportant if the co-factors required for the function of essential fatty acids are not present in the diet and if the diet is not generally well-balanced.

VISITING THE OMEGA-3 FACTOR

The idea of supplementing the diet with fish oil is neither novel nor new. A number of dietary supplements containing fish oil are sold in health food stores or pharmacies, probably as a result of increased media attention over the past decade about the health benefits of fish oil. Some of the cardiovascular benefits are well described: inhibiting platelet aggregation, reducing cholesterol levels (while raising HDL), reducing triglycerides, lowering blood pressure, and reducing blood viscosity. Unfortunately, it is not universally appreciated that people who eat large amounts of fish oil also have a lower incidence of chronic inflammatory diseases, such as inflammatory bowel disease, skin disorders, rheumatoid arthritis, and autoimmune disorders.

An important editorial in the medical journal *Lancet*, in 1983, pointed out that the high-fat, high-cholesterol, and low-carbohydrate nature of the Eskimo's diet could be predicted to cause cardiovascular disease, rather than prevent cardiovascular disease. In fact, an autopsy study of 339 Alaskan natives found that only 10 percent died of a cardiovascular cause, whereas approximately one-half of all deaths in the United States (and other Western societies) are related to cardiovascular disease. An inverse relationship between fish consumption and mortality from heart disease over a twenty-year period was reported in 1985 by Dr. Daan Kromhout and his colleagues in the *New England Journal of Medicine*. These data from European studies supported the epidemiological findings among Eskimos where the prevalence of cardiovascular disease was perceived to be far less than that among members of Western society. In this study by Dr. Kromhout and his colleagues, a twenty-year follow-up of coronary artery disease mortality was studied among men who had reported daily consumption of at least 30 grams of fish per day. In this study, the mortality due to coronary artery disease, after two decades, was half that of men who had reported no significant fish intake in their diet. This study concluded that the inclusion of a relatively small amount of fish in the diet, approximately two servings of fish per week, may confer significant protection against coronary atheroma and its consequences.

Looking from another angle, in *Fats That Heal, Fats That Kill*, Udo Erasmus has ascribed the negative observations of fish oil—to some

> ### Table 10.10: Primary Reasons Proposed as Contributing to Widespread Essential Fatty Acid Deficiency.
>
> Michael T. Murray, the naturopath who developed this list, has contributed greatly to our knowledge about the use of oils in dietary supplements.
>
> - There is "competition" within metabolic processes between hydrogenated and trans-fatty acids with essential fatty acids.
>
> - Through food processing or cooking, the health-giving omega-3 and omega-6 fatty acids are transformed into toxic, hydrogenated products, or trans isomers.
>
> - There is a relative unavailability of fresh oils that contain high concentrations of essential fatty acids, due to commercial refinement and processing of fats and oils.

degree—to the poor quality of fish oil in the diet as a consequence of untimely or poor food processing and preparation. Other factors that contribute to the widespread occurrence of fatty acid deficiency in Western countries have been proposed by Dr. Michael T. Murray in his book *Understanding Fats and Oils* (Table 10.10), but Dr. Murray seems preoccupied with flax oils as reliable source of omega-3 fatty acids.

ESSENTIAL FATTY ACIDS AND PROSTAGLANDINS—THE IMPORTANT HEALTH LINK

To reiterate, essential fatty acids are important precursors of prostaglandins and leukotrienes. Remember, too, that essential fatty acids are grouped in families, and some of these family relationships are complex. Arachidonic acid is a member of the omega-6 fatty acid family and is the prime precursor of prostaglandins and leukotrienes. Arachidonic acid is synthesized in humans from the omega-6 fatty acid linoleic acid, found in abundance in vegetable oils. When the Western diet is balanced, it is generally rich in omega-6 fatty acids and arachidonic acid, which is converted by the enzyme cyclooxygenase to a series of prostaglandin molecules, including prostacyclin and thromboxane A_2.

Thromboxane A_2 is a potent constrictor of blood vessels, and it promotes platelet aggregation and, in turn, blood clotting. In contrast, prostacyclin has opposing physiological effects. It is generally believed that the ratio of thromboxane A_2 to prostacyclin regulates vascular tone and controls the initiation of blood clotting by platelet aggregation. A variety of events may lead to a preponderance of thromboxane A_2 or a deficiency of prostacyclin, which would favor blood vessel constriction and platelet aggregation and may increase the risk of cardiovascular disorders such as heart attack or thrombotic stroke. This is why balance is so important.

In contrast, the omega-3 fatty acids, EPA and DHA, may replace the omega-6 fatty acid derivative, arachidonic acid, as a substrate for the cyclooxygenase enzyme system. This then results in a decrease in the synthesis of thromboxane A_2. If the omega-3 fatty acids in fish oils replace the omega-6 fatty acids as substrates for prostaglandin synthesis, the Type 3 series prostaglandins will be preferentially produced at the expense of the Type 2 prostaglandin series.

Remember that the Type 3 series prostaglandins are generally beneficial to health, and the Type 2 series are not always beneficial. If the Type 3 prostaglandins lead to a decrease in the production of thromboxane A_2, then the balance shifts away from vasoconstriction and platelet aggregation and towards vasodilatation and a state of anti-aggregation of platelets. When fish oils are incorporated into the diet, a different form of thromboxane is produced; this is a much weaker vasoconstrictor and platelet aggregator than classic thromboxane A_2.

As well as providing substrates for the production of prostaglandins, essential fatty acids provide material for the synthesis of leukotrienes. Leukotrienes are generally synthesized from arachidonic acid by an enzyme lipooxygenase. Leukotrienes play a significant part in promoting coronary artery disease and a variety of other common killer diseases. Leukotrienes are complex molecules and have been classified into a variety of different types, which produce a number of inflammatory effects in the body. Leukotrienes C_4, D_4, and E_4 have potent effects on constricting air passages in the lungs, and they act to increase the permeability of blood vessels. These leukotrienes increase mucus secretion. All of these factors may provoke lung disease, or exacerbate it. In addition, leukotriene B_4 causes the attraction of white cells to areas of inflammation and precipitates the degranulation of acute-phase white blood cells (neutrophil leukocytes), promoting acute inflammation in tissues. I realize this section is complex; please take a deep breath and remember the concept that omega-3 fatty acids (fish oil) push the pathways discussed to a healthier type of body chemistry.

FISH OIL SHIFTS AWAY FROM LEUKOTRIENES

The importance of the inclusion of omega-3 fatty acids such as EPA and DHA in the diet is that they will tend to interfere with the conversion of arachidonic acid to leukotrienes and result in an overall decrease in the production of leukotrienes B_4. The effects of fish oil ingestion on leukotriene production are quite complex and, in some circumstances, a different form of leukotriene may be produced. Many scientists believe that taking omega-3 fatty acids in the form of fish oil may alter leukotriene synthesis and metabolism, thereby having a beneficial effect on inflammatory processes. This has far-reaching implications for the management of a variety of disorders, including cardiovascular disease, inflammatory bowel disease, and chronic recurrent asthma.

FISH OIL AND PROSTAGLANDINS

Generating prostaglandins is a major job of EFAs, and their effects are far-reaching (see Table 10.1). Prostaglandins are very potent and versatile hormone-like substances, and more than three dozen different prostaglandin molecules have been characterized. However, the exact function and structure of many of these molecules remains underexplored. Prostaglandins are involved in a variety of important body processes; they modulate a variety of metabolic and physiological processes, and, to some degree, they modulate the effects of each other.

Three different types of prostaglandins described can be most easily defined based upon the fatty acid molecule from which they were generated. We have learned that the series, or family Type 1 and Type 2 prostaglandins are derived from the omega-6 series of fatty acids, and linoleic acid is the prime precursor of these series. The conversion process is complex. Linoleic acid is converted into gamma-linolenic acid (GLA), which is ultimately converted into arachidonic acid via an intermediary compound di-homo-gamma-linolenic acid (DGLA). In contrast, series 3, or the Type 3 family of prostaglandins, are synthesized from the omega-3 family of fatty acids, of which alpha-linolenic acid (LNA) is the prime substrate. In the human body, linolenic acid (LNA) is converted to stearidonic acid, which is then converted to EPA via an intermediary known as eicosatetranaenoic acid. The series 3 prostaglandins are then produced from EPA. The complexity of the conversion processes only serves, yet again, to enunciate the importance of balanced intake of the sources of the various EFAs.

As previously explained, overall, Type 2 series prostaglandins tend to promote disease, whereas the Type 1 and Type 3 families appear to promote health. Although this classification is somewhat oversimplified, it is useful in understanding the overall health implications of the three different families of prostaglandins.

Series 1 Prostaglandins

Series 1 prostaglandins include the prostaglandin E_1, which prevents platelet stickiness and promotes cardiovascular well-being. In addition, prostaglandin E_1 has important actions in the urinary tract, where it facilitates sodium and water excretion. Prostaglandin E_1 also tends to suppress inflammatory responses, promotes the action of insulin, improves neurological function, regulates calcium metabolism, improves immune (T cell) function, and has important cardiovascular effects. These cardiovascular effects include vasodilatation, reduction of blood pressure, and the release of arachidonic acid from cell membranes.

You may have heard about evening primrose oil (EPO), which is a rich source of gamma-linolenic acid (GLA). It has been used as a dietary supplement for many years now, and is important because it converts to prostaglandin E_1. Prior to its rediscovery in recent decades, it was a traditional remedy among some Native American groups. Interestingly, the Flambeau Ojibwe used the evening primrose plant in the form of a poultice for bruises and other skin disorders. One of the modern uses is as a treatment for eczema and psoriasis.

While linoleic acid can be converted in the body to GLA, many factors interfere with the conversion process, including an abundance of saturated fats in the diet. Since the 1970s, Canadian researcher Dr. David Horrobin has headed a group of scientists who have tested EPO for a variety of conditions, including diabetic neuropathy, benign breast conditions, premenstrual syndrome, and other problems related to menstruation, attention deficit disorder, hyperactivity, asthma—the list goes on, including such serious illnesses as multiple sclerosis and schizophrenia. Some research suggests that it can help lower cholesterol levels, reduce blood pressure, and, perhaps most striking, act as an anticlotting agent.

While I—and others—do not maintain that EPO is a cure-all, and one should never self-treat, I advise talking with your health-care provider about supplementing your diet with essential fatty acids, including EPO, because it has the potential to help reverse serious conditions. Overall, its most important contribution may be in helping the body tip the balance in favor of Type 1 prostaglandins, when this is required.

Type 3 Prostaglandins Preferred Over Type 2

The Type 3 prostaglandins are made from EPA. These prostaglandins prevent arachidonic acid release from cell membranes and interrupt the production of prostaglandin series 2. EPA is important in limiting generation of the disease-promoting Type 2 prostaglandins. Another way to say this is that Type 3 prostaglandins inhibit prostaglandin 2 production. The series 2 prostaglandins are produced from arachidonic acid. Prostaglandin E_2 promotes platelet aggregation, causes salt and water retention, promotes inflammation, and has a vasoconstrictor effect that results overall in a rise in blood pressure.

Retiring Type 2 and Emerging Types 1 and 3

You must remember that series 1 and series 3 prostaglandins both seem to regulate the production of series 2 type pros- taglandins. Together, these two prostaglandin families work to maintain balance in the body —homeostasis. Series 2 prostaglandins are important in that they help fight disease. For example, an overabundance of Type 2 prostaglandins promotes the inflammatory process in arthritis, but if we can interfere with series 2 production, then joint inflammation will subside.

Overall, EPA tends to result in the synthesis of beneficial Type 3 prostaglandins. Remember that prostaglandin production from essential fatty acids requires a number of co-factors. Fish oils should not be taken without an adequate supply of these co-factors, which include vitamin C, B3, B6, and the minerals selenium, magnesium, and zinc. The balance of prostaglandins in health and disease is an extremely complex subject, but think in terms of adding the EFAs that are not abundant in your diet. Since most diets in Western societies contain substantial amounts of omega-6 fatty acids, in general fish oils are the missing link. Just remember that omega-3 fatty acids produce predominantly the more desirable Type 3 prostaglandins. So now when you hear about the benefits of fish oils, you'll have a basic understanding of their function in bringing about the beneficial prostaglandin family.

DANGEROUS ANIMAL PROTEIN DIETS AND PROSTAGLANDINS

A variety of stimuli can accelerate the production of different types of prostaglandins. For example, inflammation in the body causes a cascade of production of Type 2 prostaglandins which, in turn, is balanced by production of Type 1 and Type 3 prostaglandins.

In order to control the potentially deleterious effects of excessive releases of Type 2 prostaglandins, the production of arachidonic acid (AA) from di-homo-gamma-linolenic acid (DGLA) occurs at a slow rate. This slow conversion rate of DGLA to AA can be overcome to some degree by supplying AA to the body in the diet. The principal dietary source of AA is animal protein. Thus, a diet high in meat contains excess arachidonic acid, which favors the production of damaging Type 2 prostaglandins. This tipping of the balance towards Type 2 prostaglandins explains in part the negative health consequences of high animal protein diets, which are associated with higher rates of heart disease, kidney problems, osteoporosis, and inflammatory conditions. Dairy products contain abundant arachidonic acid and, like meat, in their natural form are cholesterol-rich. This role of excessive animal protein in promoting prostaglandin Type 2 series is a very important, often overlooked factor that expands our understanding of the danger of high-protein diets in Western society.

Two overwhelming reasons exist to be cautious about animal protein (meat) and dairy products. First, they have a high saturated fat and cholesterol content. Second, they contain arachidonic acid, with its predilection to form the more unhealthy types of prostaglandins and leukotrienes. Animal protein–based diets can be seen to work against the omega-3 factor, as do the meat and dairy lobbies and some samples of conventional medical wisdom.

FISH OIL LOWERS CHOLESTEROL

Several studies have shown that supplementing the diet with fish oils, over the long-term, may benefit blood lipids and cardiovascular disease. These effects have been observed in cases of familial high blood cholesterol and in patients with high blood triglycerides. Fish oils also suppress VLDL (very low-density lipoprotein) concentrations in the blood, and fish oils have been shown to modify or "weaken" the cholesterol-induced rise in lipoprotein cholesterol in humans. This implies that fish oils may help prevent blood cholesterol levels from rising as a result of dietary intake of cholesterol. Overall, only a minority of studies have shown no conclusive benefits of fish oils on blood lipids.

Dr. Phillipson's Pivotal Study

In 1985, Dr. Phillipson and his colleagues reported a very important study of the reduction of plasma lipids, lipoproteins, and apoproteins by dietary fish oils in patients with raised blood triglycerides. A diet high in fish and fish oil was examined for its effect on blood lipids in twenty patients with raised blood triglycerides. The fish- and fish oil–containing diet was compared with a controlled diet composed of low-fat and low-cholesterol foods. It also was compared with a third diet, which contained a presumed health-giving vegetable-oil preparation. The diet contained approximately 30 percent fat with 325 milligrams of cholesterol as a basic content. Blood lipid levels were measured after four weeks on the respective diets. Blood lipids fell dramatically in the group taking fish oil, and there was a consistent decrease in both total cholesterol and triglyceride levels.

The importance of this study was that in the patients with a particular type of hyperlipidemia (Type V), cholesterol levels decreased by almost one-half, and triglyceride levels decreased by a factor of almost three-quarters. The 50 percent and 70 percent approximate reductions in cholesterol and triglyceride levels respectively were noted, despite the fact that the fish- and fish-oil diet was higher in fat and cholesterol than the two other diets. The group taking the vegetable-oil diet that was considered to be a "therapeutic" product had a significant and alarming rise in blood triglyceride levels. Again, the importance of the omega-3 factor surfaces.

The Eskimo Research Project

Other than consumption of fish oil in large quantities, are there other reasons that explain why Eskimos have relatively low rates of coronary heart disease? It has been proposed that there may be a protective genetic factor. However, several races with genetic similarity have many more times the risk of heart disease. Genetic factors are not irrelevant, but they do not offer substantial explanations of the differences in rates of cardiovascular disease.

In the 1970s, two Danish scientists—Dr. Jorn Dyerberg and Dr. H. O. Bang—joined with Dr. Hugh Sinclair, a nutritional researcher from Britain, to study Eskimos in their native habitat. They collected blood samples from Eskimos in northern areas of Greenland and analyzed blood lipids (cholesterol) and clotting function. The findings of these analyses were very intriguing. Within the Eskimo study group, bleeding time was found to be prolonged and clotting tendencies were diminished. In addition, LDL levels in the blood were low, coincidental with the finding of the presence of EPA and DHA in the blood.

Following these field ventures, Dr. Sinclair undertook some extremely courageous nutritional studies on himself in Oxfordshire, England. Dr. Sinclair obtained a frozen seal and used it as an exclusive food source for himself over a period of about three months. The outcome of these self-experiments was reported by Dr. Sinclair in a classic scientific paper, "The Advantages and Disadvantages of an Eskimo Diet." As Dr. Sinclair reported, his blood-clotting tendency was reduced and his body weight fell by twenty-five pounds. (He had unknowingly placed himself on a stringent, Atkins-type diet.) His blood cholesterol rose modestly by 10 mg. but LDL levels in his blood were reduced.

Coincidental with the alterations in blood chemistry, Dr. Sinclair developed bruising and nose bleeds, and his vitamin C levels fell towards zero. The explanation of the adverse effects experienced by Dr. Sinclair is consistent with our knowledge of the intricacies of the effects of omega-3 fatty acids, when supplemented in the absence of a balanced diet. These adverse events reinforce the need for Westerners to maintain balanced nutrition. Forgetting balance in nutrition is a dangerous pastime of some physicians and health-care consumers.

The beneficial effects of the omega-3 fatty acid content of the diet is apparent in races other than the Eskimo. Several elegant studies of individuals in Japan and in some Mediterranean areas who live on diets preponderant in fish show a lower incidence of cardiovascular disease, compared with people who live in urban areas. Population studies in Japan have shown conclusively that the fish-eating inhabitants of Okinawa Island have particularly low death rates from coronary heart disease, in comparison with people who live in mainland Japan. Incidentally, Okinawans are known for their longevity and some eat significant amounts of saturated fat (pork). Their longevity is probably a function of nutritional balance.

Levels of Blood Cholesterol and Amounts of Fish Oil Are Both Important

In studies where no benefit of omega-3 fatty acids is shown, it may be that the quality of fish oil or omega-3 fatty acids used in the study was not optimal. However, it seems more likely that the amount of omega-3 fatty acids used determines the outcome. The study performed in the 1980s by Dr. Phillipson and his colleagues used very large quantities of fish oil, about 20 grams per day, which may be equivalent to eating approximately three pounds of salmon or herring per day. What does this mean? On the one hand, fish oils at certain doses may have subtle physiological effects, but at high doses they may exert astounding therapeutic effects. Overall, the literature indicates that the lipid- and cholesterol-lowering benefits of fish oil are related to the dose of fish oil taken; it may also be related to the degree of hyperlipidemia experienced by the individuals. In general, the higher the cholesterol numbers, the more magnified the benefit. The same applies to lowering cholesterol with soy protein containing isoflavones (such as the supplement Genista). These are interesting observations on natural first-line options to normalize blood lipids.

Preventing Atheroma and Thrombosis

In 1978, Dr. Dyerberg and his colleagues published an important study in *Lancet* that drew attention to the role of EPA in the prevention of thrombosis and atherosclerosis. These scientists proposed that omega-3 fatty acids resulted in a state of decreased platelet stickiness, which was responsible for the observed low rate of coronary artery disease among Eskimos. A number of studies have confirmed these earlier observations and show that omega-3 fatty acid supplements may prolong bleeding time, decrease thromboxane A_2 production, and inhibit the aggregation of platelets. These effects are related to the amount of omega-3 fatty acids consumed. Studies that have failed to show much in the way of significant anti-thrombotic effects of fish oil tended to use only modest quantities of EPA as a dietary supplement.

A number of researchers have found that fish oil supplementation of the diet tends to result in a decrease of blood viscosity and a corresponding increase in the ability of red blood cells to undertake their usual acrobatics of deformation in small blood vessels. Those individuals with the highest blood viscosity appear to have the greatest reduction in blood viscosity as a result of taking fish oil, and these effects may be dose-dependent. It is notable that reductions of blood viscosity have been noted with relatively small quantities of EPA.

Lowering Blood Pressure

Omega-3 fatty acids have been investigated in detail in many clinical research studies to determine their effects on blood pressure. The most profound effect of fish oil on lowering blood pressure has been demonstrated in patients with kidney failure who are undergoing hemodialysis therapy. In addition, modest reductions of systolic and diastolic blood pressure can be observed in individuals fed a diet of cold-water fish, such as mackerel. These effects can be achieved with a daily amount of five to six grams of essential fatty acids of the omega-3 series.

The mechanism of the hypotensive (blood pressure lowering)

effect of fish oil is not entirely understood. Animal experiments suggest that omega-3 fatty acids may modify the responsiveness of arterial blood vessels to neurohormonal stimuli. In addition, hypertension induced by mineralocorticoids (steroids) can be reduced by fish oil, and the ability of catecholamines to cause contractions in isolated blood vessels is attenuated when feeding omega-3 series fatty acids to rats. Why isn't every patient who has undergone arterial bypass surgery taking fish oil?

Fish Oil for Bypass Patients

Vascular grafts are used in cardiac bypass surgery and surgery to bypass peripheral vascular disease. The effects of omega-3 series fatty acids on blood vessels may mean that fish oils in the diet help prevent occlusion—new blockages or damage—of vascular grafts. Dr. Landymore and his colleagues have undertaken extensive experiments with the use of cod liver oil in preventing the growth of the lining (intimal hyperplasia) of bypass grafts. In fact, these experiments suggest that omega-3 series fatty acids may be more effective than aspirin and/or drugs designed to stop platelet aggregation in reducing the growth that occurs in arterial bypass grafts.

Fish Oil and Angina

Conflicting evidence exists about the effects of fish oil on angina. A short-term—three-month—placebo-controlled trial of fish oil supplements failed to show much measurable benefit in patients with angina. However, in longer term trials a decrease in the number of episodes of angina and a decrease in the consumption of nitroglycerin medication to relieve angina have been noted. Further studies imply a conflicting effect of fish oil in the control of anginal chest pain, but overall the data for the general benefit of omega-3 series fatty acids in coronary artery disease are compelling.

The Focus Is on EPA

A wealth of scientific research points to eicosopentanoic acid—EPA—in protecting against cardiovascular disease by virtue of its potent and

Table 10.11: Factors That Inhibit Conversion of Alpha-Linolenic Acid to Eicosopentanoic Acid.

These factors operate by inhibiting the key enzyme delta-6-desaturase.

Diabetes mellitus or high blood glucose
Advanced age
Alcohol
Malnutrition or starvation
Low protein intake
Certain fats in the diet: high saturated fat intake, high intake of trans-fatty acids
Stress, which leads to catecholamine release
Viral disease, especially oncogenic viruses
Radiation exposure
Miscellaneous disease states

Table 10.12: Mechanisms by Which EPA Exerts Beneficial Effects on the Cardiovascular System.

Lowers blood pressure
Reduces LDL in the blood
Alters macrophage and monocyte function to act against atheromatous plaque formation
Promotes the formation of Type 3 prostaglandins
Favors the production of prostacyclins and thromboxanes that are less aggregatory to platelets

versatile effects on cardiovascular physiology. Remember, too, the importance of maintaining a balance between the intake of omega-6 and omega-3 fatty acids. Omega-6 fatty acids (cis-linoleic acid) will tend to inhibit the synthesis of EPA from alpha-linolenic acid, as will several other factors (see Table 10.11). Delta-6-desaturase is the key enzyme in the conversion of alpha-linolenic acid to EPA, and interference in the process comes from interference with this converting enzyme.

EPA can be summarized as a key heart protector in comparison with its relative, DHA, which seems to exert its maximum health benefits in the brain and nervous system. The principal mechanisms of the protective effects of EPA on cardiovascular health are shown in Table 10.12.

A Special Message for Women

The beneficial effects of fish oil on cardiovascular function and blood lipids have been shown most often in studies of male subjects. Things have changed. Researchers at the University of Guelph in Canada have studied the effects of omega-3 fatty acids on the blood lipid profile of postmenopausal women and demonstrated unequivocal benefits in altering the blood lipoprotein risk factors for cardiovascular disease. This benefit is apparent, regardless of whether or not the women are taking hormone replacement therapy. A reduced risk of cardiovascular disease can be expected by fish oil supplementation of the diet up to a factor of 34 percent. In addition, fish oil has benefits on other body functions in mature females and it may be valuable in engaging the postmenopausal onslaught of arthritis, osteoporosis, breast cancer, and decreased cognitive function.

Fish Oil Supplements

If you enjoy fish, and you can consume cold-water, oily fish in sufficient quantities to provide health-promoting amounts of omega-3 fatty acids, then you may be able to rely on fish as your source of EPA. Since this option is not practical for many individuals, concentrated fish oil supplements have several advantages.

Fish oil concentrates can be standardized for their content of EPA and DHA and are available in formats that are stable and reduced in their vitamin A contents. (Remember that vitamin A is one of the nutrients that can be toxic in excessively high doses, and it causes bleeding, liver damage, and brain disorders. Several fish oil concentrates are available in which vitamin A content is reduced, and they are considered safe and convenient to take in recommended dosages.)

There are some practical problems with taking many commercial fish oil concentrates. For example, many cod liver oil preparations are not standardized and may need to be taken in large volumes to guarantee the health benefits that can be anticipated only from specific amounts of DHA and EPA. Unfortunately, most people find cod liver oil to be unpalatable. Further, it leaves the breath with a feculent odor and, when taken in excess, it invariably causes abdominal discomfort, cramping, and diarrhea. These disadvantages have not been overcome by packaging fish oil in regular gel capsules. The best way to take fish oil is in a high concentration in an enteric-coated, delayed-release format (*e.g.*, Fisol, Nature's Way, BioTherapies). Fish oil in an enteric-coated, delayed-release format overcomes the common gastrointestinal side effects and enhances the efficiency of absorption of omega-3 fatty acids.

An increase in the level of absorption of the omega-3 fatty acid contents of fish oil has been shown when fish oils are taken in enteric-coated capsules. This also means that the dose of fish oil required to achieve the health benefits of fish oil is less when the oil is present in a delayed-release form. It has been estimated that delayed-release capsules may reduce the required amounts of certain fish oils by about one-third. Delayed-release capsules of fish oil can be made to resist gastric acid and enzymatic digestion so that the oil is preferentially delivered to its site of maximum absorption in the small bowel. (Fisol is the only example of such a product in the United States.)

The health benefits of fish oil inclusion in the Western diet is unequivocal. This underscores the value of dietary supplements in health care, since eating large amounts of food that contain the essential health-giving nutrients, in this case EPA and DHA, is not practical or often feasible.

Taking Fish Oil Is Not Fun!

The big problem for anyone wise enough to add fish oil to their diet is taking enough fish oil. The best way to get fish oil in the diet is obviously to eat large amounts of cold-water fish (*e.g.*, cod, mackerel, herring, etc.), but this is not within the reach of most people. The ideal amount of cold-water fish required for some people may be as much as three or four pounds of fish per week. Many people have selected certain kinds of fish oil supplement, but the most ideal source of fish oil is cod fish, for reasons of cost and effectiveness. Other types of oil, such as salmon oil, have no significant advantages over cod oil and they are often much more expensive.

One drawback in taking fish oil supplements is that the amount that needs to be taken is quite large. Liquid fish oil preparations generally taste rotten and regular fish oil capsules, when taken regularly, almost always cause digestive upset and foul breath. Modern science has shown us that the ideal way to take fish oil is to obtain a high concentrate of fish oil (containing EPA and DHA in a 30:20 ratio) in an enteric-coated, delayed-release format. This type of formulation of fish oil is not just a gimmick.

Fish oil, when presented in enteric-coated, delayed-release capsules, does not tend to cause digestive upset or bad breath, because the oil is protected from acid breakdown in the stomach prior to presentation to its site of absorption into the body in the intestines. Furthermore, and of major importance, is the fact that enteric-coated, high concentrations of fish oil are much better absorbed by the body.

Anyone planning to take fish oil is advised to consider the advantages of enteric-coated fish oil capsules, which will permit them to take health-giving fish oil in an optimal manner that can ensure compliance with supplementation. This is why the enteric-coated fish oil capsule has completely superseded all other forms of fish oil supplements in the market. A further important consideration relates to recent studies that have been published in the *New England Journal of Medicine*, where enteric-coated fish oil has been shown to be an optimal way of giving fish oil to suppress serious inflammation in the body. The lack of compliance with standard fish oil products is the reason why I have reiterated the advantages of enteric coating. Many people just cringe at the thought of taking regular fish oil supplements.

SUMMARY

The importance of essential fatty acids—EFAs—is too often overlooked and underestimated when discussing nutritional factors and heart disease. The omega-6 and omega-3 series of fatty acids are the two most important categories of EFAs. Omega-6 fatty acids are most often found in vegetables, and active omega-3 fatty acids are found mostly in fish and marine mammals. Omega-3 fatty acid precursors are also found in flax seeds. Within these EFA families, there are numerous types of fatty acids, but if you remember two important ones in the omega-3 series, EPA and DHA, you will be ahead of the game. EPA and DHA are the active components of fish oil, and studies have suggested that fish oil has the ability to lower cholesterol. Fish oil is a better source of omega factors than flax seed oil.

Studies of Eskimo populations, whose native diet includes mostly animal protein and fat, reveal little evidence of cardiovascular diseases, and the omega-3 series fatty acids are believed to be key in the prevention of heart disease among these populations. When Eskimos move to urban centers and their native diet becomes "Westernized," the incidence of cardiovascular disease begins to rise.

Fatty acids are efficient sources of energy for the body, and they are necessary for the production of a group of hormone-like substances, prostaglandins. There are numerous prostaglandin families that have various effects in the body. In general, Types 1 and 3 prostaglandins are considered healthful, while Type 2 is considered unhealthful. Diets that emphasize animal protein tend to lead to higher levels of Type 2 prostaglandin, and vegetable-based diets tend to favor production of Types 1 and 3.

Omega-3 fatty acid deficiencies are more common than omega-6 deficiencies because the latter is found in numerous plants, particularly seeds and soybeans, which are abundant in the Western diet. However, for most people, it would be difficult to consume enough fish to obtain fish oil in the recommended amounts. Therefore, fish oil supplements may be recommended.

What You Can Do

- Recognize that you are capable of understanding the role of EFAs in the body. The information contained in this chapter is too important to leave to the "experts."
- Deep frying is one sure way to turn a "good" fat into a "bad" fat. In addition, the value of vegetable oils, such as the ubiquitous soy oil, is lost when the oils are heated and partially saturated. All oils should be "handled with care."
- Omega-3 fatty acids can be synthesized in small amounts from fatty acids found in vegetable oils, such as safflower, sunflower, sesame, soybeans, walnuts, flaxseeds, and pumpkin seeds. Seeds are an abundant source of omega-6 fatty acids, and, therefore, have a place in your diet in *moderate* amounts. Cold-processed oils are preferred over heat-processed oils.

- Ask your health-care provider about the therapeutic use of fish oils. There is evidence that fish oils may lower blood cholesterol, particularly the LDL and VLDL (low and very low–density lipoproteins). Fish oil may also lower blood triglycerides and blood pressure, relieve angina, and may help prevent new blockages in the arteries of patients who have had bypass surgery.

- Delayed-release fish oil supplements are the most reliable source of omega-3 fatty acids, and this format has the added benefit of minimizing any gastrointestinal symptoms that may occur when fish oils are taken in supplement form. The delayed-release enteric coated formulations also increase absorption of the fish oil, which means that you may need to consume less to receive the benefits.

- Fish oil is screaming out to be used to counter the cardiovascular disease epidemic.

CHAPTER ELEVEN

SOY, THE HEART OF HEALTH

SOY AND YOUR HEART

Although in this chapter I am introducing the benefit of soy for cardiovascular health, I cannot resist expanding its overall benefits. I describe soybeans as the "heart of health" as well as the food for the next millennium. Soybeans are a relatively new discovery in the West, but in Asia this special plant has been a staple food for centuries. It is even considered a sacred plant. It is so versatile and hardy that it has helped Asian populations survive natural disasters, war, and other times of upheaval. In traditional Chinese medicine, soy foods have been considered health-promoting, and recently scientific research in the West has documented some of these health benefits. Given what we already know about the components of soybeans, I believe that it will eventually take its rightful place as the food of the next millennium. In the West, the soybean has been largely used as a source of animal feed and inexpensive oil for commercial food products, but this is changing, and the soybean is rapidly developing a new image.

In an earlier chapter, I discussed the growing trend in medicine to prescribe cholesterol-lowering drugs without first exploring lifestyle changes and dietary options. The failure to explore the full range of natural approaches, including lifestyle modifications for cardiovascular health, is an unfortunate legacy of our high-tech medical approaches. Unfortunately, the ability of soy protein to have a positive effect on cholesterol levels has been largely overlooked by the conventional medical world, even in the face of its widespread coverage in both peer-review journals and popular media. However, it has been recognized for approximately a century that animal protein may promote atherosclerosis and, conversely, that a diet abundant in vegetable protein lowers cholesterol and, by inference, decreases the risk of developing cardiovascular disease.

If I could provide only one dietary option in this book for promoting cardiovascular health in the coming decades, it would be to encourage a greater inclusion of more fruit and vegetables and less animal protein in the Western diet. I am convinced that soy offers a promise of cardiovascular health for the next generation.

A CENTRAL ROLE FOR SOY

Soy protein offers numerous advantages over animal protein, and many components—fractions—of soy have a role to play in preventing and treating several diseases and disorders. (Two of my previous books, *The Soy Revolution* and *Soya for Health*, offer a detailed look at the health benefits of soybeans. Readers who would like more complete information about soy and its important role in solving both personal and global health and nutrition problems are invited to test my reasoning in these books.) One thing I can boldly state is that unlike the need to match a cholesterol-lowering drug with one type of blood lipid disorder, soy protein in the diet is effective for most types of hypercholesterolemia.

Considerable research supports claims about the efficacy of soy protein as a cholesterol-lowering agent. For example, in 1991 K. K. Carroll, M.D., published a review of forty scientific studies of the effects of soy protein intake on blood cholesterol. Dr. Carroll's analysis concluded that thirty-four of the studies showed the positive effect of soy protein on lowering blood cholesterol by, in many cases, more than 15 percent of pretreatment levels. It is notable that soy protein significantly reduced LDL (low-density lipoproteins), the so-called bad cholesterol. This result often occurred independently of dietary fat or cholesterol intake.

Another prominent researcher, James Anderson, M.D., analyzed approximately forty major research programs on soy and heart disease. In 1995, the *New England Journal of Medicine* published his review of these studies, which show substantial reductions of blood cholesterol by supplementing the diet with soy protein or by substituting soy protein for other protein sources. The review of these studies further shows that the reductions in blood cholesterol and other lipids are similar to those achieved with maintenance doses of synthetic cholesterol-lowering drugs. At relatively high doses, these synthetic drugs produce significant reductions of blood lipids, but it is at these relatively high doses that the adverse effects of the drugs begin to appear. Therefore, it is bewildering that health-care professionals or patients with high cholesterol would choose these drugs as a first-line option instead of supplementing their diets with soy protein.

Although Dr. Anderson's work has had an impact on conventional and alternative medical practices, it still may seem as if the ability of soy to prevent or treat cardiovascular disease remains a well-kept secret! This seems particularly odd, because for nearly a century evidence has shown that vegetable-based diets, particularly soy-based diets, can lower blood cholesterol levels and protect against cardiovascular disease. My colleagues and I have been vociferous in our petition to the Food and Drug Administration to allow a claim for the cholesterol-lowering effects of soy protein containing isoflavones.

Soy Is Not Just For Rabbits!

Dr. Anderson's work is important because it flies in the face of statements issued by the Nutrition Committee of the American Heart Association, which I believe reached the erroneous conclusion that soy protein decreases cholesterol levels in rabbits but not in humans. This influential association seems to be willing to reconsider its findings given the weight of recent evidence. Dr. Anderson and his colleagues have highlighted the conclusive results of more than forty years of research showing that soy protein containing isoflavones has the ability to significantly reduce serum levels of total cholesterol, LDL cholesterol, and triglycerides. Its action on blood lipids (fats) is distinguished by its ability to cause a rise in the cardioprotective form of cholesterol (HDL).

The Genista Story

Preoccupied by my work on the effect of gel fibers on the absorption of nutrients and drugs that I published in *Lancet* in 1979, I had often recommended soluble fiber addition to my patients' diets as an adjunct to lower blood cholesterol. For several years in the 1980s, I had tried including soy in the diet of several patients and had attributed the observed beneficial reduction in total blood cholesterol to the inclusion of dietary fiber and perhaps isoflavones. I had been aware of the work of Dr. C. Sirtori in Italy on cholesterol lowering with soy, but the "penny dropped" when Dr. Anderson and his colleagues synthesized the research data on cholesterol lowering with soy in a metanalysis study. This is a statistical study that draws together results from many individuals and different studies to reach an overall conclusion.

The course of action was simple. I sought sources of high-quality soy protein in which isoflavones were present (about 2 mg./gram) and developed the product Genista, which has enjoyed five years of use as an effective dietary supplement. It provides nutritional support to promote a healthful blood cholesterol level and is designed to be used along with a heart-smart diet. Against considerable opposition, I have presented Genista to conventional medicine as a viable, first-line option for lowering blood cholesterol in a natural and safe manner. My opinion has been perceived as antagonistic by the producers of cholesterol-lowering drugs who sell billions of dollars worth of "statin" type agents (HMG co-reductase inhibitor drugs). These drugs are expensive and have worrisome side effects. I have been criticized for proposing that the use of appropriate types of soy protein could obviate the need for the prescription of more than half of all currently used cholesterol-lowering drugs.

While it is always problematic when health-care practitioners recommend products in which they have a financial interest, I acknowledge with pride my involvement in developing a natural and safe product that can lower cholesterol. I challenge any scientist to rebut claims that soy protein containing isoflavones effectively lowers blood cholesterol without unpleasant or potentially harmful side effects. In actuality, my position is being accepted in the conventional medical world, and food-producing giants such as Archer Daniels Midland and Protein Technologies have "come out of the closet" with similar health claims about their soy products. It was "heartening" when the U.S. Food and Drug Administration (FDA), in January 1999, finally gave the cholesterol-lowering benefits of soy protein a preliminary nod of approval. I hope soon to see the cholesterol-lowering claim for soy protein containing isoflavones, but fear that manufacturers of supplements will make this claim for the wrong amounts or types of soy.

HOW DOES SOY LOWER CHOLESTEROL?

Although the exact mechanisms by which soy lowers cholesterol are not fully known, there are several key components in the chemical composition of soy that are believed to play a role. In animal research, the amino acid composition of the diet seems to have a major effect on cholesterol levels, and it is possible that the same is true in humans. For example, increases in the amino acids arginine and glycine, both of which are abundant in soybeans, are associated with decreasing cholesterol levels. Compared to soy protein, animal protein is proportionately lower in these two amino acids. The amino acid lysine is proportionately higher in animal protein, and lysine raises insulin levels, which promotes production of cholesterol in the liver. The greater the lysine content of certain foods, the greater the likelihood that blood cholesterol will increase. This is one reason that vegetable protein, such as soy protein, is more effective for controlling blood cholesterol than animal-protein based diets, even those that include only lean meat, poultry, and low-fat dairy products.

It is also possible that soy protein alters the ratio of serum glucagon (a hormone involved in regulating blood sugar levels) to serum insulin levels, which, in turn, may affect production or excretion of cholesterol by the liver. In addition, soy protein may alter levels of active thyroid hormones in the blood. Thyroid hormone levels appear to be altered in varying but minor degrees in individuals who consume soy protein. I do not believe this situation is a contraindication for soy to be consumed in moderate amounts in people with thyroid disease.

Components of soybeans other than protein also may have a cholesterol-lowering effect. These include isoflavones, fiber, phytosterols, saponins, and lecithin. Lecithin, which is a natural "emulsifier," has been touted as a cholesterol-lowering agent. Because of some early beneficial observations, it has enjoyed considerable use in a somewhat purified form to reduce cholesterol levels. However, the relatively large amount of lecithin required to lower blood cholesterol and questions about its efficacy for that purpose put its value as a single agent for cholesterol lowering in question. Its use as a cholesterol-lowering agent is currently quite limited. The presence of lecithin in soy products is advantageous, but apparently not critical, at least as far as lowering blood cholesterol is concerned.

The fiber content of soybeans also helps to lower blood cholesterol. This lipid-lowering effect is shared by many different types of dietary fiber. Total dietary fiber intake is important in maintaining good health, and other efficient sources of fiber include bran, oats, and other grains that are not overrefined. Soybeans contain both soluble and insoluble types of fiber with potential health benefits, although to benefit from the complete fiber content, whole soybeans are required. Whole soybeans cause flatulence due both to fiber content and the presence of nonabsorbable carbohydrates such as stachyose and raffinose. And, as has been previously explained, it is best to increase fiber-rich foods slowly into the diet in order to partially avoid this discomfort.

Substances called *saponins,* contained within soy products, may also act to lower blood cholesterol. Saponins, which bear a chemical similarity to cholesterol, may help to block absorption of cholesterol or enhance its excretion from the body. It is interesting to note that a coincidental increase in the prevalence of cardiac disease has been observed in the populations of some countries whose overall consumption of vegetables that contain saponins has dropped. (Unfortunately, one consequence of global industrialization and urbanization has been a shift in diet consisting of relatively unrefined foods to increased consumption of packaged food and fast food. The health consequences of these dietary preferences are already appearing but keep being ignored.) Saponins may have a beneficial effect on lowering blood cholesterol, but this observation has yet to be confirmed in all studies.

Isoflavones, Estrogen's Distant Cousin

Of all suggested ways that soy protein may help lower cholesterol, looking at the role of isoflavones may be most important. Understanding the function of soy isoflavones, specifically two major types—genistein and daidzein—and a minor type, glycetein, provides further insight into the incredible versatility of the soybean plant.

Isoflavones are *phytoestrogens*, meaning that they are estrogen-like molecules of plant origin known to have effects similar to that female hormone. (Males also produce estrogen, just as females produce testosterone, so isoflavones are important for both men and women.) Isoflavones have beneficial effects independent of their ability to act as estrogens. They have particular importance for overall health because they have the ability to *modulate* the effect of estrogens. The situation is not simple because, in some circumstances, they can act as a *pro*-estrogen and, in other circumstances, as an *anti*-estrogen.

The versatility of isoflavones is further demonstrated by the fact that they appear to be effective antioxidants and can protect arterial walls from damage caused by free radicals. Isoflavones inhibit oxidation of LDL, and oxidized LDL is the form of cholesterol that is often found in the plaque that causes atherosclerosis. (Remember that other nutrients also are effective in preventing formation of the kind of plaque that characterizes hardening of the arteries and atherosclerosis.)

Studies in monkeys show that soy isoflavones account for up to three quarters of the measurable effect of lowering blood cholesterol using soy protein. Soy protein that lacks isoflavones fails to lower blood cholesterol in primates, but when soy protein containing isoflavones is given, blood cholesterol levels are reduced. Monkeys are the closest animal model to humans (they share 90 percent of our DNA), and, therefore, the results of these experiments are relevant. Besides, it has already been documented in humans that a diet supplemented with soy protein containing isoflavones produces decreased cholesterol levels.

Several other studies have corroborated the benefits of soy, and one study has shown that adding isoflavones to the diet can cause blood cholesterol to fall by as much as 35 percent. These findings provide additional support for the assertion that the isoflavone content of soy protein isolates promote general well-being and health.

SOY IN MANY FORMS

You have probably seen a variety of soy foods in mainstream supermarkets and in health food stores, too. Tofu, tempeh, soy milk, and commercial soy protein powders are becoming increasingly popular items. In addition, soy protein is used to produce such food items as soyburgers and vegetarian "hot dogs." These products vary in their composition—and their quality. When soy is consumed in these forms, some uncertainty exists about the types and amounts of the various health-giving components of soy incorporated. This is an obvious drawback for anyone who desires a stable intake of soy isoflavones for therapeutic purposes. In addition, many consumers do not find soy foods enjoyable or convenient. To counter these problems, the dietary supplement industry has developed products that can deliver certain specific fractions of soy in the dosages that provide health-promoting benefits.

Dietary supplements of any kind can arouse controversy, and some scientists have expressed concern that the supplement industry may be producing soy products with irresponsible or inappropriate health claims. There may be a measure of truth in this point of view, but many manufacturers are developing soy products with standardized content; in this form, soy fractions are nutritional supplements—nutriceuticals. The health benefits can be derived from soy in a convenient and familiar format. Millions of Westerners take nutritional supplements daily, so consuming fractions of soy in this form is not odd. The potential benefits of using soy isoflavones as a nutriceutical is well-illustrated by examining soy and the menopause. This is especially relevant because the menopause heralds the onset of cardiovascular disease in many women.

SOY ISOFLAVONES AND MENOPAUSE

One of the primary reasons that hormone replacement therapy (HRT) is recommended to women involves the mechanism by which estrogen protects against heart disease. The incidence of heart disease is far lower among premenopausal women than it is among males in the same age group. The protective effect of estrogen diminishes after menopause because the body produces less of this hormone. Estrogen may be, on occasion, a woman's best friend, but its fluctuation throughout life is the source of a variety of difficulties for some women.

Menopause and perimenopause (the years preceding the actual cessation of menstrual cycles) are not diseases, but can cause problems for some women. While menopause is a natural event, it can cause symptoms ranging in severity from barely noticeable to extremely troublesome. Hot flashes, vaginal dryness, fatigue, irritability, and increased susceptibility to urinary tract infections are among the most frequently reported symptoms. Some women suffer in silence, but many others seek relief in order to maintain a normal life. In Western societies, body symptoms and signs associated with menopause represent some of the most common reasons for women to seek health-care services.

Nowadays, millions of women take the plunge and start HRT, either in synthetic form or that derived from the urine of pregnant mares. (The latter form has become controversial because of the alleged mistreatment of the animals used to produce this product.) HRT is promoted to both treat menopausal symptoms and as a lifelong therapy to combat common diseases associated with advancing age (such as osteoporosis or Alzheimer's disease).

While the symptoms of perimenopause may be unpleasant and troublesome, the ongoing health challenges are the degenerative diseases, such as heart disease and osteoporosis, that may develop in post-menopausal women. Some individuals within the medical community assume that the majority of women will use HRT to prevent heart disease and osteoporosis, and many medical practitioners do not appear to give serious consideration to other options. Fortunately, the physician who will not address natural options for menopause is becoming a medical dinosaur because many women quite naturally balk at the notion that they will be taking powerful, synthetic hormones for twenty, thirty, or even forty years or more! Balancing estrogen with progesterone (topical or oral) has become popular, but the addition of progesterone may compromise some of the cardiovascular benefits of estrogen.

In the U.S. alone, there are more than forty million menopausal or post-menopausal women, with at least twenty-five million women who will become menopausal within the next ten years. Given these numbers, it is no surprise that HRT is a big issue—and, frankly, a big business. The proponents of synthetic or animal-derived HRT believe in its ability to control the unpleasant symptoms of menopause and help prevent heart disease and osteoporosis. However, concern about the safety of conventional HRT is increasing, too. For example, HRT brings with it an uncertain risk of breast and endometrial cancer. Frequently reported side effects include: abdominal bloating, migraines or headaches of other types, weight gain, anxiety or depression, and breast tenderness. Of course, conventional HRT is contraindicated under certain circumstances. Among those who cannot safely use HRT are women who are experiencing vaginal bleeding of undetermined cause or who have suspected genital or breast cancer, significant liver disease, or a history of thrombosis or embolism. In September 1996, the Committee on Safety of Medicines in the United Kingdom issued a warning of a three-fold risk of venous thrombotic episodes (blood clots) in women on conventional HRT. This warning received little attention in the U.S.

Obviously, the decision to use HRT or consider another option can be difficult for many women. In fact, it is one of the most important health-related decisions that women face in midlife. Given the host of mixed messages about this therapy, it is no wonder that 85 percent of postmenopausal women in the U.S. do not use HRT. Because of their concerns about safety, large numbers of women never fill a prescription they are given for HRT—the swift stroke of the prescription pen is sometimes accompanied by the rapid dunk of the prescription in the nearest garbage bin!

THE SOY SOLUTION

Simple observations often lead to simple solutions, but sometimes the obvious is overlooked. For many years, published reports have noted that many Asian women do not seem as bothered by perimenopausal symptoms as women in Western societies. A survey of Japanese women revealed that no specific word for "hot flash" exists in the Japanese language, and, furthermore, less than 10 percent of women reported experiencing them. It is interesting to note that when Asian women move to the West and begin to alter their diet to conform to the new culture, they begin to experience the same symptoms as other Western women. Recently, I have noticed a more striking trend. Korean distributors of health food products are clamoring to buy soy isoflavone supplements as soy consumption falls in the urban areas of eastern Asia.

Asian women in nonurban locations tend to consume a plant-based diet specifically rich in soy isoflavones—the "weak" estrogens previously discussed. Considerable evidence is accumulating to support the role of soy isoflavones in blocking or modulating the more potent effects of estrogens produced by the body, which are called *endogenous* estrogens. There is a lot we not know about the ability of isoflavones to alter estrogenic effects in the body. Recent research shows that the isoflavones may alter estrogen metabolism (chemical breakdown) in the body. A "blocking effect" of isoflavones on the target sites of estrogenic action (estrogen receptors) explains, in part, why phytoestrogens may be a better option than potent synthetic or animal-derived estrogens that are used in conventional HRT.

Soy isoflavones have versatile health-giving benefits and are considered *adaptogens*, meaning that they promote balance in the body. Thus, isoflavones can provide both estrogenic and antiestrogenic effects. This is what is meant by "modulating" the effects of estrogen.

One form of endogenous estrogen, estradiol, is known to stimulate breast and endometrial tissue (the lining of the uterus) and encourage cell proliferation. This is the reason estrogen is implicated in certain types of breast and uterine cancer. The incidence of breast cancer among Asian women is lower than that of Western women, and it may be that the ability of isoflavones to block the potentially harmful effects of estradiol is a factor in preventing the disease. Again, the story about isoflavones and cancer growth is not simple. Isoflavones have many effects on cancer, other than the ability to modulate the effects of estrogen. Soy isoflavones are antioxidants, they are antiangiogenic, and they interfere with enzymes that cause cancer to grow (such as tyrosine kinase and DNA topoisomerase).

Several studies have confirmed that soy isoflavones have the potential to relieve the symptoms of menopause. One important study was conducted by Dr. Gregory Burke at Wake Forest University in North Carolina. Women in the study reported that the severity of menopausal symptoms was reduced after consuming supplemental soy isoflavones, and their blood pressure was reduced in the bargain. In addition, none of the unpleasant side effects associated with HRT were noted. Unlike women using conventional HRT, soy isoflavones will not tend to cause cell proliferation in breast and uterine tissue.

Dr. Burke has noted that the beneficial effects of soy isoflavones are significant enough to warrant their use as a viable substitute for synthetic HRT or estrogens of animal origin. This extremely important development has the potential to save women from having only two choices, neither of which is particularly pleasant. Soy isoflavones represent a clear third choice, one with obvious advantages over suffering in silence or taking conventional HRT with all its attendant risks.

Dr. Susan Potter and her colleagues from the University of Illinois have performed many studies on the cholesterol-lowering effects of soy. One of their studies showed that soy protein with isoflavones had a positive effect on the lipid profiles of sixty-six post-menopausal women with high cholesterol levels, thereby decreasing cardiovascular risk among these women. Soybeans contain other antiatherogenic components, which include antioxidant properties that protect against the oxidation of LDL. Isoflavones may also act to inhibit platelet aggregation, meaning that they discourage thrombosis or abnormal blood clotting. The anti-thrombotic effects of isoflavones contrast with the thrombotic potential of conventional HRT.

A sensible approach to using isoflavones to prevent or treat mild to moderate symptoms of menopause is to take soy isoflavones in dietary supplement form. You may have seen a variety of isoflavone supplements on the market. Questions remain, of course, about the proper dosages. The dosages of isoflavones used in studies of women in perimenopause have varied considerably, from as high as 160 mg. a day in a study performed in Australia to as low as 40 mg. per day in a study performed in Boston. Based on current knowledge, dosages of 50 to 80 mg. a day appear to be quite safe, especially considering that millions of individuals in Asia routinely consume about those amounts of isoflavones in their diet. Since Asian women tend to have fewer symptoms of menopause, it makes logical sense for women in the West to ingest approximately the same amount of soy isoflavones that Asian women consume.

GOOD AND BAD SOYFOODS AND SUPPLEMENTS

Despite my strong advocacy for soyfoods and soy-based supplements, the world of soy is far from perfect. Modern food processing of soybeans, unregulated use of powerful biopharmaceutical fractions of soy (especially isoflavones), and perhaps genetic engineering are some of the future threats to the versatile health-giving benefits of the soybean. Soybean oil, which is found abundantly in commercial baked goods, is usually used in an unhealthy, hydrogenated form.

Some bulk-source suppliers of soy have created highly concentrated fractions of soy isoflavones that are sometimes used in high dosages in dietary supplements, in spite of concerns about the unknown safety of high doses of isoflavones. I am not against daily supplement amounts of up to a total of 80 mg. of mixed isoflavones per day, or higher with medical supervision. It is important that consumers understand that soy products are not standardized and, therefore, they should carefully choose their soyfoods— and supplements.

FRANKENSTEIN'S FOOD: GENETIC ENGINEERING OF SOY

The importance of soybeans in the food chain has made them a prime candidate for the practitioners of genetic engineering. Genetic modification of an organism (plant or animal) involves the taking of a gene (made from DNA) from one living source and transferring it to another living creature with a view to giving the recipient new characteristics. Examples of genetic engineering have included the taking of a "cold-resistant" gene from Arctic fish and placing it in tomato plants to make them survive frost and the production of "super fish" (especially salmon) which may, unfortunately, turn out to be deformed in a hideous manner. We now face an age of "Frankenstein's food," according to some concerned scientists and activists.

Genetically engineered soybeans have been created that contain higher concentrations of soy isoflavones and have different yields and composition of soybean oil. This practice may seem benign, but when foreign genes are introduced, no one really knows what the outcome will be as cross-pollination with other plants occurs. The development of genetically modified soybeans could result in hybridization of plants or weeds. Maybe one day we shall encounter the man-eating dandelion!

While I sound sarcastic, my attitude is tempered by the sobering thought that some problems with genetic engineering have become readily apparent. In one such venture, a gene from a Brazil nut was donated to a soybean for the purpose of boosting its protein yield. The problem was that the new soybean caused allergic reactions in individuals who had sensitivities to nuts.

In *The Soy Revolution,* I wrote that I had examined safety data on commonly used, genetically modified soybeans and concluded that they posed no identifiable human risk. In the last two years, however, my thoughts on this issue have been rapidly changing. Safety testing for genetically modified crops involves relatively simple comparisons of food components. Small chemical differences are not detectable by routine testing, but may result in profound biological effects in the organism and perhaps its neighbors in the environment. Leading developers of genetically engineered, disease-resistant soybeans have modified crops to be used with pesticides and not as an alternative to pesticide use. This situation creates real conflict when the company modifies a crop to be used with its own proprietary herbicide or pesticide. Genetic modification of plants in this manner is one of the major threats to organic farming.

RETURNING TO ANCESTRAL FOOD TECHNOLOGY

During my plenary lecture at the Korean Soyfood Association meeting in Seoul, Korea, in 1997, local food scientists told me that soyfood consumption had peaked in many Asian nations. These scientists believed that the key to enhancing the acceptability of soy to the new generation of Asians was to move away from ancestral food processing technology, which often involved fermentation, and to introduce "modern" Western-processed soyfoods. The globalization of fast food and the spread of the "double Whopper brain" may play a role in this current trend in Asia. However, when we look at the ascribed health benefits of soyfood, they are readily identifiable in population studies where ancestrally prepared (fermented) soy is consumed and not so obvious with soy processed by using modern technology.

Fermented soy probably has more to offer in some circumstances than "Western" processed soy. Fermentation will tend to produce partially digested fractions of soy, especially protein, that can be more readily assimilated. Soy isoflavones that are presented in fermented soy are present in deconjugated form, meaning that they are split from sugars and are more readily absorbed by the body. The yeast used in the fermentation process results in a residual of B vitamins and health-giving natural compounds such as beta glucan (a good stimulator of immune function).

Farsighted individuals have returned to ancestral fermentation technology to provide fermented soy for inclusion in foods and dietary supplements. Biofoods, Inc., of West Paterson, New Jersey, and BioTherapies, Inc., of Fairfield, New Jersey, are leaders in this field in the United States. These companies have produced vitamins, minerals, and biopharmaceuticals using fermentation technology. Biofoods' leading product is a nongenetically engineered, fermented, organic soybean preparation, which is a modified form of natto. This is an example of an advanced soybean product, available from organically grown sources, in the dietary supplement for women called FemSoy Plus.

FOODS VERSUS SUPPLEMENTS

I believe that soy foods are advantageous, and I encourage you to add them to your diet. Soy milk is certainly a healthful substitute for dairy milk in adults and children. Reduced-fat and calcium-fortified soy milk also are available. The versatile foods tofu and tempeh are now found in markets all over the country. However, you would need to consume a half-pound of tofu or more each day to obtain enough isoflavones for a therapeutic effect. Equally important is the fact that the isoflavone content of commercial soy foods, from tofu to soy milk to soyburgers, is not standardized. One cannot confidently say that, in general, the soybean contains a certain amount of this or that fraction. Which soybean? Grown where? Processed how? In order to receive a predictable and stable dosage of isoflavones, it is best to take isoflavones in supplement form. Isoflavone supplements are standardized and the labeling is uniform in that you can easily calculate the exact isoflavone dosage you are receiving. Remember, too, that taking a therapeutic dose of isoflavones for menopausal symptoms may have overall positive effects on your health. Soy isoflavones are antagonistic against osteoporosis, breast and prostate cancer, menopausal symptoms, and atherosclerosis.

ABOUT OSTEOPOROSIS

One of the purported benefits of HRT is that it protects against osteoporosis, one of the degenerative diseases associated with aging. Osteoporosis is the gradual thinning of the bones or, put another way, the loss of bone mass that results in "brittle" bones. Estrogen plays a role in protecting the bones in the premenopausal woman, and the risk of bone fractures increases after menopause and with advancing age. HRT is promoted as a way to slow bone loss in postmenopausal women, and so are soy isoflavones. In addition, women are advised to keep their calcium intake high (1,000–1,500 mg. a day) and engage in weight-bearing exercise (*e.g.*, walking, aerobic dancing, and weight training for the upper and lower body).

A new class of drugs, called SERMs (selective estrogen receptor modulators) mimic estrogen and are considered safer than HRT. I stress "considered" because the data to support this qualification of synthetic estrogen are not available, at least as yet. What is especially interesting about SERMs is that their composition is remarkably similar to soy isoflavones. SERMs are said to reduce LDL, the "bad" cholesterol, and so do isoflavones, but soy protein and isoflavones also help increase HDL, which SERMs are not purported to do. SERMs are not marketed to relieve the symptoms of menopause. Some studies suggest they do nothing or make such symptoms more apparent. SERMs offer protective effects against heart disease and osteoporosis. As you have seen, soy offers these benefits, without any known risks. To me, it makes no sense to take a synthetic drug that offers no advantage over isoflavones, a naturally occurring component of a common plant. Government-sponsored trials of drugs to prevent cancer started with the cancer-causing drug Tamoxifen. Government attention has now truned to SERMs. What about isoflavones?

In addition, soy is calcium-sparing, meaning that it helps the body retain and use calcium—and, by implication, it helps maintain the strength of the bones. By contrast, diets that are high in animal protein tend to cause more calcium excretion through the kidneys. Calcium intake is actually higher in Western countries whose consumption of animal protein is the highest in the world. It is ironic, therefore, that Western societies have higher rates of hip fracture than other countries, many of which are third world societies whose diets tend to be lower in animal protein as well as lower in calcium intake. One may wonder what cardiovascular disease has to do with osteoporosis. Osteoporosis underlies hip fracture in the elderly, and this event may often signal the end of life. Death following hip fracture often results from cardiovascular problems, especially pulmonary embolism.

MEN NEED THIS INFORMATION, TOO

Osteoporosis is not just a women's disease—and, for that matter, neither is hormonal fluctuation a challenge faced solely by women. I have coined the term "omnipause" to describe the midlife changes that are common to both men and women. Mature males may benefit from soy isoflavones to enhance the protective effect of calcium, thereby protecting their bones from the thinning that comes with age.

Men are also subject to hormonally dependent conditions, such as benign enlargement of the prostate gland and prostate cancer. Evidence exists that soy isoflavones may prevent prostate cancer and/or slow its growth. Epidemiological studies have shown that Japanese men develop prostate cancer, but because it grows slowly, it does not become a killer disease. In fact, the older male may not even realize he has the disease. In the 1980s, Japanese researchers discovered that the isoflavone genistein can block the signal that triggers the growth of cancer cells, which explains why prostate cancer may behave the way it does among populations for whom the soybean is a staple food. It appears that soy isoflavones also may well have a protective effect against benign prostate enlargement. So powerful is the message that soy isoflavones may be valuable for prostatic structure and function that famous scientists such as Herman Adlercreutz of Finland have proposed that every man who is serious about prostatic health should eat soy every day.

ARE SOY ISOFLAVONES SAFE?

From time to time controversies about the safety of soy supplements surface. Some of the controversy centers on questions surrounding the effects of soy isoflavones on fertility. Initially, the observations were based on fertility problems noted in sheep who were fed large amounts of alfalfa and clover, which contain high concentrations of phytoestrogens. However, no significant effects on fertility have ever been noted on human populations. The Japanese have no reported fertility problems, and the low birthrate in China is largely due to government-sponsored family planning measures, not a soy-based diet.

Across the planet, many people consume more than 100 mg. of isoflavones per day—or more—in their soy-based diets, with no harmful effects reported. Dosages of 50–80 mg. per day for therapeutic purposes are well within the safety zone.

THE BENEFITS OF SOY FOR CHILDREN

It is clear from many large international studies that high blood cholesterol levels in children may lead to symptomatic coronary artery disease in adulthood and asymptomatic artery disease in children. Furthermore, it is not unusual for children to have high cholesterol and early arterial damage. Pediatrician Charles Attwood, author of Dr. Attwood's Low-Fat Prescription For Kids, has drawn attention to studies from across the globe that highlight this alarming situation.

It is apparent that the increased consumption of dairy products, particularly cow's milk, has been a relatively recent development, particularly in third world countries. Dr. Attwood considers this growing situation quite serious, and cites statements made in 1992 by the Physicians Committee for Responsible Medicine (PCRM), a group that has been critical about the consumption of cow's milk during childhood. The PCRM contend that consuming cow's milk in infancy and childhood may be responsible for causing several major diseases, including coronary artery disease, cancer, allergies, and perhaps diabetes mellitus. Based on his clinical experience, Dr. Attwood adds anemia, asthma, sinus disease, and eczema to the list of potential problems caused by cow's milk. Because there is concern about dairy products, especially the full-fat variety, it makes sense to examine the potential role of soy milk in infancy and childhood.

In contrast to dairy milk, soy milk is an insignificant source of saturated fat and is a healthful beverage for children and adults. In addition, soy-based infant formulas have been developed and tested over the years and have been found to fulfill the requirements of a beneficial and safe food for infants. (Obviously, for infants, breast milk is preferable to soy or dairy formulas. In addition, plain soy milk by itself must not be used as an infant formula; it is inadequate for that purpose.) The protein content of soy milk is equivalent to that of cow's milk and although it is possible to be allergic to soybeans, it is not as common a condition as allergy to cow's milk. Low-fat and calcium-fortified varieties of soy milk are available, as well as a range of flavors. Concerns about isoflavones in infant formulas of soy milk remain somewhat contentious.

Soy is not the only plant basis for milk. Swedish scientists have produced palatable and healthful oat milk. There is a slow but sure move towards vegetable milk, and it is a welcome change.

ONE MORE NOTE ON THE INGENIOUS AND VERSATILE ISOFLAVONES

Soy isoflavones play a role in lowering cholesterol and increasing HDL, and they simultaneously have the potential to be a safe and effective alternative to synthetic or animal-derived hormone replacement therapy. They help the body use calcium and offer protection against osteoporosis. In addition, they may play a role in preventing hormone-dependent cancers in both men and women and have important antioxidant effects. It is easy to see that isoflavones are among nature's most ingenious substances. Soy protein and other fractions of soy also have the potential to promote healthy kidney function, play a role in preventing and treating diabetes by helping to regulate insulin, and contribute to healthy skin. Because soy isoflavones are available as dietary supplements, their benefits can be obtained in a convenient form.

The advice offered in this chapter goes hand in hand with other information presented in this book, including the need to consistently tailor your diet to promote a healthy heart. The use of soy can result in many health benefits, including its ability to promote cardiovascular health. Cardiovascular health is a primary objective, but it must not be the only goal of a heart-smart diet. Remember, too, that isoflavones are not a substitute for a healthful diet, exercise, or stress management. Although soy isoflavones are safe as well as effective, I still recommend that you discuss the therapeutic use of isoflavone products with your health-care providers.

SUMMARY

I describe soy as the "food of the next millennium" because its health benefits are far-reaching and not limited to cardiovascular disease. However, as a cholesterol-lowering agent, soy protein containing isoflavones has been overlooked for far too long. Many convincing studies have shown that soy protein containing isoflavones is a reliable cholesterol-lowering agent. In addition, as a treatment for high cholesterol levels, soy does not have dangerous or unpleasant side effects. I believe it is superior to cholesterol-lowering drugs as a *first choice* treatment option to normalize blood lipids. Soy protein also promotes healthy bone and kidney function, and because it helps to regulate insulin, it may be beneficial for preventing diabetes or as part of a treatment regimen for existing diabetes.

Components in soy other than the favorable amino acid content may help lower cholesterol and bring additional health benefits. Isoflavones are important—and extremely versatile—phytochemicals, and soybeans are nature's premiere source of these potentially important substances. Isoflavones are believed to have weak estrogen-like effects in some circumstances, and they may modulate the effects of estrogen in the body. Numerous studies have suggested that soy isoflavones may be a viable alternative to HRT (hormone replacement therapy) for mature women during the perimenopause and post-menopausal years. In addition, some evidence suggests that soy isoflavones may play a role in preventing osteoporosis in both men and women, and also may help prevent benign enlargement of the prostate and prostate cancer in men.

What You Can Do

- To lower cholesterol, or as a source of high-quality protein, choose a high-quality soy protein dietary supplement such as Genista. Avoid soy bars that allege this benefit but contain hydrogenated oils or saturated fat.
- Soybeans contain both soluble and insoluble fiber, but to obtain the benefit, you must consume whole soybeans. Add them to your diet slowly because they tend to cause flatulence. Other foods, including oats and bran, are valuable sources of fiber, too.
- Soy foods are valuable additions to your meals, but supplementing your diet with soy isoflavones may have value as well. If you are a woman approaching the menopause, talk with a knowledgeable health-care provider about the possibility of using soy isoflavones therapeutically. Isoflavones are antioxidants and interfere with the dangerous phenomenon of LDL oxidation that can cause atheroma. Strong evidence exists that soy isoflavones may prevent or relieve unpleasant symptoms associated with menopause, such at hot flashes. In addition, soy isoflavones may help prevent osteoporosis and should be part of a "heart smart" dietary plan. Unlike hormone replacement therapy (HRT), which uses synthetic estrogens or estrogens from an animal source (mare urine), soy isoflavones do not carry the uncertain risk of increased breast and uterine cancer.
- Men also should take heed. Soy isoflavones may play a role in preventing benign enlargement of the prostate gland, and in addition, these versatile substances may help prevent prostate cancer.

CHAPTER TWELVE

THE HEALING PLANTS

For centuries, extracts from plants have been used to prevent and cure an enormous number of human health complaints, from minor indigestion and the common cold to heart disease and cancer. It may seem strange, but despite this worldwide history, relatively few scientific studies of merit are available to support the use of plant-based remedies. I hope some practitioners of alternative medicine hear this wakeup call.

Fortunately, this situation is changing as research from other societies is recognized in the West and new research projects are initiated. The terms "medicinal herbs" or "botanical remedies" should never be used lightly. Some of our powerful modern pharmaceuticals are derived from plants or base their action on known properties of plants. Pharmacognosy is a well-developed science that studies the development of medicine from herbal and botanical sources. However, this subject has been dropped from the teaching curriculum of many pharmacy schools, and many modern physicians are complete strangers to this scientific discipline.

The idea that nature has provided a pharmacy for humans is not new and is by no means revolutionary; precedent for using botanical products to treat cardiovascular disease exists. For example, an extract derived from foxglove was once popularly described as a "heart tonic" or "cardiac stimulant." This extract is, of course, known as digitalis, and it is the basis of one of the most commonly prescribed medications for cardiac disease. The basis of modern-day synthetic drug therapy largely developed from knowledge about and use of plants. It is easy to forget that more than one-quarter of all current prescription drugs are derived from plants.

PROCEED WITH CAUTION!

You should *never* experiment with herbal remedies for significant illnesses on your own. Not only do many botanical remedies act in a powerful way on the body, but commercial herbal products do not necessarily contain predictable ingredients; few are presented in standardized formats or dosages. This means that the type and amount of the active ingredients may vary considerably from one brand of dietary supplement to the next—or even within the same brand. The problems inherent in using nonstandardized products have been overcome to some degree in countries such as Germany, where standardized botanical formulas—herbal remedies—are frequently prescribed for common health problems. Chinese, Korean, and Japanese medicine also rely heavily on botanical compounds in treatment programs. I have traveled extensively in China and Korea and have first-hand experience of the application of traditional Chinese and Korean medicine and some of its benefits. However, many countries lag behind Germany and several eastern Asian countries in regulating botanical health products by providing clear guidelines for their use.

Some people believe that herbal remedies are safe because they are "natural." This is a serious mistake. Some of the most potent toxins known to man are of plant origin. Plants that can heal when used correctly can be harmful when misused; *i.e.*, taken in amounts larger than the recommended doses or over a longer period of time than recommended. The safest option is to seek the advice of a health-care giver who is qualified and experienced in herbal or botanical treatments before these remedies are even considered. Unfortunately, many physicians know very little about botanical remedies, and some alternative health-care providers who claim knowledge about plant medicinals are actually inexperienced with their use. Conventional medical literature is full of reports of serious and sometimes fatal adverse effects of medicinal herbs. These reports tend to be played down by some of the new generation of alternative medical practitioners and herbalists. This situation has led many conventional medical practitioners to suspect that many herbs are dangerous and are of dubious benefit anyway. This is part of the damaging dichotomy that exists between alternative and conventional medical practices.

The issue of the potential danger of herbal remedies must be put in perspective. In the January/February 1999 issue of *New Age* magazine, Dr. Andrew Weil responded to an editorial published in the *New England Journal of Medicine* that was critical of "risky and untested" alternative therapies. Dr. Weil was disappointed (to say the least) in the disparaging tone of the editorial, particularly because of what he calls the "double standard" used to discuss alternative therapies. According to an article published in the April 1998 *Journal of the American Medical Association* (*JAMA*), adverse reactions to *prescription drugs* has been found to be the fourth to sixth leading cause of death in the United States. That means that it falls just after heart disease, cancer, and stroke!

Overall, reported incidents of adverse reactions to botanicals or nutritional supplements are far fewer than adverse reactions to prescription drugs. Admittedly, physicians argue about reporting bias because herbal side effects are not routinely documented the way drug side effects are. So, if you hear alarming reports about herbal remedies, remember that prescription drugs are not, by definition, safer—and, in fact, also must be used with great care. All disciplines of modern medicine live in glass houses, but they remain eager and willing to throw stones.

Despite potential problems inherent with their use, more than twenty different botanical extracts or formulations have been used with some frequency in Western countries to combat atherosclerosis. I recommend *Botanical Influences on Illness*, by Melvyn R. Werbach, M.D., and Michael T. Murray, N.D. Their book contains a discussion of botanical influences on cardiovascular disease. Dr. Murray has also written *The Healing Power of Herbs*, which offers valuable information about botanicals. My book *Miracle Herbs* (coauthored with Linda Comac), is another resource for readers interested in learning more. A few plants appear to stand out from the rest in their ability to have a positive influence on cardiovascular wellness. While some of these plants may be familiar to you, the healing power of others may come as a surprise. You will also notice that some are found in many corners of our planet and even make appearances in centuries-old folklore.

THE MAGIC OF GARLIC

Through the ages, garlic has been one of the special plants to which magical powers have been ascribed. Midwives in ancient Greece used it to protect newborns from evil spirits and witches. Ancient Egyptians used it to swear oaths, the way modern Westerners use the Bible in a court of law. Various cultures have called it an aphrodisiac and a source of power for males in battle. Hippocrates, the father of Western medicine, named it as one of the most important of his four hundred remedies. In Ayurvedic medicine it was used to treat leprosy, and in China a legend about wild garlic holds that it was an antidote to poison. Far from being relegated to legend, however, the modern Chinese use up to five cloves of garlic per person per day in their cooking. And what would Mediterranean cuisine be without it? Moving forward to our scientific age, Dr. Erich Block of the State University of New York has referred to garlic as the "spice of life." This is a modest statement, especially when we look at the versatile therapeutic benefits of this common and, in many places, revered plant, whose botanical name is *Allium sativum.*

After reviewing extensive scientific information about garlic, I find support for its health-giving benefits so convincing that I strongly recommend you include it in your diet. Five cloves a day may not be necessary, but some lesser amount will help. While it is true that the taste and odor of garlic and its cousins in the allium family, onions, do not appeal to all tastes, there are now odorless dietary supplements containing the health-giving components—fractions—of garlic, especially those that are known to have a positive effect on cardiovascular health.

Garlic is widely acknowledged as a relatively safe and effective therapeutic agent for arteriosclerosis, sharing many of the advantages of fish oil. There is unequivocal evidence that garlic—and some of its fractions—reduce blood cholesterol and triglyceride levels. It has an antihypertensive effect, meaning that it may have a role in preventing high blood pressure. It also has anti-thrombotic actions, which means it may work against the formation of blood clots in the blood vessels.

At least forty clinical studies have been performed on the effects of garlic preparations on total blood cholesterol. Only eight of these studies showed no significant effect of garlic on total blood cholesterol readings. Thirty-two studies showed statistically significant percentage reductions of blood cholesterol, ranging from –6 to –29 percent. The effectiveness of garlic to reduce serum triglyceride levels is equally impressive. In more than thirty-two clinical studies, only eleven showed no significant effect and the remaining studies reported significant percentage reductions of serum triglycerides ranging from –7 to –34 percent. When the study protocols are examined, the differences between the low to high percentages can be accounted for by the variable types and amounts of garlic preparations used. The actual mechanisms that cause the beneficial effects have not been fully explained. To date, most evidence seems to suggest that *allicin* is the active constituent, or agent, that causes the cholesterol-lowering effects.

You are probably wondering just how much garlic you should consume to bring about these positive results. Based on clinical studies, to achieve the lipid-lowering result, the optimal dose of *allicin* is on the order of 0.05–0.1 mg./kg. of body weight. Translated, this represents two to three grams of fresh garlic per day, taken for a period of four to eight weeks. You cannot add a clove or two of garlic to a prepared dish a couple of times a week and expect to see positive results. I do not discourage you from using garlic liberally in your cooking, but you will not see immediate results using a haphazard approach.

The positive effects of garlic on blood pressure are complex, but well-documented. These effects are believed to be related to the ability of garlic to relax blood vessels and expand their diameter (vasodilate). Overall, clinical studies show a significant reduction in both systolic and diastolic blood pressure (both numbers in the blood pressure reading) with daily doses of different garlic preparations ranging from 18 mg. to 1.2 grams. The actual components of garlic that lower blood pressure are still not known.

Garlic and some related compounds enhance a process called fibrinolysis, by which blood coagulation is impaired and blood flow is enhanced. Fibrin is a protein in the blood that is involved in blood coagulation. Arteriosclerosis is associated with measurable decreases in fibrinolytic activity, meaning that there are decreases in the activity necessary to dissolve blood clots. To some degree, garlic can reverse this process.

About a dozen clinical studies of the effect of garlic on fibrinolytic (clot-dissolving) activity show conclusively that different garlic preparations in doses ranging from 4 mg. to 1.5 mg. per day result in significant and rapid enhancement of this process. As adjunctive therapy, meaning a secondary treatment that accompanies a primary treatment, garlic has been used for thrombotic (clotting) disorders and thromboembolic conditions with variable success.

Remember that platelets (thrombocytes) play a major role in causing atheroma. When circulating platelets clump together, they stick to blood vessel linings and release substances that promote adverse changes in the lining of blood vessels. These changes create an environment favorable to cholesterol deposits and blockages in the vessels. It is significant that many studies demonstrate that garlic preparations inhibit the process of platelet adhesion—in other words, garlic may discourage platelets from sticking together. This is the fundamental reason why garlic can be used therapeutically to prevent arteriosclerosis. The active constituents in garlic that inhibit platelet function include allicin, allyl sulfides, and adenosine. Overall, allicin seems to be the most important element.

As you can see, more than one element in garlic accounts for its cardiovascular benefits. This is not surprising—it is a complex plant that contains a number of health-giving substances. Many of these constituents may act synergistically. (It's no wonder that both soybeans and garlic have, in the past, been considered miracle foods—the more that is known about their chemical complexity and versatility, the more they prove that their reputation has been well-deserved all along.)

It is clear that *allicin* is a key health-giving fraction of garlic. If you want to use a dietary supplement containing garlic, you should be reasonably sure that any preparation you choose contains allicin (or *alliin* in concentrations of at least two times more than allicin; alliin is an element found in garlic oil). If it does not contain allicin, don't buy it—it will not provide the desired cardiovascular and other health benefits.

Understand, however, that the amount of a certain component of garlic required to bring about the health-giving effect may vary considerably, depending on what it is being used for. One could logically conclude that the best way to use garlic would be in its natural form, but several hundred species of garlic plants exist and each has differences in its active chemical components. Furthermore, growing conditions alter the health-giving components and contents of plants, even within the same species of garlic plant. (This principle applies to virtually all plant life.) The demand for odorless garlic products adds to this already complex situation.

Thankfully, garlic is as popular now as it has ever been and can easily be found in its various forms. I encourage you to use fresh garlic in your cooking. To date, there is no such thing as the "ideal" supplemental garlic product because our knowledge of the biopharmaceutical effects of all garlic fractions is quite incomplete. However, as a guideline, a daily dose of garlic powder that is standardized to contain approximately 1.3 percent alliin or 0.6 percent allicin, which is approximately equivalent to 3.6 to 5.4 mg. of allicin, can achieve the lipid-lowering effect.

The process of standardization has been hampered because there is a relative lack of pure standard garlic compound to use as a reference. The two main types of garlic preparations come in powder form or as extracts of garlic oil. Based on current knowledge, garlic powders that contain a standardized content of allicin are preferable to other products. This is largely because most evidence to date is based on results of research using garlic powder. Aged garlic extracts (*e.g.*, Kyolic, Kyoleopin, Leopin-Five) and odorless garlic extract (*e.g.*, Tolstat) have little to offer over standardized garlic powder preparations that contain adequate allicin (or alliin). I am most impressed with the garlic preparations made by Nature's Way, a company based in Utah. Nature's Way is one of a handful of dietary supplement companies that have made a firm commitment to "standards" in herbal products.

To summarize, you will gain the health benefits of garlic if you daily consume about 3.5 to 5.5 mg. of allicin. This corresponds to 0.6 to 1.8 grams of fresh garlic (containing 0.3 percent allicin-releasing potential). In terms of garlic powder products, these figures translate to 0.3–0.9 grams of garlic powder per day, which will yield 0.6 percent allicin. In Europe, four grams per day of fresh garlic is considered necessary to gain the potential health benefits. Based on current literature, I believe that about 2.5–3 grams per day is adequate.

THE MYRIAD FLAVONOIDS

Organic chemists may like to toss around names such as "oligomeric proanthocyanidins," but I do not expect that you want to be become bogged down in chemistry lessons. The term is important, however, referring to a group of flavonoids that are abundant in plants and contribute to overall health in ways that we are only beginning to understand. Flavonoids are the chemicals responsible for the yellow, red, or deep blue color in some fruits, herbs, vegetables, and flowers. There are more than fifteen classes of flavonoids, and one class, *bio*flavonoids, is found in citrus fruits. An important class of flavonoids is also found in soybeans (soy isoflavones). Procyanidolic oligomers include or, in some cases, are considered to be synonymous with other biochemical elements such as pycnogenol, leukocyanidins, and complexes of polyphenols or flavonoids. Do not be put off by these terms. The importance of these substances will be clear as we move along, so please don't skip this discussion just because it contains some unfamiliar concepts!

A group of chemicals called *polyphenols* are cancer-fighting substances, and flavonoids, including bioflavonoids, are one type of these naturally occurring polyphenols. These substances are found in a wide variety of plants. Polyphenols are powerful antioxidants; thus, bioflavonoids are believed to be capable of preventing a variety of diseases, including cardiovascular disease, viral infections, and cancer. In addition, these compounds may play a role in regulating blood glucose.

Dr. Albert Szent-Gyorgyi, the 1937 Nobel Laureate in medicine/physiology, called bioflavonoids "vitamin P" and demonstrated that they act like a vitamin in the body. Conventional medicine will not recognize or acknowledge the term vitamin P. It is apparent that many of these polyphenolic compounds work synergistically, or in a mutually protective manner, with vitamin C, and they are known as vitamin C "helpers."

Numerous studies show the health benefits of bioflavonoids, especially in promoting cardiovascular wellness. Bioflavonoid compounds such as hesperidin, rutin, and quercetin, which are found in citrus fruits, are examples of the most widely researched

Table 12.1: Metabolic Effects of Flavonoids and Certain Procyanidolic Oligomers.

Facilitates phospholipid metabolism
Vitamin C helper effects
Antioxidant effects
Vitamin E–like activities
Free radical scavengers
Protein phosphorylation
Effects on arachidonic acid metabolism
Potent effects on redox reactions
Influence gene expression
Affects calcium ion transport

bioflavonoids. It is known that hesperidin, rutin, and quercetin protect the structure and integrity of capillaries, and they have an important role in stabilizing cell membranes. These compounds also contribute to cardiovascular wellness by helping to lower cholesterol and by inhibiting platelet aggregation—the "clumping" phenomenon in the blood that was discussed earlier.

Bioflavonoids are available in dietary supplement form in health food stores and some pharmacies. They are frequently mixed with vitamin C, which both facilitates their effect and prevents them from degrading. (This is an example of synergistic, additive action.) Recommended daily intake of these substances varies, but some guidelines go as high as one gram (1,000 mg.) per day or more. The ideal dose is unknown and is probably quite variable. In the mixed supplements, a popular source of active bioflavonoid elements is often algae (from which quercetin is sometimes derived) and buckwheat (from which rutin is obtained).

Many different natural sources of bioflavonoids exist, and it is difficult to make a specific recommendation about the best type to take as a dietary supplement. There is no question that a mixture of bioflavonoids is preferable, so if you are interested in supplementing your diet with bioflavonoids, examine the label for specific information about the amount of these agents that are standardized in the dietary supplement product. Several classes of herbal products contain polyphenols and bioflavonoids as their active constituents. The bioflavonoids are one very good reason to reach for fruit and vegetables.

PYCNOGENOL

In recent years, considerable interest has been focused on extracts of the European coastal pine, a tree that is native to the island of Corsica. It has been noted that extracts of the bark of the tree *Pinus maritima* have potent antioxidant effects. This extract has been marketed under the name pycnogenol, or the plural, pycnogenols. The general class of flavonoids to which pycnogenol belongs is *oligomeric proanthocyanidins*, mercifully shortened to OPCs. The antioxidant effects are what has drawn attention to these extracts and the OPC family. Pycnogenol may strengthen blood vessels and, because of its antioxidant effect, is believed to have a role in preventing heart disease, perhaps by diminishing cholesterol deposits within blood vessels. Like bilberry, pycnogenol (and grapeseed extract) may also enhance vision.

Extracts from grapeseeds also contain OPCs, and there is increasing indication that grapeseed extracts containing bioflavonoids may be as effective as extracts from European coastal pine. Using grapeseed, a readily renewable agricultural resource, is ecologically sound, whereas the European coastal pine is a rather rare tree that could be depleted. In any case, pycnogenol is expensive, which is why alternative sources of OPCs are actively sought.

Table 12.2: Potential Health Benefits of Pycnogenol.

Modified from Passwater and Kandaswami (1994).

Anti-inflammatory action
Anti-arthritic effects
Reduces oxidative stress
Potential longevity benefit
Maintains normal capillary function
Improves red cell membrane flexibility
Improves skin elasticity and smoothness
Anti-allergic action, *e.g.*, hay fever
Reduces diabetic retinopathy
Enhances immune function
Beneficial in stomach ulcers
Reduces risk of phlebitis and varicose veins
May reduce tissue edema

The flavonoids within grapes are found mainly in the skin and seeds, and a variety of cancer-fighting compounds have been isolated from grapes, including catechins, anthocyanidins (as found in bilberry), and proanthocyanidins. Other important sources of these agents are the popular beverages green tea, red wine (especially young wine), and red grape juice. The importance of flavonoids in red wine has been exemplified by much recent research, which stresses moderate wine intake (one to two glasses of red wine per day) as beneficial for health.

THE RED WINE ISSUE: REVISITING "THE FRENCH PARADOX"

The story of the health benefit of red wine and grapes involves observations that the death rate from cardiovascular disease in France, particularly coronary artery disease, is much lower than it is in Britain or North America. The reason for this lower death rate from coronary artery disease may be due in part to the higher rates of consumption of red wine and grapes in France. Studies of the nutritional profile of French people versus British and American citizens indicate that the intake of saturated fat in the diet is quite similar. A famous study that was published in the British medical journal *Lancet* in 1979 implied that the lower heart disease rate in France was most notable in regions of the country where red wine was the primary type of wine consumed.

The results of this study have caused some argument. On the one hand, it is known that moderate alcohol intake may tend to normalize blood lipids and increase HDL levels. Thus, some scientists have attributed the lower death rates from coronary artery disease in the French to a higher rate of moderate alcohol consumption among the population. It is possible that alcohol itself may have a protective effect because it relieves stress and anxiety. However, many individuals maintain that the powerful bioflavonoids in red wine may account for this improvement in cardiovascular wellness in several regions of France where wine consumption is prevalent. Red wine also shows anti-thrombotic effects that are not noted in individuals who consume white wine.

Despite the many advantages that seem apparent, there are also disadvantages. The incidence of liver cirrhosis in France is much higher than it is in the rest of the world, and excessive consumption of any alcoholic beverage cannot be considered healthy.

Many individuals find the alcohol issue quite incongruous. Alcohol promotes formation of free radicals, which cause disease, but when taken in moderation there are beneficial effects. *Moderation*, of course, remains one of the universal secrets of good health and longevity. After publication of the epidemiologic studies that showed a lower incidence of cardiovascular disease among French red wine consumers, there was an almost immediate rise in the sale of red wine throughout the Western world.

Some detailed laboratory research has confirmed the proposed rationale for the use of red wine containing bioflavonoids. It appears that the bioflavonoid quercetin, which is found in abundance in red grapes, may exert effects similar to aspirin. Bioflavonoids in red wine appear to enhance immune function, at least in drunken mice! Unfortunately, the news for white wine drinkers is not as good, because white wine contains a lesser amount of bioflavonoids than red wine. On the other hand, red wine may tend to cause heartburn more often than white wine. These symptoms of heartburn are not necessarily benign and may simulate or stimulate episodes of angina for individuals with coronary artery disease. For this reason, I recommend that individuals who want the health benefits from the bioflavonoids contained within red grapes take the bioflavonoid complex that is produced from the grapes, rather than use red wine as the source of the bioflavonoids. Another important component of grapes that has potent and versatile effects is resveratrol, which is found in abundance in grape skins. Resveratrol has been synthesized and is available as an expensive dietary supplement. Resveratrol is one example of synthetic agents that masquerade as natural therapies.

The interest in pycnogenol and OPCs stems from their reputation as highly effective antioxidants that have the ability to scavenge free radicals. They share this reputation with other flavonoids (The potential health benefits of pycnogenol are summarized in Table 12.2). It is important to note that the lower the flavonoid intake, the higher the incidence of heart disease. This relationship was found to be present in the Zutphen Study even after correcting for other lifestyle or dietary influences on the incidence of heart disease. The potential beneficial effect of pycnogenol has been likened to the observed beneficial effects of vitamin E supplement. It is believed that pycnogenol and other OPCs prevent oxidation of LDL. These flavonoids also inhibit platelet adhesion.

Overall, procyanidolic oligomers have promise for the prevention and perhaps therapy of coronary heart disease, but the argument for their use seems to be outweighed by the evidence to support the dietary incorporation of other botanical products, such as soy protein containing soy isoflavones, omega-3 fatty acids (predominately fish oil) taken in a correct ratio with omega-6 fatty acids, and garlic preparations.

GINKGO

You have probably seen advertising on television and in print for ginkgo products. Until a few years ago, you might have thought that ginkgo was just an attractive tree, but now you are being told that a daily dose of extracts from ginkgo could improve your memory and increase your sense of well-being. Since virtually everyone worries about lapses in memory, it is easy to see why over-the-counter ginkgo products are becoming increasingly popular. Ginkgo products are also promoted for their alleged antidepressant effects and their known benefits of promoting blood flow in the body.

It appears that ginkgo enhances blood flow to the brain, thereby increasing the supply of nutrients and oxygen that nourish the brain cells. Ginkgo has an overall beneficial effect on blood circulation and some preparations contain quercetin and other bioflavonoid compounds, such as flavone glycosides. The presence of these bioflavonoids may add to the health benefits offered by ginkgo.

In both animal and human studies, ginkgo has been shown to inhibit platelet aggregation and it directly inhibits the platelet-activating factor, the factor that starts platelets sticking together. In other words, ginkgo inhibits the formation of blood clots, thereby offering a direct advantage for maintaining a healthy heart. As with many remedies of natural origin, the effects of ginkgo are not immediate. In the experience of many health-care providers who use ginkgo in their practices, it may take up to three or four months before any beneficial effect is noted, especially if the desired effect is improved blood circulation. Furthermore, anecdotal clinical observations indicate that it can take from nine months to a year to show improvement in blood circulation. Persistence with ginkgo (and other natural remedies) is required for its use to pay off. As a general rule, remedies of natural origin almost never give the "quick fix" that we have learned to expect from pharmaceuticals.

To date, the optimal dose of ginkgo is not known. If you are going to take ginkgo supplements, 40–50 mg. of a standardized flavoglycoside (the active compound) in a concentration of approximately 20 percent or more is recommended. If the overall content of flavoglycoside listed on the label is not 20 percent, then look for another product. Remember that all herbal products are not created equal! "Grass clippings in a can" may be found all too often in "bargain" dietary supplements.

BILBERRY: FRUIT FROM EUROPE

Bilberry (*Vaccinium myrtillus*) is grown throughout Europe. It can be used to make a delicious fruit pie, which is, unfortunately, often overbaked, causing the heat to damage its nutrient content, which may promote health. Bilberry fruit is dark blue or purple, and the active flavonoids are anthocyanidins. It is believed that these anthocyanidins are capable of lowering blood cholesterol and triglyceride levels, at least in a modest manner.

Heart disease aside for a moment, bilberry has been used for its beneficial effect on vision. The finding that bilberry could enhance the ability of the eye to adapt to the dark was noted serendipitously by pilots of the Royal Air Force in World War II during their nighttime bombing missions over Germany. I have noted that some individuals with coronary artery disease who have taken bilberry extracts report spontaneous improvement in their vision, especially during twilight hours. Some preparations of bilberry also contain chromium, and they have been used with alleged success to prevent or treat diabetes, although this application is not widely known.

It is difficult to obtain enough anthocyanidins from fresh bilberry; concentrated extracts are required to provide optimal amounts. Several dietary supplements are available containing standardized amounts of anthocyanidins to a level of between 20 and 25 percent.

HAWTHORN MAY BE GOOD FOR YOUR HEART

Hawthorn (*Crataegus species*) is quite rich in the polyphenols quercetin, catechin, and vitexin. In various studies, these substances have been shown to lower serum cholesterol and *sometimes* lower blood pressure. Certain beneficial effects have been noted on some cardiac arrhythmias (abnormal heartbeats).

Some authorities believe that extracts of hawthorn can dilate blood vessels, and fractions of the plant other than polyphenols may have an effect on improving cardiac muscle function. Although this has not been confirmed in controlled experiments, it suggests that hawthorn extracts can help reverse atherosclerosis and may act as a diuretic.

It is unlikely that all the alleged health benefits of hawthorn can be attributed to the mix of bioflavonoids in the extracts. The scientific research on the cardiovascular effects of hawthorn is incomplete; fractions must be isolated, characterized, and further studied in order to assess their therapeutic value.

Please note that you should *not* use hawthorn in any self-medicating regimen, especially if you are taking heart medications such as digitalis, digoxin, or lanoxin. The potential toxicity of hawthorn is unclear, especially in higher doses. Vitexin is the component of hawthorn that is usually suggested to be of the most value. Vitexin should be standardized to approximately 2 percent or thereabouts in dietary supplements of hawthorn, which are best used under medical supervision.

HEALTH-BUILDING GREEN TEA

Green tea has become increasingly popular because of its alleged ability to prevent thrombosis—a blood clot in a blood vessel—and its ability to lower cholesterol. Note that I am not talking about just any kind of tea. Only green tea has the special, beneficial effects on cardiovascular health. So, what is the difference between green and black tea?

Black tea is consumed in great amounts throughout the world, and it is produced by drying, fermenting, and roasting the leaves of the tea bush *Camellia sinensis*. Green tea is processed in a different manner, whereby the fresh leaves from the tea plant are treated with heat to prevent fermentation. By not fermenting the leaves, the residual content of health-giving—and cancer-fighting— compounds are preserved. (The disadvantages of fermenting green tea is in contrast with the advantages of fermenting soy.) Green tea, when appropriately processed, contains significant quantities of vitamin C and E, together with a reasonable range of minerals.

The active constituents of green tea appear to be related to *catechin*, a substance that has effects similar to aspirin, in that it inhibits formation of clots. It appears that catechin has a direct effect on the regulation of the production of platelet-aggregating factors. Other compounds in green tea may also have a similar effect. Among its multiple benefits, green tea is believed to have a role in lowering cholesterol and normalizing blood pressure. In one Japanese study, consuming green tea was associated with a lowered risk of stroke; the Japanese government has endorsed green tea (more than ten cups per day) as a cancer-preventive agent.

The benefits of green tea are so convincing that some dietary supplement manufacturers have produced capsules and powders of green tea extracts that contain standardized polyphenol contents, which may be equivalent of up to five cups of tea per day. In capsules where there is a content of approximately 50 percent polyphenols, an average daily dose may be up to 200 mgs.

For many people, taking decaffeinated green tea extracts is more convenient than drinking the brewed tea. This a sensible approach because many green teas contain significant amounts of caffeine. Individuals with coronary artery disease should avoid excessive caffeine, especially if they are susceptible to irregular heartbeats.

Many people find green tea quite delicious and choose to brew the tea, but selecting the right kind of green tea is quite an exercise. The teas vary greatly in terms of their processing and source, which makes them a unreliable way to receive a consistent dose of polyphenols. Furthermore, if the tea is not prepared correctly then the polyphenols can become damaged or oxidized. The best varieties of green tea include gyokuro, sencha, and gumpowder teas, all of which are available in natural food markets and some mainstream supermarkets as well. People are often advised to drink no more than four or five cups a day, especially if the selected variety contains a significant amount of caffeine. However, the health benefits of green tea are only apparent when intake is high. For example, the anticancer benefits of green tea are experienced with an intake equivalent to ten cups of the tea per day. Therefore, decaffeinated green tea supplements are a practical way for many Westerners to enjoy the benefits of green tea.

GINGER

Ginger is a common herb, and it is very safe for general use in the diet. You may think of it primarily as an ingredient in cooking, particularly baking, but it also has medicinal uses. For example, in parts of Europe, ginger extracts are used to control nausea and vomiting, and they are sold as a safe alternative to over-the-counter motion sickness remedies.

In the Ayurvedic healing tradition of India, ginger is considered a digestive stimulant and also is used as a "body cleansing" or detoxifying agent. Because of its stimulating effect, an Ayurvedic practitioner might recommend a ginger tonic as a weight-loss aid. In many traditions, ginger has acknowledged health benefits, such as improving digestion, and it is a home remedy for indigestion.

In classic Chinese medicine, ginger is a "heat-producing" plant; it is therefore thought to have a stimulating effect on internal organs and helps adjust metabolism, as well as acting as a diuretic, thereby removing excess fluids from the body. When used with other herbs and spices, ginger becomes an ingredient in tonics intended to "stimulate" the heart (cardiotonics). Other ingredients of these heart-stimulating tonics may include Chinese aconite, Chinese sage, licorice, poria, and Chinese angelica.

Animal experiments in Japan indicate that ginger has the effect of slowing the heartbeat but it also increases the force of cardiac contractions. In these experiments, extracts of ginger were also shown to lower blood pressure for a period of several hours. We still do not know the mechanism for these effects, but one theory is that ginger may have a direct action on the adrenal glands and modulate the release of adrenaline.

Although the research is limited, some animal experiments in India and China have shown that ginger may have a cholesterol-lowering effect. When ginger was added to meals rich in cholesterol, it appeared to have a protective effect against the rapid rise of blood cholesterol levels in laboratory animals. Although the mechanism is unknown, an important study published in 1980 in the *New England Journal of Medicine* confirmed earlier observations that ginger may reduce blood cholesterol. Ginger is also believed to contain an anti-thrombotic agent, in that it interferes with platelet aggregation. Current research on the use of ginger extracts as anti-clotting agents centers on the development of a substance called Shogoal. Ginger extracts may reduce platelet stickiness and prevent blood clots from forming in much the same way as garlic or aspirin do. (For this reason, do not self-medicate, especially if you are taking anticoagulant drugs or are using aspirin.)

While ginger in the diet is safe in any reasonable amount that a person could ingest in meals, the toxicity of high doses of the extract remains unclear. Use ginger for medicinal purposes only with the guidance of a person knowledgeable about its effects.

GUGGUL

Guggul, which contains many different types of compounds, is extracted from the resin of the mukul tree (*Commiphora mukul*). The gum within the resin is used to produce purified extracts called guggulipids. Within guggulipids there are several steroid compounds that are called guggulsterones, steroids that are believed to be the active agents.

Guggul has been extensively researched in India for its use in promoting cardiovascular wellness. Several studies have indicated that it is able to reduce blood cholesterol and triglyceride levels by a factor of up to 30 percent when taken over a period of about twelve weeks. Extracts have been shown to both reduce LDL cholesterol and increase HDL cholesterol.

Guggul has not been used in Western medicine for cardiovascular wellness to the same degree as other botanicals. However, some authorities have argued that it may have as much therapeutic potential as garlic and other lipid-lowering agents, such as soy protein containing isoflavones. A number of laboratory experiments have indicated that its extracts may reduce platelet stickiness. Obviously, with the potential dual effect, guggul could provide an additional natural treatment available to heart patients. Clinical observations imply that guggulipids can act synergistically (in an additive manner) with soy protein and isoflavones to lower cholesterol. The addition of vitamin C to guggulipids makes them more effective dietary supplements for lowering blood cholesterol.

Guggul has become known in North America very recently, so Western medicine can provide very few favorable reports about its use. However, it appears to be quite safe and without significant toxicity, even when given in daily doses of up to 5 grams. Much more research is needed to determine if this interesting plant resin has the potential to become an important remedy in preventing and perhaps treating coronary artery disease.

CONTRIBUTIONS FROM THE AYURVEDIC TRADITION

Ayurveda is one of the oldest healing traditions in the world, and it is not surprising that in the search for "pluralistic" health care, it would make its way to the West. It is a complex system, but like traditional Chinese medicine, it emphasizes balance and synergy between elements in nature. Prevention methods are preferred, of course, and remedies are created to help the body heal itself. Many of the healing plants used in Ayurvedic medicine have the potential to help in a quest for cardiovascular health.

Amrit kalash is the name of an ancient herbal formula with its origins in India. It is a mixture of herbs that are believed to have powerful antioxidant properties. The interest in this formula has centered around its ability to protect the body against damage caused by free radical activity. In many circumstances, it unwise to make a claim about a combination of herbs. However, amrit kalash is an ancient remedy and has been passed down through the generations as a single entity. Its antioxidant properties may have a positive effect on cardiovascular disease because it prevents oxidation of LDL and it has anti-thrombotic effects.

Amalaki (or amla) is a fruit that is an ingredient in well-known formulas used in Ayurvedic medicine. This plant distinguishes itself by having one of the highest known concentrations of vitamin C among the edible plants. It is used as an anti-inflammatory remedy and to promote good digestion, but its role in cardiovascular health appears to be as both an antioxidant nutrient and as an agent to stimulate circulation. Studies have shown that it can lower blood cholesterol. It is possible that the vitamin C content favorably affects cholesterol metabolism. Again, I stress that the addition of vitamin C to many herbals used to lower cholesterol can often enhance their effects.

In the Ayurvedic tradition, the bark of the plant *arjun* (or arjuna) is one of the most commonly used substances for a wide range of cardiovascular diseases. It is reported to have the ability to lower blood pressure and improve the common symptoms of congestive heart failure (CHF). Patients experiencing the common shortness of breath associated with CHF reported improvement, and this plant appears to strengthen the contractions and pumping action of the heart. One study showed that after three months of taking arjun, patients with coronary artery disease had the beneficial effects of fewer bouts of anginal pain, reduced blood pressure, and an improved blood lipid profile. It is believed that arjun is a powerful antioxidant, which may account, in part, for its beneficial actions.

GINSENG ACROSS THE GLOBE

In the West, ginseng has an image that is somewhat exotic, but in Asia it is one of the most commonly used health tonics. The word itself means the essence, "sing," of man, "gin." It is the root of the ginseng plant that is used as the source of herbal concoctions. To some degree, the shape of the plant resembles the shape of the human body. In ancient Chinese medical writings, this resemblance led to the belief that the root of the ginseng plant represented "the essence of the earth in the shape of the human." This led to many of the health benefits ascribed to ginseng, including its powers of healing, recuperation, rejuvenation, and general revitalization. Others have argued that it resembles the shape of the penis; of course, ginseng has also enjoyed use as an aphrodisiac.

Worldwide, ginseng is one of the most popular herbal tonics. (I have summarized the potential health benefits of ginseng in Table 12.3.) However, ginseng should not be viewed as one entity. In fact, the ginseng commonly available in health food stores comes in three distinct types. The first is *Panax ginseng*, often called Chinese or Korean ginseng; it is distinguished from *Panax quinquefolium*, which is known as American ginseng. Chinese, Korean, and American ginseng belong to the Panax *genus* of plants. Siberian ginseng, the third type of ginseng, does not. However, Siberian ginseng and the other two types belong to the same *family* of plants, *Araliaceae*.

The Araliaceae family produces different types of ginsengs which, overall, appear to have similar effects. The health-giving compounds within ginseng have been isolated to some extent, and many have chemical compositions that resemble the structure of human steroids and hormones. It is said to contain a good range of vitamins, amino acids, and trace minerals. Its active components are generally regarded to be *ginsenosides* and related compounds. The health-giving fractions of ginseng are begging to be defined by science.

There appears to be major variations in the health-giving potential of different types of commercially available ginseng. Some analytic pharmaceutical studies have shown that the constituents of commercially available preparations vary to a major degree. For example, it is known that the ginsenoside content of ginseng supplements can vary from zero up to approximately 10 percent. Therefore, if you are considering taking a ginseng product, it is important to look for a supplement that has a standardized ginsenoside content.

Table 12.3: Beneficial Health Effects Ascribed to the Use of Ginseng.

Enhances physical performance and endurance
Improves sexual function
Lowers blood cholesterol
Enhances energy
Increases alertness
Exerts a protective effect on cellular damage from radiation
   or toxins
Improves memory and other psychomotor functions
Has anti-stress effects
Promotes general homeostasis

Several studies have shown that fractions of ginseng can reduce blood cholesterol levels and also have anti-thrombotic effects, in a manner similar to garlic and guggul. Although the mechanism is not completely understood, it appears that ginseng directly affects the transport and metabolism of cholesterol; overall, LDL cholesterol levels decrease, and HDL cholesterol levels increase. So, in today's popular terms, ginseng favors the so-called good cholesterol while it discourages the so-called bad cholesterol.

Unfortunately, ginseng has an unpredictable effect on blood pressure, and some studies have shown that certain ginseng extracts may cause elevations. For this reason, anyone with established heart disease should take ginseng only under the supervision of a qualified health-care provider.

Overall, ginseng is thought to be quite safe, but some researchers have described a syndrome (a collection of signs and symptoms) that may occur as a consequence of excessive dosing of ginseng, or ginseng abuse. I realize that identifying such a syndrome sounds bizarre, and some experts dispute its occurrence. However, I believe that "ginseng abuse syndrome" may occur when individuals take extremely large amounts of ginseng supplements. This syndrome is characterized by general excitability, including feelings of anxiety, nervousness, and an inability to sleep.

Although not yet well-described, this syndrome does make pharmacologic sense when we understand the effects of ginsenosides on the central nervous system. Ginsenosides are known to effect the release of neurotransmitters, the chemical messengers in the brain, and they may alter blood flow to the brain. Despite the fact that some deny the reality of the ginseng abuse syndrome, it seems prudent to avoid taking ginseng if irritability and/or anxiety are experienced—*and especially in the presence of uncontrolled hypertension.*

Siberian Ginseng

Siberian ginseng is popularly called "eleuthero" because of its origin from the shrub *Eleutherococcus senticosus*. The active constituents of Siberian ginseng are eleutherosides, which differ chemically from the ginsenosides found in Panax ginseng. Regardless of these differences, Siberian ginseng appears to have the beneficial effects similar to those reported with the use of Korean or American ginseng.

Based largely on studies performed in Russia, the term "adaptogen" has been applied to Siberian ginseng. The term adaptogen implies that an agent can enhance, modulate, or normalize functions within the body. Thus, adapotgens promote homeostasis within the body.

The beneficial effects of Siberian ginseng on cardiovascular function are not as well-described as they are for Panax ginseng. Siberian ginseng is often cheaper than Panax ginseng, but there is even more variation in the quality of dietary supplements made with it. Therefore, it is important to attempt to find Siberian ginseng that has some standardization of its eleutheroside content.

Ginseng is sold in a variety of forms, including encapsulated extracts, ground whole root, tablets, tea, liquid preparations, and even chewing gum. Despite the widespread use of ginseng, there is still relatively little known about the full scope of response to varying concentrations of ginsenosides or eleutherosides in dietary supplements.

Some health-care practitioners use varying doses of ginseng extract for different disorders. On average, when used as an agent to assist in cardiovascular wellness, a dose of approximately 150–500 mg. of ginseng extract contained in tablets or capsules are recommended, providing that they are standardized to contain somewhere between 4 and 9 percent ginsenoside. Products that contain higher concentrations of ginsenosides or eleutherosides can be taken in smaller doses. One recommendation is to attempt to increase or lower the dose of ginseng as needed to achieve an optimal effect. Unless you are under close medical supervision, it is unwise to exceed a dose of 700 mg. of capsules or tablets that contain up to 10 percent ginsenoside on a daily basis. Little bottles of ginseng tonic have appeared in abundance at the checkout counter in grocery stores. They are not standardized, and many must be considered worthless.

FO-TI: PLANT FROM CHINA

Fo-ti is a traditional Chinese medicine that is used for a variety of medical purposes, but it is most famous for promoting longevity and overall wellness. Research performed in China has shown that in relatively large doses, fo-ti reduces cholesterol levels and helps prevent atherosclerosis.

The active components of fo-ti include lecithin, which has been associated in some studies with reduced cholesterol levels. Fo-ti seems to be safe when taken in relatively large doses, but its beneficial effect on cardiovascular health is not as clear as the benefit of agents such as soy, garlic, or essential fatty acids.

CELERY FOR HIGH BLOOD PRESSURE

Celery, when taken as the whole vegetable or as the seed, has been used for many years in traditional Chinese and Ayurvedic medicine. It appears that celery seeds have a diuretic effect, but caution is required with their use because in high doses they appear to be toxic. They are contraindicated in excess during pregnancy.

Essential oils derived from celery also have been used to lower blood pressure, and they are believed to help "relax" the smooth muscle found in the wall of blood vessels. The active constituent of this essential oil is believed to be *butyl phthalide,* which is known to cause modest reductions in systolic blood pressure and exert some effects on lowering cholesterol.

I emphasize that you should not experiment with high doses of celery and its seeds on your own, but only use these extracts with the advice of a health-care provider. Celery extracts are available in health food stores in a variety of formats but, unfortunately, their contents are not always standardized. I believe that three or four whole stalks of celery per day is probably very safe and the caloric value is very low, making it a valuable vegetable for those who are on weight-loss plans.

COMBINATION REMEDIES IN DIETARY SUPPLEMENTS: MIXED BLESSINGS?

If you look on the shelves of your health food store or peruse one of the many nutritional supplement catalogs, you will probably see a variety of dietary supplements that contain mixtures of compounds.

These combination supplements may claim to benefit cardiovascular function directly, or perhaps indirectly, by lowering cholesterol. Several of these combination dietary supplements are sold with supporting literature that is anecdotal and sometimes based on questionable scientific evidence of safety and efficacy. In particular, be aware of marketing literature on dietary supplements that promise that the supplement will prevent sudden death or heart attack. *Anything* that is described as a quick method to prevent or reverse cardiovascular disease should be treated with skepticism.

A variety of botanical extracts are available in combination with some simple products such as sugar or dietary fiber, but claims for using such combinations in the treatment or prevention of heart disease cannot be substantiated by credible observations of their effects. Mind you, I am not rejecting the importance of some evidence that individual constituents in certain herbal concoctions may have some benefit. Obviously, the botanicals mentioned in this chapter may have these favorable effects. I am objecting to the combination formulas or any individual herbal remedy that makes untested claims. Combination formulas are, for the most part, not standardized; few have been subjected to any well-controlled, clinical research. Statements that indicate that natural cures can rapidly reverse atherosclerosis with the result that cardiac surgery can be avoided are unworthy claims. This kind of outrageous hope contributes greatly to an appropriate rejection of that segment of the dietary supplement industry that behaves unscrupulously in marketing supplement products. That said, widely available botanical remedies may emerge in the not-too-distant future as a standard treatment offered to patients. Nature offers us an amazing pharmacy, and we should use it—and preserve it—with care.

SUMMARY

Herbal or botanical medicine is making a comeback in the West. For many thousands of years, humans have made use of "nature's pharmacy," but the advent of synthetic drugs drew attention away from the healing power of the vast variety of healing plants. However, we should always remember that some of our most valued modern drugs are either derived from plants or are designed to "mimic" the known action of plant constituents.

Among the plants that have a positive effect on cardiovascular health, garlic is a "standout." It appears to share many of the advantages of fish oil, it is cheap and abundant, it has a role in lowering cholesterol, and it may help prevent high blood pressure.

Flavonoids also are important chemical substances, and more than fifteen classes of flavonoids exist. *Bio*flavonoids are one class, and they are found in citrus fruits; soy isoflavones are another class. OPCs, an additional class of flavonoids, include pycnogenols (which are found in the bark of the European coastal pine tree), and grapeseed extract. Pycnogenols are powerful antioxidants. The connection between heart health and red wine comes in part from their OPC content.

Other plants with proposed ability to prevent cardiovascular disease include: ginkgo, which promotes blood flow in the body; bilberry, the extracts of which may help regulate cholesterol and triglyceride levels; hawthorn, which may help lower cholesterol and reduce blood pressure; green tea, which has anti-thrombotic properties and may help lower cholesterol; ginger, used in many parts of the world for its stimulating effects; and guggul, known in India as a cholesterol-lowering agent.

Ginseng is one of the world's most common health tonics. The three major types of ginseng are: Chinese or Korean, American, and Siberian. The chemical composition of ginseng is not completely defined, nor have the potential health-promoting properties been completely investigated. However, some of the major active components of commonly used ginseng are ginsenosides, which may have a beneficial effect on cholesterol levels.

What You Can Do

- Realize that botanical remedies may have great value in your quest for cardiovascular wellness, but do not self-medicate with herbal preparations for heart disease. When used correctly they are safe, but their contents are not necessarily standardized in many dietary supplements, and their effects vary among individuals. Use herbal remedies *only* under supervision of a qualified practitioner.

- Garlic is generally a safe product, and I advise using it liberally in your cooking. The Chinese recommend using five or more cloves of garlic per day. You may not want to consume that much, but begin experimenting with garlic to enhance your meals—and your health.
- Commercially available garlic supplements may also be beneficial for lowering cholesterol levels. The use of garlic along with soy and fish oil may be among the safest and least expensive treatments for elevated cholesterol.
- Although red wine has beneficial compounds known as OPCs, if you choose to drink red wine, use it in moderation.
- Many common plants such as ginseng, green tea, ginger, ginkgo, and so forth may contribute to cardiovascular wellness. When used appropriately, they are safe. Green tea and ginger, for example, can be consumed as part of your daily diet.
- I do not recommend using the combination herbal formulas that are fast filling drugstore shelves. However, interest in botanical treatments is making a welcome comeback, and I encourage your interest in the potential value of "nature's pharmacy."

CHAPTER THIRTEEN

HOSPITALS AND DANGEROUS DRUGS

By now you have a good idea about the array of important elements of a heart-smart lifestyle, including the kinds of foods that promote optimal health. In addition, you are now familiar with some health-promoting botanical therapies that come to us from many healing traditions and philosophies. Although I consider appropriate diet and the judicious use of nutritional supplements critical components of any plan designed to prevent cardiovascular disease, stress management and giving attention to your emotional and spiritual health are significant, too. I included the information about behavior modification and stress management because they are so important in building and maintaining a healthful lifestyle. By now, you also understand that the ideal diet and lifestyle for cardiovascular wellness promotes overall health, too.

Before rounding out this book, I thought it wise to remind you about the consequences of *not* following a plan that builds cardiovascular health, which as I have said, is the true fountain of youth. In a society that prides itself on its technological advances in all areas, including medicine, it is too easy to fall back on the notion that all these advances will "save" us. However, to understand the reality of heart disease and the available treatments for this group of disease, it is important to paint a more complete picture.

CHELATION THERAPY

Chelation therapy does not fit into a neat category. In the next few years, this treatment has the potential to become part of standard treatment practice for heart disease, yet it is still quite controversial. In fact, a war has raged among doctors and government regulatory agencies about the application of chelation therapy.

Chelation therapy was originally developed as a technique to remove toxic chemicals from the body. It comes from the Greek word *chele*, which means "claw" or "bind"; if you prefer a visual description, imagine a substance circulating through the body in a liquid solution, and as it makes this journey, molecules of various minerals bind to it and are eventually removed from the body through the kidneys. Calcium, for example, is part of plaque formation, and chelation therapy theoretically removes it from the bloodstream, thereby preventing it from attaching to arterial walls. In this way, atheroma is prevented or existing plaque formations are reduced—though I have to admit that this is an oversimplified explanation of the theory of chelation.

The circulating agent used most often in chelation therapy is EDTA (ethylene-diamine-tetra-acetate), which is a synthetic amino acid originally developed in Germany for use in the dye industry. In the 1950s, a physician in the U.S. discovered that EDTA was an effective treatment for sailors who showed signs of toxicity after exposure to lead-based paint used on naval ships. In addition to being an effective method of treating the toxic effects of heavy-metal accumulation in the body, it was observed serendipitiously that symptoms of arteriosclerosis improved as well—a positive side effect.

The FDA (Federal Drug Administration) has approved chelation therapy only as a treatment for heavy-metal toxicity, but nonetheless, over a thousand physicians in the U.S. use chelation therapy for a variety of heart-related conditions. For example, peripheral vascular disease affects circulation in the extremities and, as it progresses, it causes cramping and discomfort in the legs. In severe cases, ulcerative sores can appear on the feet, and over time the extremities can become gangrenous.

Proponents of chelation therapy maintain through their documentation that the treatment can improve circulation and can even reverse atheroma (blockages in the blood vessels). Considering that conventional treatment in severe cases of peripheral vascular disease can include amputation, it is not surprising that many people consider chelation therapy—if they are aware that the option exists. Government-sponsored health-care programs such as Medicare do not pay for chelation treatment, and private insurers do not reimburse patients for it either. Therefore, the treatment is available only to those who can pay for it themselves. This is a good example of how lateral thinking is commonly discouraged and physicians are constrained in their treatment.

How Chelation Works

Chelation therapy usually involves a series of as many as twenty to thirty treatments, usually taking place over a period of several months. It is expensive and often uncomfortable. Chelation is done most often on an outpatient basis in the office of the treating physician. Currently, only medical physicians (allopaths and osteopaths) are qualified to perform chelation therapy. It is essentially a painless treatment, requiring only an intravenous line through which the solution enters the body. However, the treatment is cumbersome, time-consuming, and not without some potential hazard due to acute alteration of body chemistry in some recipients.

The Chelation Answer by Morton Walker, D.P.M., and Gary Gordon, M.D., is one of the most complete books about chelation therapy, and it offers a variety of case studies in which patients show improvement after a course of treatments. The book includes information about the costs of the treatment and a more extensive discussion of the way chelation may improve a variety of conditions, including diabetes. At this writing, some anecdotal reports are very favorable, while other reports claim no benefit at all. Chelation therapy remains mired in controversy. It has been the focus of legal battles between U.S. government agencies and medical societies, such as the American College for the Advancement of Medicine. This professional organization, which advocates chelation therapy, has approximately one thousand members and many more followers.

I contend that chelation therapy should be studied and more complete documentation amassed in order to give it a fair assessment. It is not unusual for a treatment to produce positive results for some individuals, while it may have no such effect on others. This does not make the therapy invalid, which is what is often claimed about chelation, and wide variation in results is not in and of itself a sufficient reason to reject a treatment. However, more controlled studies are needed to document the benefits over time.

Dr. Walker and Dr. Gordon also discuss oral chelation therapy, in which varying amounts of certain nutrients are combined in supplement form. Fundamentally, oral chelation therapy is allegedly a form of "detoxification therapy," and some nutrients—vitamin C, for example—are described as natural chelating agents and antioxidant nutrients. Some of these supplements contain a small amount of EDTA. However, EDTA is not absorbed when given orally and it is not a substance you can simply use on your own, so I do not recommend any unsupervised use of supplements containing EDTA.

The idea of an oral chelation agent is very appealing, however, because it would obviate the need for expensive intravenous treatments with intravenous chelating fluids, with their attendant risks. My colleague, Nikolaus J. Smeh of the National Skincare Institute, and I investigated the possibility of oral administration of EDTA using special ways of delivering it to the body in orally administered liquids in which EDTA is contained within delivery molecules, called liposomes.

Liposomes are essentially envelopes of fatty acid molecules, which can form a kind of bubble that can be used to engulf the chelating agent, EDTA. These tiny bubbles—liposomes—are able to pass through the intestinal walls to a variable degree, and they can carry the EDTA into the body. Smeh and I engaged in some self-experimentation to show that this is possible.

Using ourselves as "guinea pigs," we first took a hefty drink of EDTA and proceeded to experience painful abdominal cramping and diarrhea. Because EDTA is not absorbed, it plays all sorts of games with the bowel when taken in substantial amounts. Smeh then substituted the simple EDTA "cocktail" with a liposome EDTA cocktail. We learned that the lipsome delivery system enabled the EDTA to be tolerated when given orally. Our findings are subject to a patent, and work has started to investigate further, at a major university medical center, the option of oral chelation therapy with liposome delivery. If our findings are confirmed, oral chelation therapy could be around the corner. I see the real value of oral chelation as a first-aid measure in industrial settings where accidental heavy metal poisoning can occur.

You may notice that some mineral supplements are labeled "chelated," meaning that the minerals are bonded with another substance in order to enhance their use by the body. Ascorbic acid or amino acids are sometimes used as the chelation agent. Chelated minerals are useful in isolated circumstances, but this process is not the same as intravenous chelation therapy.

Dr. Walker and Dr. Gordon make an important contribution by explaining that chelation itself is a natural process, meaning that it is a physiological process that goes on in the body—and in nature—all the time. Many nutrients have the ability to act as chelating agents, serving to remove toxins from the body and acting as free radical scavengers. The idea of detoxification of the body is deeply rooted in several traditional medical disciplines, including Ayurvedic medicine and traditional Chinese medicine. Detoxification is often scoffed at by conventional medicine, but thousands swear by it.

HOSPITALS AND CORONARY CARE UNITS

Advances in pharmaceuticals and technology have led to a greater survival rate in patients suffering from myocardial infarction—heart attack. This fact alone has offered hope to millions of individuals who have suffered a cardiac event. The next step, of course, is helping individuals not only survive but recover and begin to again live a normal life. Unfortunately, the same environment that can help victims of cardiovascular disease survive may also be a dreary and rather frightening place.

During my years as a medical student, I was never more nervous in a hospital setting than I was in a coronary care unit (CCU), where each patient was surrounded by "gadgets" and electronic equipment. All this instrumentation was considered essential, so I was naturally surprised when, in my last year of medical school, I became aware of research that compared home and hospital treatment for patients who were recovering from an uncomplicated heart attack. This study, performed in England and published in a British medical journal, showed that the death rate was about the same for patients cared for at home *and* in an intensive care unit.

In the face of increasing litigation in the United States, the idea of having a heart attack patient cared for at home would be unacceptable because it is not usual and customary medical practice. Therefore, the issue is essentially moot in the U.S. However, this research raises legitimate questions about the setting of the modern coronary care unit. It appears that a CCU precipitates anxiety in some patients and may even worsen or exaggerate cardiovascular response to an already stressful situation. There is also evidence that some patients, particularly the elderly or those suffering from dementia, will not adjust well to the tense environment of the coronary care unit. These are patients for whom home care would appear ideal.

In his book *Medical Care Can Be Dangerous to Your Health*, Eugene D. Robin, M.D., highlights the drawbacks of the coronary care unit as a healing environment. CCUs were first developed in Western Europe in the 1950s, because it was recognized that early death following a heart attack may be prevented by using certain interventions. The ability to continuously monitor individuals at risk following a heart attack thereby made appropriate interventions possible. However, this has also led to overtreatment or overinvestigation, and, in addition, subjects almost all heart attack patients to increased stress and anxiety. According to Dr. Robin, patients should attempt to take control of their situation to the extent they can and to limit their time in the CCU. (This assumes, of course, that there are no special complications that warrant extensive monitoring.) Dr. Robin also discusses the misuse of intensive care units for patients who are dying, those for whom treatment may involve needless discomfort, and loss of dignity. These are very hot political, social, legal, and medical issues that are best addressed by health-care recipients, not lobbies with vested interests.

A CLOSER LOOK AT MEDICATIONS

There are several classes of medications used to treat hypertension, all of which carry risk and have disadvantages. For example, the diuretics, designed to efficiently eliminate excess sodium from the body, may also deplete the body's supply of minerals, particularly magnesium and potassium, both of which are critical for cardiovascular functioning. This may occur even when these drugs are designed to be "potassium-sparing." These drugs may also cause fatigue and muscle spasms. Another class of drugs, known as "beta blockers," may lead to depression and/or adverse sexual function, and some patients report dizziness and fatigue. The so-called "vasodilators," which open the arteries and relax blood vessels, can have a negative effect on heart functioning and increase the heart rate. These drugs should not be taken casually—fatalities have occurred with several blood pressure–lowering drugs!

Eric Braverman, M.D., has outlined a nutritional approach to controlling blood pressure in his book *Hypertension and Nutrition.* The book discusses the role of beneficial fats in regulating blood pressure, and you will find that many of his dietary and lifestyle recommendations are similar to those presented in this book. Dr. Braverman's book presents a sound self-care program that has the potential to build overall health. However, while I agree that natural approaches to preventing and treating hypertension are valuable and preferable to drug therapies when possible, *do not stop taking blood pressure medications without consulting your health-care provider.*

TREATMENT AS SAVIOR

It is unfortunate that today's typical medical practice emphasizes treatment for health problems rather than prevention of disease. Medical news tends to favor publicity about "miracle" surgeries and drugs. The downside is that some of the media attention surrounding the development of important procedures such as bypass surgery and angioplasty, as well as cholesterol-lowering drugs, may lead to a false sense of security. For many people, the question ends up being: What are my treatment options *when* I develop heart disease? The real question should be: How can I *prevent* the disease in the first place?

Simple prevention techniques may not be as glamorous as the image of surgical teams operating in an "every-minute-counts" surgical theater. After all, television medical dramas seldom have episodes that revolve around scenes in which dieticians or nurse practitioners discuss the negative features of saturated fat and hydrogenated oils or good dietary practices.

Although cardiac bypass surgery seems quite common, even mainstream opinion still remains somewhat divided about the benefits of using it to effectively treat angina, prevent cardiac ischemic episodes, and enhance longevity. The technique of coronary artery bypass grafting is based on simple principles. Blockage of coronary arteries results in compromised blood supply to the heart muscle. When these obstructions are identified, the surgical procedure called bypass grafting may be recommended. This procedure uses blood vessel grafts, often taken from peripheral veins in the body, to bypass the areas where blockages exist. There are many variations of bypass surgery, and it is individualized based on the severity of the arterial obstructions in the coronary arteries.

Bypass grafting became popular in the 1960s, and today it is one of the most common surgical procedures performed in the U.S. To say that bypass surgery is a multibillion dollar business is not an exaggeration. The high cost of bypass surgery is one of the principal reasons that alternatives have been proposed.

One such alternative is angioplasty, which is popularly known as "balloon surgery." The latter term is actually descriptive of the procedure. A thin catheter tube with a tiny inflatable balloon at its tip can be passed backwards into vessels and lodged in locations such as the coronary artery. When the uninflated balloon is placed into the site of narrowing, the balloon can be inflated and the area of the blockage dilated. The technique can be controlled by watching the progression of the catheter by x-ray screening.

The advantages and disadvantages of bypass surgery and angioplasty are beyond the scope of this book, but you should be aware that these common procedures are not without controversy or risk. The bottom line is that one or two of every hundred patients die from bypass surgery itself. Up to one in twenty patients may develop some sign of compromised blood flow in the body. Unfortunate potential complications include the occurrence of stroke or decreased brain function, which are more common in elderly patients undergoing bypass surgery.

On the other hand, it has been documented that cardiac bypass surgery may prolong life, and, beyond that, improve quality of life and provide relief from angina and the pain associated with angina. The surgery has the ability to help patients return to a normal life, including the ability to go back to their jobs or professions. When these treatments are successful, cardiac patients no longer need to think of themselves as invalids. However, universal beneficial outcome is not always present.

It is not my purpose to advise you about the efficacy of bypass surgery or angioplasty in your case. Instead, my reasons for including this information are related to my hope that you can adopt the kind of lifestyle that will help you *avoid* the CCU and these treatment decisions in the future.

Drug therapy for high cholesterol, angina, first heart attacks, and the bypass or angioplasty decision all come after heart disease has been established—and this process may take many years. Many of the natural options discussed in this book can be initiated before heart disease has developed. Cardiac or vascular surgeons often raise their eyebrows when the possibility of avoiding surgery with remedies like fish oil are proposed. It is apparently "too simple" for them to grasp, but I have personally witnessed reversal of angina and diminished "rest pain" in the legs of people with peripheral vascular disease who have taken enteric-coated fish oil in large doses. Can we try at least to expand our thoughts about remedies of natural origin?

Western societies have tended to put great stock in new drugs to treat a variety of problems that are directly or indirectly related to cardiovascular disease. Recent experience tells us, however, that we should proceed cautiously. The following information illustrates exactly what I mean.

IS VIAGRA REALLY A WONDER DRUG?

In 1997, few laypersons had heard of Viagra (sildenafil citrate), but by spring of 1998, this new drug was being hailed as a "panacea" for male impotence. Viagra was touted not only as a miracle drug and a literal "godsend" to men, especially older males—it was viewed as having potential political and social significance as well. Days within becoming available, psychologists and marriage counselors joined in the public debate as they tried to determine if Viagra would enhance marriage or lead to divorce! Insurance plan administrators were challenged to quickly state their policies about covering the cost of the drug—and how many of these magic pills their plans would pay for. This provoked women to challenge their insurance companies about the wisdom, not to mention the justness, of covering Viagra, but persistently refusing to cover prescriptions for birth control drugs or other contraceptives.

It is ironic that with all the hype around Viagra, very few people heard that it was a drug first developed as a potential treatment for angina pectoris. You will remember that angina is pain that occurs as a result of blockage of the arteries supplying the heart, and this blockage is usually caused by atherosclerosis. Viagra was found to be ineffective for this use, but, moreover, *the clinical use of Viagra has been associated with cardiac problems, including heart attacks!*

In order to understand the potential negative effects of Viagra, it is important to understand how the drug works. Contrary to popular belief, Viagra does not act directly to cause erections but rather, helps initiate and maintain an erection. Many circumstances, other than penile blood flow, need to be optimal if Viagra is used to enhance sexual activity. It will not enhance sexual activity when sexual performance already is optimal for an individual. The notion that the drug will turn an ordinary, healthy man into a sexual "superman" is a myth. If your sexual function is good, by all means leave Viagra alone.

Viagra works mainly by enhancing the relaxation of smooth muscles that are found in the walls of arterial blood vessels. Relaxing the wall of an arterial blood vessel will enhance blood flow. This rush of blood fills the "caverns" within the spongy tissues of the penis and helps to cause an erection.

When sexual stimulation occurs, substances are released in the body that cause blood vessels supplying the penis to relax. One such substance is nitric oxide, which is released locally in various regions of the penis during sex. Viagra enhances the action of nitric oxide, and thus the blood vessels are enlarged (vasodilation), thereby allowing blood to fill penile tissues and form pools that stiffen the penis.

Not long after the initial hype about Viagra began, serious cardiac problems were linked to its use. The wonder drug has an apparent downside after all. About four months after Viagra became available, the Food and Drug Administration had received sixteen reports of individuals who had died after taking Viagra. The deaths were attributed to heart attacks occurring in association with sexual intercourse or often as a result of a proposed lethal interaction between Viagra and nitrates. Nitrates are commonly used to treat angina. Viagra must be used with caution in patients using nitrates. (Nitroglycerin, a common drug used for angina, is an example of a nitrate-based medication.) Poor blood flow to the penis is the most common cause of erectile impotence, and this results from poor cardiovascular function. Thus, the target population for Viagra may be the very people who stand to suffer the possible side effects of this drug.

Viagra directly affects the blood vessels, so it stands to reason that there are potential adverse interactions with other cardiovascular medications. There are warnings about these interactions on the labels of some Viagra prescriptions, but not everyone reads or understands these warnings. The real question is: Why are these individuals, who are already at increased risk of cardiac events or drug interactions, receiving prescriptions for this drug in the first place, especially given the very responsible behavior of the manufacturer of Viagra (Pfizer)?

Unfortunately, mounting evidence suggests that one of the biggest problems with Viagra is its inappropriate use. This is not unusual when a drug is hailed as a panacea—a potion, if you will—that will cure a painful personal problem. Some people flocked to get the popular drug Prozac, not because they were clinically depressed, but because the idea of avoiding normal fluctuations of mood is seductive.

Aside from the potential cardiovascular risks, the American Academy of Ophthalmology has issued a stern warning to people using Viagra. An increasing number of individuals who take the drug have reported sensitivity to light or a visual distortion that results in seeing a bluish tinge in their visual fields. This side effect is predictable when one considers that at higher doses Viagra can occasionally cause up to a 50-percent drop in retinal function. The retina is the light-sensitive receptor at the back of the eye. Therefore, eye specialists have suggested that individuals with retinal disorders, which includes a large number of elderly people, should be cautious about using Viagra. The visual disturbances last about five hours or longer, which of course has implications for driving or operating any kind of machinery where optimal vision is essential. Other common side effects include acid indigestion, headaches, and nasal congestion. Some individuals report sleep disturbances and drowsiness.

More than 50 percent of cases of impotence are related to abnormal blood flow to the penis, and this is the problem that Viagra corrects to some degree. The blood flow that is required for erection can be obstructed by "hardening" and narrowing of the blood vessel that supplies the penis. This narrowing is most often due to atherosclerosis. If you concentrate on a healthful lifestyle that prevents atherosclerosis, then the need for Viagra may be diminished.

This discussion of Viagra has two purposes. The first is to remind you that the drug has some obvious and, according to some physicians, potentially lethal side effects. It most certainly should be used with extreme caution by men who already are taking medications for cardiovascular disease or who have retinal disorders. The second purpose is to reinforce the idea that the best medicine is prevention. If you want to look forward to continued sexual health, then *protect your heart*. (For additional information about natural ways to enhance your sexual health, refer to my book *The Sexual Revolution*.)

PHEN-FEN: ANOTHER WEIGHT-LOSS MIRACLE?

As previously discussed, obesity is a significant health concern and—despite the proliferation of low-fat diets, health clubs, and exercise programs—it is epidemic in our society. When the drug known as Phen-fen arrived on the scene, many people had great hopes for it as a treatment for obesity. Phen-fen is actually a combination of two drugs, phentermine (phen) and fenfluramine (fen). (Sometimes the sequence is reversed and the drug is known as Fen-phen.) Prior to Phen-fen, the primary weight-loss drugs were amphetamines which, in addition to having unpleasant side effects and causing rapid heartbeat and raised blood pressure, are also addictive.

Phen-fen and similar medications appear to work by means of modulating serotonin, a chemical in the brain that influences, among other things, appetite. At one time, about eighteen million people in the U.S. were taking Phen-fen, and there is no question that in the majority of cases, weight loss resulted, at least in the short term. Unfortunately, Phen-fen was overprescribed and used too often to achieve "cosmetic" weight loss. In other words, this drug combination was prescribed for individuals who had a small amount of weight to lose and were not struggling with the health consequences of chronic obesity.

The immediate side effects of Phen-fen were considered mild, particularly when viewed from the perspective of individuals who knew only too well the painful reality of being an obese person in our society. Dry mouth, constipation, drowsiness, and fatigue were considered tolerable and offset by the steady short-term weight loss many experienced.

Unfortunately, there was a downside to this particular miracle, too. Serious heart-valve problems were the side effects that led to the drug's removal from the market. It appeared that the heart-valve problems were not present prior to taking Phen-fen.

It was documented in one report that twenty-four women experienced serious problems and five of these women have undergone surgery to replace damaged, leaking valves. The damage to the heart valves was not typical, meaning that it was not the type associated with common causes of valve problems, such as rheumatic fever and bacterial endocarditis. Surgery revealed valve changes that are usually associated with a type of tumor that secretes chemicals, called a carcinoid, and also with damage associated with some drugs used to raise serotonin levels. This type of heart-valve damage is not associated with obesity. The symptoms of this type of damage to the valves resulted in congestive heart failure: shortness of breath, fluid retention, fatigue, and so forth.

Primary pulmonary hypertension (high blood pressure in the blood vessels of the lungs) is a less-publicized but even more serious risk associated with Phen-fen. Of the twenty-four women with heart-valve damage, eight also developed the potentially fatal complication. This condition damages blood vessels, thereby impairing the transfer of oxygen to the blood. The stress on the heart then leads to heart failure.

Millions of individuals were told to immediately stop taking Phen-fen. Unfortunately, many of these patients had not fundamentally changed their diets nor had they modified their destructive behavior with food, and so they regained the weight they lost. Again, this is an additional case of placing great hopes in a so-called miracle cure that turns out to bring with it great risk. The information about weight loss presented previously is still your best hope for achieving permanent weight loss. To date, no diet drug has ever really been shown to be effective in anything other than the short term.

To balance our own perspective, the dietary supplement industry has its own examples of serious adverse events. Ma Huang (ephedra), the popular component of "natural" slimming supplements (Metabolize and Save, Metabolife, etc.), has significant cardiovascular side effects, and death has been reported with its misuse.

THE STRANGE CASE OF TAMBOCOR

Tambocor (*flecainide acetate*) is the name of one of a family of drugs used to treat irregular heartbeat—arrhythmia. Irregular heartbeats are distressing to patients, but they also signal problems with the electrical mechanisms of the heart, which are linked with sudden cardiac death. The group of drugs used for irregular heartbeat are designed to be taken continuously in order to prevent cardiac arrest; discontinuing the drug means that the irregular heartbeat will return.

In his book *Deadly Medicine*, investigative reporter Thomas J. Moore describes a situation in which Tambocor, and other drugs in the same family, were greeted with great hope and fanfare. Because patients with irregular heartbeats are at a high risk for cardiac arrest, physicians naturally hoped that these drugs represented a true breakthrough. Tragically, it took several years and considerable controversy in the medical, academic, and political communities to prove that these drugs actually *caused* the very condition they were designed to prevent. In fact, it is estimated by some that fifty thousand people died as a result of taking these drugs—and they died from cardiac arrest.

Deadly Medicine is a detailed look at the way Tambocor and other medications are developed, tested, approved, and marketed. This class of drugs is listed in reference books designed to present information about prescription drugs in language the layperson can understand. Recent editions of these books warn that one potential side effect is new heartbeat abnormalities or an increase in severity of the arrhythmic condition. The lists of potential side effects are long and detailed. However, the first patients using these drugs had no such warning. One striking issue emerges from looking into Viagra, Tambocor, and Fen-phen. It often takes a long time and a lot of patient experiences (or deaths) before side effects are ascribed to new drugs. The same may be true about some dietary supplemens!

The important thing to understand here is that when we look at our high-tech medical system, which prides itself on its reliance on science and "provable" medicine, we must remember that today's miracle may turn into tomorrow's tragedy. There are no guarantees in life, and prevention cannot promise longevity and happiness. However, the latest pharmaceutical developments cannot make these promises, either. It may not be perfect, but prevention and the judicious use of safe, natural remedies are still among the best-known pathways to continued good health.

SUMMARY

You now realize the importance of a heart-smart lifestyle, and you have probably examined many areas of your life and discovered changes you can make. One of the most important concepts in this book is the fact that the available treatments for heart disease are not free from risk. In fact, despite demands from patients for natural therapies, many physicians still seem to be wearing earmuffs.

Chelation treatment is emerging as a potential treatment for heart disease, although it is not yet approved by regulatory agencies and, for the most part, the conventional medical world does not believe in its efficacy. Briefly, chelation involves using EDTA as a circulating agent designed to help remove minerals such as calcium from the bloodstream, thus preventing plaque formation. The idea behind chelation, which is detoxification, is a part of many healing traditions. In the future, oral chelation agents may be developed, and intravenous chelation may become an accepted treatment. To date, however, the jury remains out on this issue.

While cardiac procedures such as bypass surgery and angioplasty are valuable in many cases, they should never be regarded as panaceas. They carry their own risks, as do the common drugs used to treat hypertension. Too often, however, medical news is dominated by reports of the latest miracle drug or "cure." However, high-technology approaches have great merit. We are witnessing advances in noninvasive (safer) types of surgery. Keyhole bypass surgery is around the corner.

In the presence of significant heart disease, extreme caution should be used with particular drugs such as Viagra, which was first developed as a treatment for angina pectoris. It is now considered a "miracle" drug for male erectile dysfunction, but it has potential cardiac side effects, including heart attacks. Phen-fen, another highly touted "miracle drug," has been taken off the market because heart-valve problems occurred in some patients. Even more serious, the potentially fatal condition, primary pulmonary hypertension, occurred in some of the patients with or without heart-valve problems. Tragically, the drug Tambocor, used to treat arrhythmia, is an example of drug that may cause the very problem it is intended to fix. It appears that many thousands of deaths have resulted from the use of this drug, according to some reports. Though pharmaceuticals can be unsafe, "natural" altenatives, such as Ma Huang (ephedra), are not necessarily any safer.

I believe there is a place for all the standard treatments for heart disease and other diseases as well. However, they do not come without risk and, furthermore, they should *never* be considered as complete substitutes for the natural ways to a healthy heart. Would anyone really prefer treatment over prevention? We are all looking for safer, simpler, gentler, more natural health-care options.

What You Can Do

- Always be aware that there are likely consequences of not following a heart-smart lifestyle. Consider all the components, from diet to stress management to exercise.
- Many drugs and surgical procedures are valuable and must be used when necessary. However, these treatments are not without risk. Educate yourself about treatments for heart disease.
- Viagra, a drug used in the treatment of erectile dysfunction, has been associated with cardiovascular and visual side effects. The evidence suggests that it has more problems than hitherto supposed. Consider the risks involved before taking it, and if your sexual function is good in the first place, then absolutely leave it alone.
- Never be pulled into the hype around so-called "miracle drugs" or "miracle herbs" (even though I have used this title myself to make a point about remedies of natural origin). When the media report about medical issues, they sometimes fail to adequately explain the potential dangers of new drugs and treatments. Unfortunately, the dietary supplement industry is not entirely blameless!

CHAPTER FOURTEEN

PULLING IT TOGETHER:
THE CARDIOPLAN

You have no doubt noticed that this book has not presented a series of pretty pictures—one that promises exotic cures or tells you to adopt a weird, radical lifestyle. It is apparent that there are many natural ways to promote a healthy heart, and even more apparent that many of these ways to health are based on simple common sense. During my extensive travels in Southeast Asia, I spent considerable time trying to understand the factors that would promote longevity. The Chinese revere the statue of "the longevity man" with his charismatic smile. Having spent some time with monks in several Buddhist temples, I began to learn that their secret to a long, healthy, and happy life was not a great secret, but more a function of lifestyle. You will probably say that it is not possible for you to live the cloistered existence of a Buddhist monk. That is no doubt true, but it *is* possible to learn from their experience.

A central attribute of the Buddhist monk is his harmonious existence with nature. Anxiety, stress, and depression are not permitted to color the monk's life, although these emotions present themselves to him in the same way as they present themselves to everyone in society. The monks do not subscribe to a single or secret cure for illness, but they direct their attention to total body wellness by achieving a peaceful mind combined with thoughtful personal care and nutrition. The answer to the modern, chronic diseases that plague society rests in combining nutrition, natural healing processes, and the power of the mind over the body.

As you have seen, there is a bouquet of risk factors that are not amenable to a single intervention. Anyone who promises restored health or guarantees that diseases can be prevented—if only you would use a single herb or vitamin—is at least as guilty as the physician who prematurely prescribes a synthetic medication. No, five cloves of garlic per day, along with two packs of cigarettes, will not result in cardiovascular health. My "CardioPlan," a holistic approach to cardiovascular health, is actually a summation of the information in this book. It includes the following key recommendations:

- Maintain an optimal weight.
- Control elevated blood pressure.
- Engage in physical activity.
- Do not smoke or inhale secondhand smoke.
- Reduce your dietary intake of saturated fat and cholesterol by moving towards more vegetarian sources of protein.
- Pay special attention to your psychological well-being.
- Do not use dietary supplements as a way of supplementing a lousy diet.
- Remember the mirror principle in life: your input is your return.
- Moderation in most pleasures is advisable.
- Use natural substances to promote cardiovascular well-being.
- Conventional medicine, when applied appropriately, has immense advantages for health.

While diet is of great importance, I also want you to consider an overall lifestyle plan. If obesity is a problem or if you have difficulty maintaining a healthful weight, then you know that diets are impositions or deviations from normal eating patterns and habits. The term habit is important because without motivation and considerable behavior modification, all diets will fail. You can read tomes about behavior modification, but they all come down to this: Get to know yourself, recognize your "tricks," and catch yourself before you engage in what you know is destructive behavior. This applies to those who are trying to change unhealthful eating patterns, even if their weight is normal.

BEING CLEAR ABOUT YOUR GOALS

When you plan your diet—and I use the term generically here, and not to apply only to weight loss—you must understand your objectives and goals. Look at Table 14.1, which summarizes how certain selected dietary interventions may work in cardiovascular disease prevention

Table 14.1: Dietary Changes That Both Prevent and Treat Heart Disease Directly and Indirectly.

NOTE: (x) signifies lowers cholesterol; (y) signifies beneficial cardiovascular effects independent of lowering cholesterol; and (z) signifies direct or indirect effect on lowering blood pressure.

Dietary Maneuver	Health Outcome	
	Treats Heart Disease	Prevents Heart Disease
Incorporate balanced omega-3 and omega-6 fatty acids in diet	Yes (x, y, z)	Yes (x, y, z)
Add soy protein containing isoflavones	Yes (x, z)	Yes (x, z)
Lower calorie intake (except under-weight)	Yes (y)	Yes (y)
Lower cholesterol intake	Yes (x)	Yes (x)
Lower saturated fat intake	Yes (x)	Yes (x)
Lower salt intake	Yes (y)	Yes (y)
Switch from animal to vegetable protein; *e.g.*, soy	Yes (x, z)	Yes (x)
Move from simple to complex carbohydrate sources	Yes (x)	Yes (x)
Lower alcohol intake and stop smoking	Yes (x, y, z)	Yes (x, y, z)

or treatment. Note the multiple benefits, direct or indirect, that simple dietary changes may make on cardiovascular wellness.

I am not a great supporter of "prescribed" meals. It is better for you to plan your own meals around foods you currently enjoy, taking into account the healthful foods you want to add to your day-to-day menus. Physicians are not often equipped to provide you with guidance about specific meal plans, but a dietician or nutritionist may be of great help to you. Many health-care offices, both conventional and pluralistic, have access to qualified nutritional counselors. Direct marketing companies like Cyberwize.com and Brain Garden have powerful health messages involving nutrition.

For those who enjoy cooking, the number of health-oriented cookbooks is vast, including vegetarian cookbooks and those that provide information about using soy foods. Experiment on your own and plan your meals according to your tastes, not someone else's. The list below provides the characteristics your diet should have:

- The right diet has the right objectives for you.
- It should provide balanced nutrition, if possible.
- The benefits should be obvious.
- For weight loss, the diet must supply less energy than your energy requirements.
- When calorie intake is below 1,800 calories per day, mineral and vitamin supplements are required.
- The diet must have a high degree of acceptability; monotony spells failure.
- It should be part of a lifestyle adjustment or behavior modification regimen.
- Its success is equally dependent on food exclusion and healthy food substitution.
- Goals should not be focused in one wellness domain alone.

You are aware that significant weight loss should always be supervised by a health-care provider. However, the respective roles of soy protein and essential fatty acids are the most underestimated nutritional interventions for cardiovascular health, and I hope you will attempt to bring this information to your health-care providers. I believe that a diet that provides adequate essential fatty acids and soy will make a real difference to cardiovascular health in Western society. Listed below are some simple guidelines that include specific foods and food groups.

- A special health role exists for soy, essential fatty acids, and fiber.
- Your diet should include low saturated fat, a normal intake of vegetable protein of your preference, low simple sugars, high complex carbohydrates, and low salt. Be cholesterol conscious. Varying foods is recommended.
- Calorie intake reduction is the key to weight loss. Calorie intakes of less than 1,800 calories per day require supervision of a health-care professional.
- Avoid diet pills or dietary supplements with false claims.
- Educate yourself about calorie counts and nutritional values of foods. Read labels on food.
- Train yourself to eat properly—*e.g.*, eat only when hungry, chew well, make a meal an occasion.
- Decrease intake of: animal foods, fried foods, and especially beef, cheese, butter, and margarine. Watch for more "unhealthy" types of fruits; *e.g.*, avocado, coconut, and nuts high in saturated fat. Avoid excessive alcohol, food colorants, additives, or too much refined sugar.
- Increase intake of: vegetables, fish, grains, and low-fat, unsalted, fresh nuts. I believe that aspartame (NutraSweet, Equal) is safe, but stevia (an herbal sweetener) may be preferred.
- Supplement diet with fiber (more than 25 g/day), soy protein containing isoflavones (more than 25 g/day), and omega-3 and omega-6 fatty acids from foods and dietary supplements. Fish oil is a savior for cardiovascular and general health. Garlic and grapeseed extract offer additional help.

Remember that the plan you will create is meant to unravel your bouquet of risk factors and lead you to greater health. The following questions apply to everyone, and will help you put some order in your plan.

Answer the following questions.

- Am I obese? (Don't let the question be clouded by emotion.)
- Am I a cardiovascular "time bomb"?
- How fat and how much at risk may I be? (Consult a health-care giver.)
- What are my dietary objectives and goals, and what is my timetable? (Ask a health-care giver to help you.)
- Have I eliminated some cardiovascular risk factors—*e.g.*, smoking, excessive stress?
- Can I *commit* to lifestyle changes and do whatever it takes to modify my behavior accordingly? (It's make-your-mind-up time!)
- Do I know enough about food facts and fallacies? (Ask a health-care giver; read credible sources of information, preferably written by experienced health-care givers with training and credentials to give advice.)
- What foods will I eat for a healthier lifestyle? (Look below for a good start.)
- How can essential fatty acids and soy help me? (Ask a health-care giver who took the time to find out the answer.)

Then—

- *Create* your plan.
- *Work* your plan.

THE KEY FOODS

I have recommended that you think in terms of what healthful foods you can add to your diet rather than focus on what must be removed. Of all the natural agents used to promote cardiovascular wellness, soy protein with isoflavones, garlic, essential fatty acids (omega-3 series, fish oil), and an adequate intake of specific vitamins and minerals and polyphenols stand out as most important. While this list of recommendations of natural treatments for cardiovascular well-being is not complete, it is a list of recommenda-

Table 14.2: Natural Substances Recommended for Inclusion in the CardioPlan.

This CardioPlan is not recommended to substitute for a healthy balanced diet. Individuals with significant cardiovascular disease are advised to seek the attention of an experienced health-care giver.

• Soy protein (at least 25 grams per day) contains isoflavones. At least 50 to 80 mg. per day is recommended to lower cholesterol and exert important antioxidant effects that can prevent atherosclerosis.

• Garlic, which has versatile cardiovascular effects, can be taken in doses of 600 mg. to 1 gram of pure or concentrated garlic or garlic extract powder, or 1.8 to 3 grams of fresh garlic equivalent, or 1,800 to 3,600 mcg. of allicin per day.

• A cardiac-specific vitamin supplement is recommended that contains adequate amounts of vitamin C, E, and B-complex, together with chromium, magnesium, and the addition of coenzyme Q10. This is useful for reducing homocysteine levels.

• Essential fatty acids, especially omega-3 fatty acids from fish oil in a delayed-release format such as Fisol.

• A polyphenol-containing supplement with active bioflavonoids to deliver approximately 50 to 100 mg. of mixed bioflavonoids daily.

tions for which there is scientific evidence to support the use of these agents alone or in combination.

Even if you take medications for an existing cardiac condition, using these natural agents is generally safe. However, your health-care provider should be aware of what you are adding to your health-building plan. Dangers do exist with some natural therapies if multiple medications are used. Drug interactions with herbal and other dietary supplements is a neglected area of research and science. For example, the omega-3 family of fatty acids may enhance the effect of anticoagulant medication, so monitoring is required if higher doses of fish oil are taken. In addition, several botanical agents may act synergistically or counteract synthetic drugs. Table 14.2 includes the list of natural substances and some recommended quantities (remember, some recommendations for natural therapies are inferences and not based on scientific fact or dose-response studies in humans).

IS THE USDA FOOD
PYRAMID A GUIDE?

At one time, a balanced diet was described in terms of food groups—
i.e., dairy, meat, grains, fruits, and vegetables. Today, these food
groups are still relevant, but there is greater emphasis on the percentage of the diet that should be chosen from various groups. The
New Food Pyramid, endorsed by the U.S. Department of Agriculture
(USDA) can serve as a rough guide for your food choices. I say rough
because individual needs vary considerably, and if weight loss is a goal
the serving numbers may vary. In addition, the food pyramid does not
emphasize beneficial fats and oils, which I consider a primary weakness of this approach. One danger of looking at pictorial demonstra-
tions of the Food Pyramid is that it encourages refined foods (bread,
pasta) and is heavily weighted toward carbohydrates. Do not interpret the Pyramid as a license to eat junk food! However, for the first
time in the U.S., vegetables and grains and plant proteins take on
more importance in a government-endorsed diet.

The bottom of the food pyramid, obviously the largest section,
emphasizes grains, cereals, rice, and pasta. Food pyramid guidelines
recommend six to eleven servings per day. (One piece of bread is considered a serving, as is one-half cup of pasta or rice.) Soy-based cereals,
such as "soy flakes," fall into this category (but few people eat them!).

The next tier of the pyramid includes fruit, two to four recommended servings, and vegetables, three to five servings per day. Some
individuals may choose to include more vegetable servings, particularly if weight loss is a goal.

In the next tier, dairy products, including cheese and yogurt—two
to three servings per day—and poultry, fish, meat, beans, eggs, and
nuts and seeds—two to three servings per day. As I have said, soy milk,
tofu, and soy protein products are heart-healthy substitutes and should
be included. I recommend that any dairy products you choose be the
low-fat variety, which reduces their saturated fat content. Of course,
dairy products and other animal proteins are optional. Vegetarian eating is generally healthful, but only in the hands of a knowledgeable person. Most people find that "going vegetarian" is either a gradual
process, allowing for a learning curve, or a partial change, allowing for

lean animal proteins, particularly poultry and fish.

The final tier of the pyramid includes fats and oils, which, according to the guidelines, should be "used sparingly." This is all well and good, but it ignores the importance of the omega-3 fatty acid family and the potential benefits of monounsaturated fat in the form of olive oil. And while these fats should be used carefully, they are as important as other foods on the pyramid. The majority of the small amounts of fat you include in your diet should come from healthful fish and vegetable oils, not from saturated animal fats.

I recommend adapting Food Pyramid guidelines, recognizing that they are not written in stone but can be used as a tool to help you design a weight-loss plan—a plan suitable for individuals with diabetes, and of course, a cholesterol-lowering, heart-healthy food plan. One could say that in general, a heart-healthy diet is good for general health and for the whole family. Frankly, the whole family needs the benefits of a diet that promotes general health and cardiovascular wellness. I recommend that you try to broaden your dietary horizons and think of your diet as part of a life-long, health-promoting lifestyle. I would like to see the Food Pyramid move toward more vegetable protein (especially soy), and have more emphasis on essential fatty acids (fish oil) and less acceptance of refined carbohydrates. Organic sources of food, especially vegetables and fruit, should be stressed more. These small changes may make a huge difference to the health of a nation.

SOME ALARMING FACTS ABOUT CHILDREN

No book on heart disease—or wellness—would be complete without mentioning the effects of a less than healthful diet on our children. Throughout this book I have urged you to consider limiting the sources of unhealthful fat in your family's diet, as well as view lifestyle issues as extremely relevant in children's lives.

In the book *Healthy Kids For Life*, Dr. Charles Kuntzleman presents an excellent analysis of some of the health problems that appear in childhood. In the first chapter, he gives some alarming statistics on the health and well-being of children in North America. I have summarized some of this information in Table 14.3, and if you are a par-

Table 14.3: Some Facts on Fitness, Lifestyle, and General Health Issues Among Children in the United States.

Based upon data presented by Dr. Charles Kuntzleman in his book *Healthy Kids for Life* (1988).

- Average duration of vigorous exercise is less than fifteen minutes per day.
- Greater than 20 percent of calories come from simple sugars.
- More than one-quarter may have high blood pressure.
- One-third have elevated blood triglycerides.
- One-half of all children may have high blood cholesterol.
- Two-thirds eat too much salt.
- Three-quarters eat excessive fat in their diet.
- Sixty-seven percent of all children have three or more risk factors for cardiovascular disease.
- Almost 100 percent of all children have at least one major risk factor.
- Sixty-four percent of all children may fail to meet minimum physical fitness criteria.

ent, it is likely that you will find these observations alarming.

Support for these statements comes from the National Health and Nutrition Examination Survey (HANES). The HANES implies a direct relationship between a child's weight and the amount of time he or she may spend watching television. Looking at this another way, based on implications from the HANES data, it is estimated that childhood obesity increases by approximately 2 percent for each additional hour a day that a child watches television. Besides TV, kids are often mesmerized by video games and the Internet. Actually, these factors appear to operate in adults much to the same degree that they operate in children. Sitting on a couch and sharing cigarette smoke and eating simple sugars, excessive salt, and fat are obvious examples of behavior that should be avoided. The sad situation is that children tend to take their lead from adults.

While the causes of childhood obesity remain poorly understood, several factors are known to make a contribution. Yes, there are some known genetic predispositions to obesity. But beyond those factors, there are recognized contributions coming from emotional factors, family eating habits or behavior, lack of activity and exercise, and misguided attitudes about food. Unfortunately, overweight children often suffer from social isolation and are even objects of cruel remarks and unrelenting teasing about their weight. This may lead them to seek comfort from food, and their condition worsens.

In an ironic tone, Dr. Kuntzleman writes about children "eating to lose," and draws attention to the fact that 99 percent of American children eat sweet desserts on at least six occasions in a week and that they may, on average, drink about twenty-four ounces of soda per day. Since eating meals in restaurants is commonplace today, diets inadequate in fiber and essential nutrients are often the norm. Our kids are strangers to essential fatty acids and vegetable protein (especially soy). Although Dr. Kuntzleman's book includes information about eating in fast food restaurants, I advise that for the most part you avoid this type of food as much as possible. As you know, the dietary habits of average kids are often dominated by burgers and fries, or "fried anything"—foods loaded with cholesterol, saturated fats, and damaged unsaturated fats. These foods are guaranteed, when taken in excess, to break any heart! I realize that parents who deny their children access to fast food are likely to have a revolt on their hands, so why don't we try to view fast food as an occasional treat rather than one of life's staple foods?

The most striking portion of Dr. Kuntzleman's book discusses exercise—or the lack of it. I was astounded to learn that only about one-third of all American school children receive daily physical education classes. In Dr. Kuntzleman's experience, these classes provide only about one to three minutes of rigorous exercise. As I have said elsewhere in this book, walking or even cycling is no longer part of daily life for adults or children, and this should ring some alarm bells. It is about time that more attention is focused on promoting lifestyle changes among children in Western communities. Although many will take issue with this, perhaps it is time for the more affluent populations to understand that economic security and even the relative opulence millions of our children experience do not guarantee health—and, in fact, may lead them away from healthful choices.

Early preventive interventions to enhance wellness are more important than previously recognized. Although substance misuse or abuse and sexual risks are readily identifiable as immediate problems for youngsters, poor diet is not addressed effectively in many educational programs for children. In terms of overall public health significance, education about healthy eating should be given priority. Hypercholesterolemia is much more common in children than most medical professionals have recognized. Our epidemic of heart disease starts with our children.

How does one tackle this problem? Children are receptive to positive attitudes about healthy food choices and the implications of those choices for weight control, athletic performance, and for an overall feeling of well-being. Hypercholesterolemia and abnormal blood lipid profiles should be taken seriously in childhood, at least when children reach school age. However, drug therapy with lipid-lowering drugs should be avoided in childhood. Strategies designed to control high blood lipids in children are not complex. Ideally, children should not be allowed to develop bad habits. As any adult smoker will attest, if they had never smoked in the first place, they would never have had to struggle with putting cigarettes down for good. What we do not know about, we do not miss.

Dr. Attwood's Twelve Common Myths

Another authority on children's health is Charles R. Attwood, M.D., a pediatrician from Louisiana and author of the book, *Dr. Attwood's Low-Fat Prescription for Kids*. Drawing on more than thirty years of experience in pediatrics, this book provides parents with sound dietary advice for children. Dr. Attwood subscribes to the theory that cardiovascular disease has its roots in childhood, and a proper diet can result in reduced death rates from cardiovascular disease and increased longevity.

Dr. Attwood's work revolves around a description of twelve common myths that have percolated over the past few decades. His twelve myths, shown in Table 14.4, have resulted in an unhealthy diet, but the same myths can be turned around to produce practical recommendations for changing to a healthier diet for children.

Dr. Attwood recommends that an ideal diet has just approximately 10 to 15 percent of its calories derived from fats. Obviously then, children's diets must be quite selective, especially in quantities of meat and dairy and, of course, snacks. Typical children's snacks are notoriously packed with large amounts of saturated fat, hydrogenat-

Table 14.4: Twelve Myths Proposed by Dr. Charles R. Attwood.

The comments are taken in part from my interpretation of Dr. Attwood's writings in *Dr. Attwood's Low-Fat Prescription for Kids*.

Myth	Comment
Controlling cholesterol can wait	Emphasis is placed upon cholesterol screening in childhood and intervention with diets to correct blood cholesterol levels of over 150 mg.
Controlling obesity can wait	Obesity must be controlled in childhood because even if weight is lost in later life, residual health risks exist.
"The Fat Taste" is natural and inborn	A taste for fat food is learned behavior and associated with rewards and social events in childhood. Fat taste is learned by conditioning and is not innate.
Small reductions in dietary fat will do	Scientific evidence exists that major reduction in dietary intake of saturated fatty acids and cholesterol are required for optimum health.
Children's diets are getting better	The food industry has presented more high-fat food based upon consumer demand.
Meat is needed for protein and iron	Vegetables can provide complete ranges of essential amino acids, and meat is not necessary to ensure a dietary supply of complete protein.
Milk is needed for calcium and protein	Dairy products are rich in saturated fats and cholesterol. Vegetable-based diets contain adequate calcium and protein, and milk is not necessarily the best source of calcium. In Southeast Asia, soy milk has overtaken dairy milk, and it is "ideal."
Low-fat diets lack vitamins and minerals	Calories from fat that are replaced by vegetables, fruits, grains, and legumes can provide adequate sources of vitamins and minerals.
A low-fat diet means limited choices	Dr. Attwood indicates that children's diets that exclude meat and dairy foods have a greater variety of foods.

(continued on page 314)

Myth	Comment
Low-fat diets retard growth	There may some flaws in studies that have reported growth retardation in children on low-fat diets. Excluding the need for essential fatty acids in early life, there is little evidence to suggest that elimination of saturated fat and cholesterol poses any negative health effects, unless this elimination is not replaced by an adequate range of healthy food.
It's obvious which foods are high in fat	Fat is available in food stuffs in a disguised manner. Close attention should be paid to food labels.
No one knows what is really best for my child	Children eat too much fat and not enough complex carbohydrates. Modern diets are low in fiber. Unequivocal evidence now exists that low-fat diets in childhood may be preventative against coronary artery disease in later life.

ed oil, and sometimes, dangerous trans-fatty acids. Dr. Attwood, and others cited by him in his book, have been somewhat critical of the U.S. Department of Agriculture's new Food Pyramid. I share many of their concerns.

Dr. Attwood believes that the Food Pyramid was adopted in part because it is "politically expedient," in that it satisfies a variety of food producers who are an important segment of the total economy. I have gone further in criticizing the Food Pyramid because of the inadequate recommendations about beneficial fats, such as fish oil, and its liberal viewpoint of refined carbohydrates.

Dr. Attwood's recommendations also differ from those of the American Heart Association (AHA), in that they are much more stringent in recommendations concerning the control of saturated fat intake. Because he is sympathetic to difficulties parents face when they change a child's diet, he defines four stages to reach an ideal diet.

In Stage 1 of Dr. Attwood's dietary recommendations for children, he proposes that the AHA guidelines are followed by consuming up to 30 percent of calories from fat. He believes that the allowance of fat proposed by the AHA is too liberal, but this is a sound introductory stage because it is a readily attainable initial goal. Many children eat a much higher percentage of calories from fat sources, so gradually withdrawing it makes sense. In Stage 2 he recommends reduction of fat intake to 20 to 25 percent of total calories. Stage 3 and Stage 4 recommendations lead to a transition from 15 to 20 percent of calories from fat down to less than 15 percent of calories from total fat in the diet. According to Dr. Attwood, Stage 4 represents the ideal diet, and it contains only about 3 to 5 percent of calories from *saturated* fat.

The taste for fat is a key concept in Dr. Attwood's work. He is convinced that there is a phenomenon, which he has termed the "fat taste," that appears to be the basis of poor nutrition in childhood. I would add the "sweet taste" that makes junk food attractive, with its generous supply of refined sugar and hydrogenated oils. He believes that after reaching a Stage 4 diet, children may lose their taste for fatty foods—high-fat sweets and fried foods simply lose their appeal. He does recommend that children be provided with sources of vitamins, especially the vitamin B series and other multivitamin supplements.

Overall, Dr. Attwood's recommendations mean moving from a meat-based diet to a more vegetarian type of diet. He draws on experiences from Southeast Asia to explain the importance of moving towards a vegetarian diet. For example, the China Health Study, conducted over a six-year period beginning in 1983, was a collaborative research effort between the Chinese government, Oxford University in England, and Cornell University in New York. This study measured lifestyle issues and the diets of 6,500 Chinese individuals and showed much less coronary artery disease and cancer among individuals who had the lowest fat intakes. Dr. Attwood believes these beneficial outcomes are related to greater physical activity and the consumption of low-fat, low–animal protein diets. Other factors that may have played a role include dietary fiber intake, the presence of soy foods in the diet, and other differences in lifestyle habits.

Dr. Attwood's recommendations are innovative, quite sound, and close to ideal. Unfortunately, it is difficult for a child in Western societies to avoid excessive fat in the diet, not to mention being sure to include only the right kinds of fats. I believe that working towards the ideal by vigilant modification of our children's diets is beneficial; an inability to comply with the strict recommendations proposed by Dr. Attwood and others should not discourage you from making some changes. Moving toward a more vegetarian mode is a positive step in itself.

Adolescents and Their High Blood Pressure

Adolescents with hypertension are a difficult group to manage because they are less likely to believe that high blood pressure is serious and needs attention. Hypertension among teenagers often goes undetected because it is considered rare in this age group. However, young people with hypertension usually fit a recognizable profile. They often have a family history of hypertension, they may be obese, and they may have a tendency to avoid physical activity. These children appear as "normal kids," and sadly, many kids match the profile—a poor reflection on our supposedly "advanced" society. Adult screening for hypertension has overshadowed the importance of the early detection of high blood pressure in childhood.

Substance abuse is an important underlying factor in the cause of elevated blood pressure among teens. This substance abuse ranges from overdoses of caffeine-containing soft drinks to illicit drug use. Health-care providers and parents should be vigilant in spotting drug abuse and take immediate steps to help the young person correct this type of adverse lifestyle.

THE ELDERLY ARE A SPECIAL GROUP

Mature and elderly individuals are typically the groups in which strategies to lower blood pressure are often undertaken, and the health risks associated with hypertension increase as an individual gets older. In fact, blood pressure rises with age and is a function of age. In the past, this knowledge unfortunately led to a *laissez faire* approach to the treatment of hypertension in the elderly. Interventions are beneficial even among people of very advanced age. Recent clinical trials have shown benefits of reducing diastolic blood pressure in people over the age of sixty-five to levels below 90 mmHg. In addition, it is worthwhile to reduce systolic blood pressures in excess of 180 mmHg in elderly people to levels that are less than 160 mmHg.

Recent evidence suggests that the elderly are the group for which natural options may be among the most ideal treatment approaches. Natural options or lifestyle interventions, rather than drug therapy, should always be considered for elderly people with *mild* hypertension. The reasons for this are obvious. Elderly people may not tolerate the side effects of antihypertensive medication, and the benefits of strict blood pressure control of mild hypertension in the elderly are not as well-defined as they are in younger people.

Clinical evidence exists to show that reduction of isolated systolic hypertension or reductions in combined elevations of systolic and diastolic blood pressure can result in reductions in morbidity and mortality in mature individuals. Studies have shown that in fairly long followup periods of five years or more, older adults can substantially reduce their risk of heart attack, stroke, and kidney failure by appropriately managing high blood pressure.

Several special factors are important when treating an elderly individual with high blood pressure, and treatment interventions are only appropriate when these factors are carefully considered. The aging process results in a situation where reflexes in the body diminish. Even in the absence of high blood pressure or antihypertensive medications, elderly individuals may become faint when they move quickly from lying or sitting to an upright position. This is called *orthostatic hypotension* and is quite common in the elderly—and, of course, it is often made worse by many prescription drugs that lower blood pressure.

Unfortunately, a host of factors may contribute to a situation in which elderly people are less attentive to their diets. They may add too much salt to their food in an effort to enhance taste. Pouring salt on food may be an unconscious response to diminished ability to enjoy the taste of food; remember that acuity of all the senses diminishes with age. Elderly people may consume more alcohol than they are able to safely metabolize. Frankly, substance abuse in the elderly is much more common than once believed. Social isolation is at the root of unhappiness and substance abuse in the elderly, and we need to think about the way in which our fast-paced Western society often ignores its elderly population. Adults dumping grandmother or grandfather in an emergency room has become a problem in acute medical care settings.

Self-reliance (or ordinary stubborn behavior) may increase with age, and you may know that some elderly people are resistant to discussions about their lifestyle habits. In some individuals, advanced age leads to a tendency to relax vigilance about their behavior, which may lead to errors in judgment. For example, it is widely recognized that errors in taking medication are quite common among the elderly. For this reason, health-care providers should periodically ask their elderly patients to bring their medications to the office. From my own experience, it is quite surprising what elderly people may take in terms of over-the-counter remedies. It is even more surprising these days that people will mix dietary supplements and prescription medications without any concern or consideration for their potential interactions. By the way, while more common among the elderly, these problems certainly are not confined to that age group. "Polypharmacy," as it is formally called, is a major and underestimated health concern.

Finally, and very important, as we age, the body has a decreasing capacity to handle both synthetic and natural medications, and, therefore, it may necessary from time to time to adjust dosages of some medications or dietary supplements. Diminished kidney function occurs with age, and this means that compounds cannot be excreted or metabolized by the body in a normal manner. Concerns about health care in the elderly are of increasing significance as the elderly population increases.

It should be clear that no age group in the population is irrelevant to a discussion of cardiovascular wellness. You may be concerned about your own health, but also have a desire to do what you can to give your children—and maybe your grandchildren—a healthy start or new beginning. Perhaps you are concerned about the health of your parents as they age. As you know by now, the bouquet of risk factors is important to every person—no one can afford to be complacent.

DO NOT FORGET THE MIND/BODY CONNECTION

Regardless of your age, I hope you are aware that you are far more than just your physical body. One of the reasons mind/body medicine has become so important in modern medical life is that we know how important it is to treat the whole person. It is just as important that you do the same. The quality of your relationships, how you spend time alone, and your spiritual connections are as important as learning about good fats and bad fats. In your quest for improved health, remember to treat yourself as a whole person.

Even if you have established coronary artery disease, you may improve your prognosis—and your sense of well-being—by changing your lifestyle and combining conventional medical approaches with the use of safe natural substances. Fortunately, almost all medical practitioners are becoming increasingly aware of natural medical options and are beginning to believe much more in the importance of mind/body interactions. I have attempted to give you the tools you need not only to avoid heart disease, but to enhance the quality of your life. The rest is up to you.

SUMMARY

The bouquet of risk factors for heart disease must be untangled one factor at a time, and all must be addressed. Unfortunately, risk factors form a bouquet of barbed wire. It is time to set goals for your new lifestyle. This chapter is, in essence, the basics of your life-long "CardioPlan."

If you have children, realize that heart disease often has its roots in childhood, perhaps even in utero. Your children should have a "heart-smart" diet, too. In addition, the lifestyle issues such as exercise and stress management are important in childhood, and unfortunately, children in our society tend to be less active than ever before. Exercise is an antidote to poor physical and mental health. It is not surprising that childhood obesity is increasing, and too many children are living on fast food meals and highly processed, sugary, fat-laden commercial snacks.

The elderly are another group that can benefit from natural therapies. In addition, drug interactions and adverse side effects are common among the older population. Lifestyle issues should be addressed as well. No matter how many years we live, we all can benefit from relationships with others and a rich social life. Tragically, loneliness and depression are too common among our elderly population.

What You Can Do

- Review the "Cardio Plan," and evaluate where your lifestyle and that of your family and friends need the greatest attention.
- Use Table 14.1 to help plan your diet. It will help you see which changes will bring the greatest benefits. See the other tables in this chapter for additional suggestions about making your meals health-building and enjoyable.
- Consider using the USDA's Food Pyramid as a basic guideline for your diet, but avoid the "white foods" and add fish and other beneficial oils in moderation. Consider the appropriate use of such foods and supplements as fish oil, soy, garlic, and all fruits and vegetables.
- If you have children, pay special attention to advice given by Dr. Charles Kuntzleman and Dr. Charles Attwood about food and lifestyle choices in childhood. The findings are shocking but revealing, and change is required if we are to escape the cardiovascular time bomb.
- If you are elderly or you are involved in the care of elderly parents, watch for symptoms arising from drug interactions. In addition, watch for signs of social isolation, depression, and changes in eating habits. Recognize that the components of the CardioPlan are for everyone.
- Treat yourself as a whole person with physical, psychological, and spiritual needs. This book has given you the tools that comprise a holistic plan for cardiovascular wellness. Use these tools and reap the benefits.
- Pull together and we can defeat the cardiovascular epidemic.

Attwood, Charles. *Dr. Attwood's Low-Fat Prescription for Kids.* New York: Penguin, 1995.

Cheraskin, Emanuel, Neil Orenstein, and Paul Miner. *Lower Your Cholesterol in 30 Days.* Perigree, 1986.

Chopra, Deepak. *Ageless Body, Timeless Mind.* Harmony Books, 1993.

Erasmus, Udo. *Fats That Heal, Fats That Kill,* 2nd ed. Alive Books, 1993.

Firshein, Richard. *The Nutriceutical Revolution.* Penguin, 1998.

Ford, Norman. *Eighteen Ways to Lower Your Cholesterol in 30 Days.* Keats, 1992.

Frankel, Paul, and Fred Madsen. *Homocysterine through the Methylation Process.* The Research Corner, 1998.

Goldstrich, Joe. *Healthy Heart, Longer Life.* Ultimate Health Publishing, 1996.

Holt, Stephen. *Soya for Health.* M.A. Liebert, 1997.

———. *The Soy Revolution.* New York: M. Evans, 1998.

———. *The Sexual Revolution.* Wellness Publications, 1999.

———. *The Weight Control Revolution.* 1999.

Holt, Stephen, with J. Banlla. *The Power of Cartilage.* Kensington/Zebra Books, 1998.

Holt, Stephen, and Lindon Camac. *Miracle Herbs.* Carol Publishing, 1998.

Kabat-Zinn, Jon. *Full Catastrophe Living.* City: Delacorte Press, 1990.

McCully, Kilmer S. *The Homocysteine Revolution.* Keats, 1997.

Messina, Mark, and Virginia Messina. *The Simple Soybean and Your Health.* Avery, 1994.

Mindell, Earl. *Earl Mindell's Soy Miracle*. Simon & Schuster, 1995.

———. *Earl Mindell's Anti-Aging Bible*. Simon & Schuster, 1996.

Moyer, Ellen. *Cholesterol & Triglycerides*. People's Medical Pharmacy, 1995.

Ornish, Dean. *Dr. Dean Ornish's Program for Reversing Heart Disease*. Ivy Books, 1996.

Schmidt, Michael. *Smart Fats*. Frog, Ltd., 1997.

Shreeve, Caroline. *A Healthy Heart for Life*. City: Thorsens Publishing Group, 1988.

Shute, Evan. *The Heart and Vitamin E*. Keats, 1977.

Sinatra, Stephen, T. *Heartbreak and Heart Disease*. Keats, 1996.

———. *The Coenzyme Q10 Phenomenon*. Keats, 1998.

Susser, Arnold J. *How Did We Get So Fat?* BL Publications, 1994.

Walker, Morton, and Garry Gordon. *The Chelation Answer*. Second Opinion Publishing, 1994.

Weil, Andrew. *Spontaneous Healing*. Knopf, 1995.

———. *8 Weeks to Optimum Health*. Knopf, 1997.

Wilen, Joan, and Lydia Wilen. *Garlic, Nature's Super Healer*. Prentice Hall, 1992.

Information about Soy and Dietary Supplements

Biotherapies, Inc.
9 Commerce Road
Fairfield, NJ 07004

1-800-700-7325